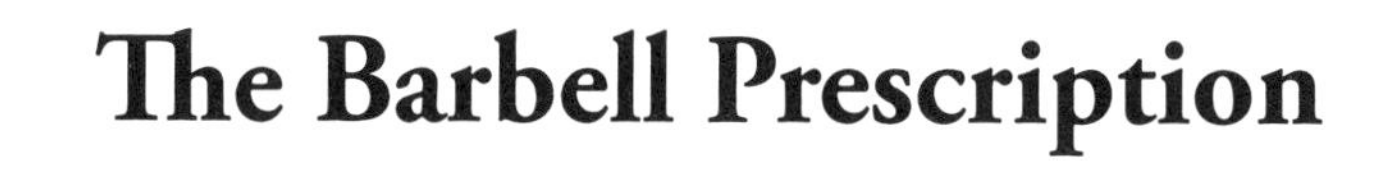
The Barbell Prescription

# The Barbell Prescription

## Strength Training for Life After Forty

Jonathon M. Sullivan MD, PhD, FACEP, SSC

Andy Baker, SSC

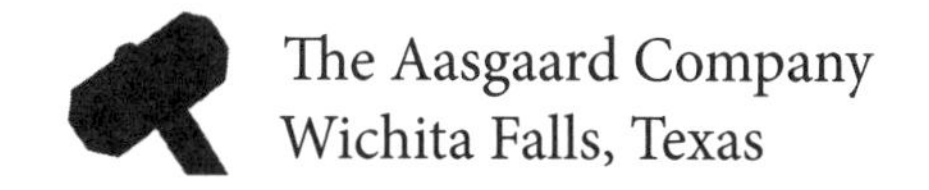
The Aasgaard Company
Wichita Falls, Texas

Indexing & Proof – Mary Boudreau Conover
Editing, Layout & Proof – stef bradford
Illustrations Chapters 1-6 by Simma Park, Chapter 7 by Jason Kelly, and Chapter 15 by stef bradford.
Photographs by Thomas Campitelli except Figures 8-3 & 11-5 by Steve Brack and 12-1 & 21-1 by Nick Delgadillo.

20 19 18 17 2 3 4 5 6 7 8 9 10

ISBN-13: 978-0-9825227-7-6 (paper)
ISBN-13: 978-0-9825227-8-3 (electronic)
ISBN-10: 0-9825227-7-0 (paper)
ISBN-10: 0-9825227-8-9 (electronic)

Printed in the United States of America

**The Aasgaard Company**
3118 Buchanan St, Wichita Falls,TX 76308, USA
www.aasgaardco.com
www.startingstrength.com

**JONATHON SULLIVAN:**

**For Kirk Bishop**

Who gave me a barbell. I miss you.

And

**For Marilyn**

Who rode a bike to work in the snow. I love you.

**ANDY BAKER:**

**For All My Clients, Past and Present**

You have taught me more than I'll ever teach you.

And

**For My Wife, Laura**

For your unending patience, love, and support. Without you, none of what I do would be possible.

# Contents

# Foreword: Learning from the Tails

I was honored to be asked by Mark Rippetoe to write the foreword of this book. But the reader may ask the following: What does someone whose research is on the risk of random events, particularly extremes, have to do with strength training?

Well, the Starting Strength approach is precisely about extremes, what people in my business call the "tails," the rare events that are consequential though of low probability. Just as systems learn from extremes, and for preparedness, calibrate themselves to withstand large shocks, so does the human body. Indeed, our body should be seen a risk management system meant to handle our environment, paying more attention to extremes than ordinary events, and learning from them.

You will never get an idea of the strength of a bridge by driving several hundred cars on it, making sure they are all of different colors and makes, which would correspond to representative traffic. No, an engineer would subject it instead to a few multi-ton vehicles. You may not thus map all the risks, as heavy trucks will not show material fatigue, but you can get a solid picture of the overall safety.

Likewise, to train pilots, we do not make them spend time on the tarmac flirting with flight attendants, then put the autopilot on and start daydreaming about vacations, thinking about mortgages or meditating about corporate airline intrigues – which represent about the bulk of the life of a pilot. We make pilots learn from storms, difficult landings, and intricate situations – again, from the tails.

So when it comes to physical training, there is no point engaging in the time-consuming repetitive replication of an active environment and its daily grind, unless you need to do so for realism, therapy, or pleasure. Just calibrate to the extreme and work your way down from there.

The other reason Rip asked me to write this foreword is because I am myself engaged in a variant of his exercise program – and the ethics of skin in the game dictate that one should be eating his own cooking, tell us what you think and what you do. I learned that what you do for training needs to be separate from what you do for pleasure. I enjoy hiking, walking, ocean swimming, riding my bicycle, that sort of things; but I have no illusion that these activities will make me stronger. They may be necessary, but for other reasons than the attainment of strength. I just consider walking necessary therapy, like sleeping.

It also happened that part of my research in risk overlaps with complexity theory. The first thing one learns about complex systems is that they are not a sum of body parts: a system is a collection of interactions, not an addition of individual responses. Your body cannot be trained with specific and local muscle exercises. When you try to lift a heavy object, you recruit every muscle in your body, though some more than others. You also produce a variety of opaque interactions between these muscles.

This complex system method applies to all situations, even when you engage in physical therapy, as I did for an injured shoulder. I discovered that doing the more natural barbell presses and (initially assisted) pull-ups, works better and more robustly than the complicated and time consuming multi-colored elastic bands prized by physical therapists. Why don't physical therapists make you do these robust barbell exercises? Simply, because they have a rent to pay and, just as with gyms, single-exercise machines look fancier and more impressive to the laity.

Further, muscles are not the whole story. In a line of research pioneered by Gerard Karsenty and his colleagues, the skeleton with its few hundred bones has been shown to be endocrine apparatus, regulating blood sugar, fertility, muscle growth, and even memory. So an optimal exercise would need to work, in addition to every muscle in your body, every bone as well, by subjecting the skeleton to weight stressors in order to remind it that the external world exists.

Finally, the body is extremely opaque; it is hard to understand the exact physiological mechanisms. So we would like to make sure our methodology is robust and can stand the judgment of time. We have had theories of how muscles grow; these come and go. We have theories of nutrition; these come and go – the most robust is the one that favors occasional periodic fasts. But we are quite certain that while theories come and go, the phenomenologies stay; in other words, that in two thousand years the method of whole-body workout in the tails will still work, though the interpretation and "scientific" spin will change – just as two thousand five hundred years ago, Milo of Croton carried an ox on his shoulders and got stronger as the ox grew.

Nassim Nicholas Taleb

# Introduction:
# Resistance is not futile

A quiet revolution is transforming the way we think about fitness and health in the aging adult. It's changing our concept of what aging is, how it should be approached by doctors and patients, how its worst effects can be blunted – how it should be *lived.* Recent research has turned old assumptions about exercise in healthy aging inside-out. We've always known that exercise is important for health. But we have new ideas about the type and intensity of activity that can be tolerated and will best promote health in aging adults.

We can sum up these new ideas simply: *healthy aging is strong aging.* After decades of equating exercise with aerobics and fitness with endurance, *strength* has made a comeback. Martial artists, surfers, dancers, cyclists, rowers, skiers, and even a few savvy runners have joined football and rugby players in the weight room. A growing recognition of the importance of strength for performance, mobility, everyday functioning, injury prevention and health has led to a rediscovery of weight training and new interest in exercise selection and technique, programming, and strength-oriented nutrition. In short, fitness professionals, athletes, the general public and even a few alert doctors have rediscovered ***resistance training*** – training for strength and power.

The impact is arguably most profound for those in middle age and beyond. Lifting weights has always been viewed by most as a young person's game, more particularly as a young *man's* game. That's changed. In recent years, we've seen an explosion of published biomedical evidence on resistance training in the aged, in women, in children, and in people suffering from a broad spectrum of health conditions, ranging from diabetes to hypertension to congestive heart failure to Parkinson's. What this growing body of data tells us is that everybody who *can* lift weights *should* lift weights. This most emphatically includes those in their 40s and beyond.

Strength training can slow, arrest or even reverse many of the degenerative effects of aging: loss of muscle and strength, brittle bones, floppy ligaments, dysfunctional joints, and the decline of mobility and balance. Instead of losing lean mass and replacing it with fat, healthy aging can be characterized by the retention or even addition of healthy, functional tissue. You can think of every bout of strength training as a prudent deposit into a "Physiological 401K": saving strong muscle, hard bone, and full mobility for your retirement. As with retirement savings, the benefits are greatest for those who start early and keep at it. But recent research makes it clear that even the very old can get stronger and more powerful, improving their health and quality of life.

This book is a comprehensive treatment of resistance training for those in their 40s, 50s, 60s, and beyond. It is intended for everybody in this age range, for everybody who hopes to live through this age range, and for their doctors, coaches, friends and family. In Part One, Dr. Jonathon Sullivan will present the evidence that *strength training is essential for healthy aging in the modern era.* The most effective and rational method of strength training is a program consisting of just a few multi-joint barbell and conditioning exercises that will build strength, increase power, add functional tissue, optimize metabolic and cardiovascular fitness, and improve quality of life. In Part Two, Dr. Sullivan and Coach Andy Baker will present an overview of these exercises, specify the essentials of performance, explain the rationale for their use, and describe how they may be varied or supplemented to meet the needs of trainees in their fifth decade and beyond. In Part Three, Coach Baker and Dr. Sullivan will present detailed training programs for adults over forty, and demonstrate how the underlying structure of the Stress-Recovery-Adaptation cycle permits these programs to be tailored to the needs of any individual, no matter how old, weak, or deconditioned they may be.

*It is not the purpose of this book to instruct you in the performance of these exercises.* Although these exercises can be learned by motivated individuals through reading, study and practice, the movements are best learned on the platform under the direction of a competent coach. In any event, an exhaustive treatment of these exercises would be a book in itself, and that book has already been written. But we will provide readers with a description, explanation, and rationale for these movements, and direct you to resources for learning to perform them properly. You will see why a program of barbell-based resistance training is worth the effort involved in learning the exercises, and why it is far and away the most powerful, rational, simple, safe, and effective approach to fitness. You'll learn how such a program can be accomplished in two or three days a week, and how it integrates exercise, sleep, and nutrition into a complete and healthy lifestyle for the aging adult.

This book is both a prospectus and a training manual. It is theory and practice, an evidence-based case for *why* you should invest the time and effort to learn a few basic barbell and conditioning exercises, and a practical examination of exactly *what* must be done and *how* these exercises can be incorporated into a complete, lifelong training program.

Most of us grew up surrounded by a model of aging we would be well-served to jettison. Even the healthier, relatively active people we knew in their 50s and 60s were nevertheless weak, with thinning muscles and brittle bones. Most of them weren't even *that* well off. For too long, aging has been an excuse to take it easy, to avoid the "dangers" of over-activity, to act your age, to resign to the inevitability of decline, and to consider yourself fit for your age if you could get through a few holes of golf or hobble around the park twice a week.

Weight lifting? At my age? *Are you crazy?*

It's time to change all that. There's a different type of aging available. We're not promising perfect health, or even longevity. Getting strong won't bring back your eyesight, restore your bald spot, shrink your prostate, or smooth your wrinkles. Aging *always* ends in decline and death. Bad luck and disease can strike down even the strongest, just as a bad market can ruin a rich man who has invested wisely. But getting old, even *very* old, doesn't have to guarantee frailty, loss of independence, weakness and misery. It is possible, in fact it is *essential,* to save strong healthy tissue for the years when we'll need it most. With discipline, hard work, and a little luck, we can compress the morbidity of aging into a tiny sliver of our life cycle, remaining strong and resilient well into our final years. Instead of dwindling into an atrophic puddle of sick fat, we can make our ending like a failed last rep at the end of a final workout. Strong, vigorous and useful, to the last.

Time always wins in the end. But we hope to convince you that resistance is not futile.

# Part I: WHY

## From Exercise Prescription to Training Program

# 1

# The Sick Aging Phenotype

Getting older has never been easy, but if you had to choose one epoch of history in which to embark on the fourth, fifth or sixth decade of life, the current era would be your best option. Never before has it been possible for so many people to live so long, in so much comfort, in security against so many ancient horrors, and with so many teeth. Of course, every silver lining has a cloud. Aging in the postmodern era can result in either the healthiest "seniors" the world has ever seen, or a ghastly and increasingly common syndrome of maladaptive aging, which we shall call the Sick Aging Phenotype. The Sick Aging Phenotype is a complex of interrelated and synergistic processes, in which the metabolic syndrome, muscle and bone loss, frailty, loss of function and independence, and an ever-growing stew of pharmaceuticals conspire to destroy the health and quality of life of the aging adult. In this chapter, we'll see just how badly things can go wrong for the aging adult in a world of wonder drugs, leisure, plenty, and peace.

## Wellness Will and Phat Phil

***Phenotype*** is an unfamiliar but useful word. It's a biological term, a construction from the Greek: *phainen* + *typos*, or "show" + "type." It's the "show type" of an organism: the appearance, traits, behaviors, and overall structural and biochemical peculiarities we observe when we look at that organism. The phenotype of a creature is to be distinguished from its ***genotype***: the inherited instructions (genes) encoded in its DNA. Two organisms of the same species with identical or nearly identical genotypes will tend to have very similar phenotypes. But their phenotypes can also be very different.

Allow me to give you an example. Consider a pair of identical twins, Will and Phil. Will and Phil both develop from the same fertilized egg. One sperm, one egg, one blueprint for one baby. But at some point early in development, the zygote splits, resulting in two embryos with exactly the same DNA sequences in every gene. Genetically speaking, Will and Phil are completely identical: *They have the same genotype*. When they're kids, they look exactly the same. Their parents have trouble telling them apart, they engage in untoward capers that exploit their identical appearance, their Mom dresses them in the same funny rabbit suit every Easter, and they even seem to have similar temperaments. In other words, during development, childhood, and adolescence, Will and Phil demonstrate astonishingly similar phenotypes. Because their phenotypes are heavily influenced by their genotypes, this is not surprising. It is the genes, after all, that provide the source code for our biological development and overall constitution.

Let's fast-forward about 55 years. What has happened to the genotypes of Will of Phil? *Nothing*. They still share exactly the same genotype (a few cosmic rays, transposons and viral infections notwithstanding). But when we step out of our time machine, we find that their phenotypes are vastly different.

Will has the more uncommon phenotype. He's an avid sportsman. Somewhere along the line, he took up fishing, hiking, and rock climbing. He's planning on going to the Grand Tetons next summer...for the fourth time. To keep his edge, Will goes to the gym, where he works on his strength and conditioning. He's a bit of a health nut, and he eats a lot of lean meat, fish, green vegetables and fruit. He likes to cook with fresh ingredients. He has about 17% bodyfat, and he weighs a very solid 210 lbs. He's strong, and he looks it. He gets regular checkups with his doctor, although the only medicine he's on is a daily baby aspirin, occasional acetaminophen for pain, and sildenafil for his mild erectile dysfunction. His sex life is awesome. He's got a touch of arthritis, and he had a melanoma removed from his arm in 2007. Overall, he's in excellent health. Barring a car accident, pandemic, or the odd asteroid, he will enjoy three more very robust decades before he dies suddenly of a hemorrhagic stroke, age 88, while hiking in the Scottish highlands with his 67 year-old girlfriend.

Will's twin brother Phil displays the more common phenotype. Somewhere along the line, he took up smoking, drinking, and lots of quality time with his big screen TV. He's planning on watching the entire third season of *Battlestar Galactica* this weekend...for the fourth time. To keep his edge, he drinks lots of Pepsi, and keeps scrupulously up to date on his Netflix queue. He's a fiend for Domino's Pizza and Doritos. He likes to cook with frozen ingredients and a microwave. His bodyfat is through the roof – he's about 48% fat by weight – and he tips the scale at 283, about 70 lbs on his twin brother. He doesn't like doctors, although he's known to make frequent trips to the ER for chest pain, fatigue, sore joints, or a skin infection. He hasn't had a real erection since the start of the Obama Administration. He has Type 2 diabetes, arthritis, messed-up serum lipids, and high blood pressure. He doesn't know it yet, but he also has a ticking time bomb in his left anterior descending coronary artery. Three years from now, this lesion will clamp off the blood flow to Phil's left ventricle in the middle of a *Die Hard* movie marathon. He'll breathe his last in the cardiac ICU 6 weeks later, age 58.

Same genotype. Very different phenotypes.

More specifically, Will and Phil have different *aging phenotypes* and different *death phenotypes*. Phil's aging phenotype is an unsightly and miserable catastrophe, while his brother's is an exemplar of healthy aging. Will's death phenotype is be envied: he's healthy, vigorous, active and happy until the minute a tired, tiny vessel in his brainstem switches him off in the middle of a great final adventure at the end of his ninth decade, many years from now. Will is going to pack all of his dying into about 7 seconds.

*Phil is already dying*, and he will spend six painful weeks in the hospital after his heart attack, battling cardiogenic shock, pneumonia, a nasty bedsore, sepsis, and all manner of wickedly invasive and painful medical interventions. *His* great final adventure comes to an end on his 43rd hospital day, when a thrombus breaks loose from the deep veins in his fat-laden, chronically underused legs. The clot takes the vena cava express to the right side of his heart, lodges in his main pulmonary artery, induces Total Vapor Lock, and mercifully dispatches him from his miserable existence. Fortunately Phil has Blue Cross. So his family doesn't get the $185,000 bill, which means Will can afford to go hiking in Scotland some 30 years later.

Both Wellness Will and Phat Phil are *modern* phenotypes. In ages past, war, famine and infectious diseases were the scourge of mankind. Smallpox, diphtheria, cholera, measles, dysentery, plague, malaria, influenza, pneumonia, meningitis, cellulitis, pink eye, tooth abscess, and other microbial diseases devastated individuals, populations, and even entire civilizations.[1] Today, the organisms that cause diphtheria, measles, and a host of other infectious diseases are held in check by vaccination. Herd immunity protects even those who haven't had their shots. Sanitation and simple oral hydration have reduced cholera and the dysenteries from monsters that sweep through entire populations to isolated outbreaks that are survived by most victims. Pneumonia, meningitis, cellulitis, and pink eye wither in the face of antibiotic therapy.[2] Infectious diseases are no longer leading causes of mortality in industrialized societies,[3] although a few idiot busybodies are working hard to undo these advances.[4] *Modern* aging and death phenotypes are increasingly the product of abundance, longevity and idleness, with the major cardiovascular diseases (including stroke) being by far the number one cause of mortality.[5] Cancer runs second, while diabetes, Alzheimer's, and respiratory diseases bring up the rear. When infectious diseases do kill us, they tend to do so at the extremes of age and ill health.[6]

Wellness Will and Phat Phil are excellent icons for the spectrum of aging and death phenotypes in modern industrialized societies, staking out the two extremes. Unfortunately, the distribution of phenotypes across this spectrum does not occupy a classic bell curve, with most people somewhere in the middle. Instead, the distribution is skewing away from Will and toward Phil.[7] The "average" human genotype has not changed *substantially* in many thousands of years, but in the postmodern era, the human phenotype of industrialized nations has undergone a staggering and destructive transformation.[8] Will's Healthy Aging Phenotype is more achievable than at any time in human history. But Phil's ***Sick Aging Phenotype,*** as defined below, is well on the way to becoming the norm.

Because this is a phenotypic transformation, and not a genotypic one, most scientists and physicians have concluded that the blame for this slow-motion public health catastrophe falls squarely on environmental and behavioral variables.[9] I believe this conclusion is correct in general, although there remains considerable controversy about the particulars, especially with regard to the role of cultural influences, medical interventions, and diet.[10] It appears the modern aging phenotypes are profoundly sensitive to a number of external and behavioral variables. Obviously, this book is focused on one of those variables: physical exercise. But before we get into that, let's take a closer look at what we're dealing with.

## The Sick Aging Phenotype

The Sick Aging Phenotype is complex, but it can be summed up in a few words: ***metabolic syndrome, sarcopenia and osteopenia, frailty,*** and ***polypharmacy***. Each of these imposing terms invokes a monster lurking in a grim and altogether likely future for all of us. In this section, we'll take a brief look at how these components of the Sick Aging Phenotype develop and work together to create a living nightmare.

## The Metabolic Syndrome

The ***metabolic syndrome*** is a key driver of unhealthy aging in developed countries[11] (and some undeveloped countries, bad lifestyle choices being one of the West's more profitable exports).[12] This plague affects 25–30% of the population of North America.[13] In medicine, a *syndrome* is a constellation of symptoms, findings, and disorders that tend to occur together. Metabolic syndrome has different definitions and clinical criteria for diagnosis, depending on where you're from and who you read.[14] But the generally recognized *physiological* components of metabolic syndrome are listed below.

### Components of the Metabolic Syndrome

1. ***Visceral obesity*** – accumulation of fat around the internal organs. This change is highly correlated with the more visible ***truncal obesity***, variously defined by the (rather crude) metrics of waist-hip ratio or BMI.

2. ***Insulin Resistance*** and ***Hyperglycemia*** – loss of cellular sensitivity to insulin signaling leads to numerous derangements. This includes diabetes or a pre-diabetic state characterized by poor serum glucose control.

3. ***Hypertension*** – elevated blood pressure.

4. ***Dyslipidemia*** – derangement in serum triglyceride (fat) and HDL/LDL (cholesterol) levels.

5. ***Inflammation*** – This is not a *classical* component of the metabolic syndrome, and is *not* used in most established definitions. I include it here because of the increasing recognition that metabolic syndrome involves chronic over-activation of cellular and biological defense mechanisms that cause pain and damage to tissues.[15]

These miseries fill my days as an emergency physician. People who get sick and come to the emergency department are disproportionately fat, hypertensive, and diabetic. That's because people who are fat, hypertensive, and diabetic are more likely to get sick, and in a vast variety of unpleasant ways. People with metabolic syndrome or its components are more likely to become frail,[16] to suffer from stroke, cardiovascular disease and heart attack,[17] to develop heart failure,[18] to develop kidney failure,[19] and to suffer from erectile dysfunction,[20] depression,[21] loss of independence, and premature death.[22]

How does this happen? The development of metabolic syndrome is complex, and research into this nightmare is ongoing. A complete examination of the biology of metabolic syndrome is beyond the scope of this book, but it is worth getting an overview of how this disaster develops. Most authorities focus heavily on ***obesity***,[23] so that's where we'll begin.

**Obesity.** The role of obesity in the development of metabolic syndrome is complex, and complicated by the question of whether obesity *itself* has a causal role, or whether obesity is a ***biomarker***, an indicator of abnormal energy balance in overfed, sedentary individuals. It does not appear to be the case that *being fat itself* always leads to the metabolic syndrome. We all know people with some fat on their frame who are nevertheless active, vital, and vibrant. They carry some weight around, but they glow with good health. Moreover, obesity is itself multifactorial, encompassing genetic, lifestyle, environmental, psychosocial, and cultural issues. These complex associations are worthy of a book or two in themselves, but for our purposes it really boils down to how our behavior affects our weight, because our genetics and our cultural milieu are more or less beyond our control.

The behaviors that affect our weight are *what* we eat, *how much* we eat, and *how much energy we burn off* through physical work and exercise.

Obviously, we're going to talk a lot about exercise, not nearly as much about diet, and virtually not at all about factors beyond our control. The point I want you to come away with right now is that truncal obesity – a big waistline, a spare tire, a beer belly, a *fatbody phenotype* – is strongly associated with the development of the metabolic syndrome. This is so well-established in the epidemiological literature, and the putative mechanisms leading from visceral and truncal fat accumulation to metabolic syndrome are well-enough described, that there *really is no argument here*, obesity apologists please take note.[24]

So Phil's sedentary, overfed lifestyle creates a derangement in energy balance, leading to the accumulation of unhealthy visceral fat and a reduction in the sensitivity of his body's tissues to insulin. This ***insulin resistance*** is at the core of the metabolic syndrome.[25]

**Insulin Resistance and Hyperglycemia.** Insulin is a peptide (a short protein) secreted by specialized cells of the pancreas, and is known to most of us as the hormone that regulates blood sugar. In response to a meal, insulin is secreted into the bloodstream. In circulation, insulin interacts with receptors on the surfaces of cells, as a key interacts with a lock. Insulin trips these locks, opening up ***glucose transporters***, which shuttle ***glucose*** (a simple six-carbon sugar) from the bloodstream to the interior of the cells.

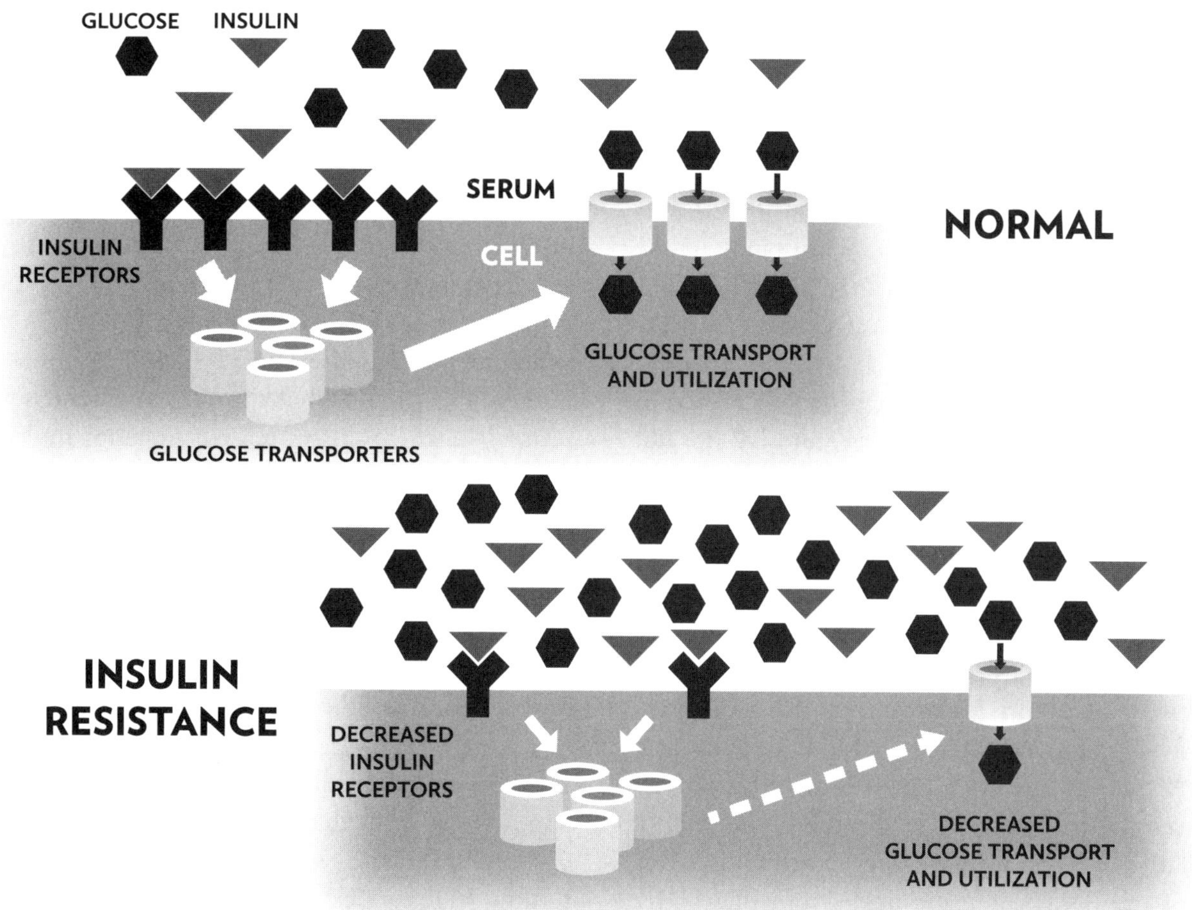


***Figure 1-1.*** Insulin signaling in health and disease. In the normal state (*top*), an increase in serum glucose triggers the release of insulin. Insulin binds to abundant receptors (Y shapes) on the cell membrane, triggering an insulin signal that sends glucose transporters to the membrane. This results in glucose transport into the cell. In insulin resistance and Type 2 diabetes (*bottom*), insulin receptors are "downregulated"; that is, removed from the membrane. Fewer insulin receptors means less insulin signaling and less glucose transport, even though serum insulin and glucose levels are abnormally high.

Obviously, a decrease in blood insulin level will prevent glucose from being taken up by cells, leading to an accumulation of sugar in the blood. But the same effect can be achieved by *decreasing the sensitivity of cells to insulin signaling*. In this condition, blood insulin levels can be normal or even elevated, but blood sugar will remain high because the response of cells to insulin signaling is blunted (Figure 1-1).

This is what's happening in the metabolic syndrome. Notwithstanding the role of genetics and environment, it appears that *lifestyle alone* is sufficient to trigger this state of insulin resistance.[26] Increased energy intake and sedentary lifestyle (eating too much and sitting on your butt all day, not to put too fine a point on it) upset the energy balance of the body. Obviously, weight gain will ensue, but the body's metabolic response is even more insidious. The constant supply of excess food energy overwhelms insulin signaling systems, resulting in the so-called "downregulation" of insulin receptors. In this model,[27] insulin receptors are removed from cell membranes, so there are fewer locks to accept the insulin keys, and fewer glucose transporters available to remove glucose from the bloodstream.

This is even more catastrophic than one might think, because insulin isn't just a glucose-regulating hormone. Its effects are far deeper and more fundamental than that. Insulin is a ***growth factor.***[28] When it binds to its receptor it triggers not just glucose uptake, but also a network of powerful growth and survival responses, both in cellular chemistry and at the genetic level. Insulin signaling tells tissues that they are in a fed state, and it tells the body that the circumstances are ideal for growth, development, and repair. Insulin resistance in the setting of overeating and sedentary lifestyle sends an inappropriate and paradoxical message that the organism is *unfed*.[29]

The wide-ranging and catastrophic effects of insulin resistance are outlined in Figure 1-2. It's not a great leap to see how insulin resistance will lead Phil to hyperglycemia, and thence to full-blown diabetes. The other consequences are less obvious, but no less devastating.

**Elevated Blood Pressure.** Decreased insulin sensitivity helps drive changes in the biology of Phil's vascular tissues (blood vessels). This includes the cells which form the inner lining of his arteries and veins, and comprise almost the entire wall of capillaries.[30] Derangements in insulin signaling inhibit the release of nitric oxide from these cells. Nitric oxide is an important signaling molecule involved in the regulation of vascular tone. In short, it tells blood vessels to relax, which has the effect of lowering vascular resistance and decreasing the blood pressure. In the setting of metabolic syndrome, nitric oxide release is depressed, blood vessel tone is increased, and blood pressure goes up.[31] The result is ***hypertension***, the silent killer. High blood pressure puts a strain on Phil's heart, which must work harder to "push" against the increased load. With every heartbeat, the increased pressure causes insidious, cumulative damage to his brain, retinas, kidneys, and arteries. It bears pointing out that the derangement in nitric oxide release is also a contributing factor in the development of Phil's erectile dysfunction.[32]

**Inflammation.** Recent work reveals that the metabolic syndrome is strongly associated with an increase in systemic inflammation. Inflammation promotes the development of atherosclerosis and degenerative changes in many tissues,[33] promoting the development of the Sick Aging Phenotype.

One of the principle sources of inflammatory products in the setting of obesity and metabolic syndrome is the fat itself. We now know that fat cells (*adipocytes*) can release a number of products with untoward effects, including TNF-alpha, interleukin-6, and C-reactive protein. Fat cells also release abnormal amounts of other so-called ***adipokines*** (signaling molecules of fat cell origin), which further aggravate the interlocking, interactive processes of the metabolic syndrome.[34] This sort of process, in which a tissue releases signaling molecules into the blood to affect physiology (for good or ill), is what a physiologist would call ***endocrine*** activity. In other words, in the setting of his obesity and metabolic syndrome, *Phil's fat tissue behaves like an abnormal gland*, producing an unhealthy adipokine "hormone" profile that accelerates the pathological processes at work throughout his body.[35]

**Dyslipidemia.** Finally, the metabolic syndrome appears to contribute to the development of dyslipidemia, the increase in blood levels of serum triglycerides (fat) and "bad cholesterol" (LDLs), which are widely believed to be major contributors to the development of vascular disease, leading ultimately to heart attack and stroke. The relationship between dyslipidemia and vascular disease is more controversial than it used to be, in part because drugs designed to correct dyslipidemia have had mixed results,[36] in part because low-fat diets have only a moderate effect, if any, on the rate of heart disease in populations,[37] and in part because the scientific literature on this topic appears to be a big mess.[38] I believe that metabolic syndrome does indeed lead to the development of vascular disease, but not simply because serum triglycerides and cholesterol levels are elevated. Biological systems are complicated, and any particular phenotype is always the result of multiple factors. So it seems far more likely that vascular disease results from several primary effects of the metabolic syndrome *working together*.[39] Dyslipidemia *and* hypertension *and* inflammation *and* deranged insulin signaling acting *in concert* lead to the development of vascular disease and all the wickedness it will rain down on Phil's life.

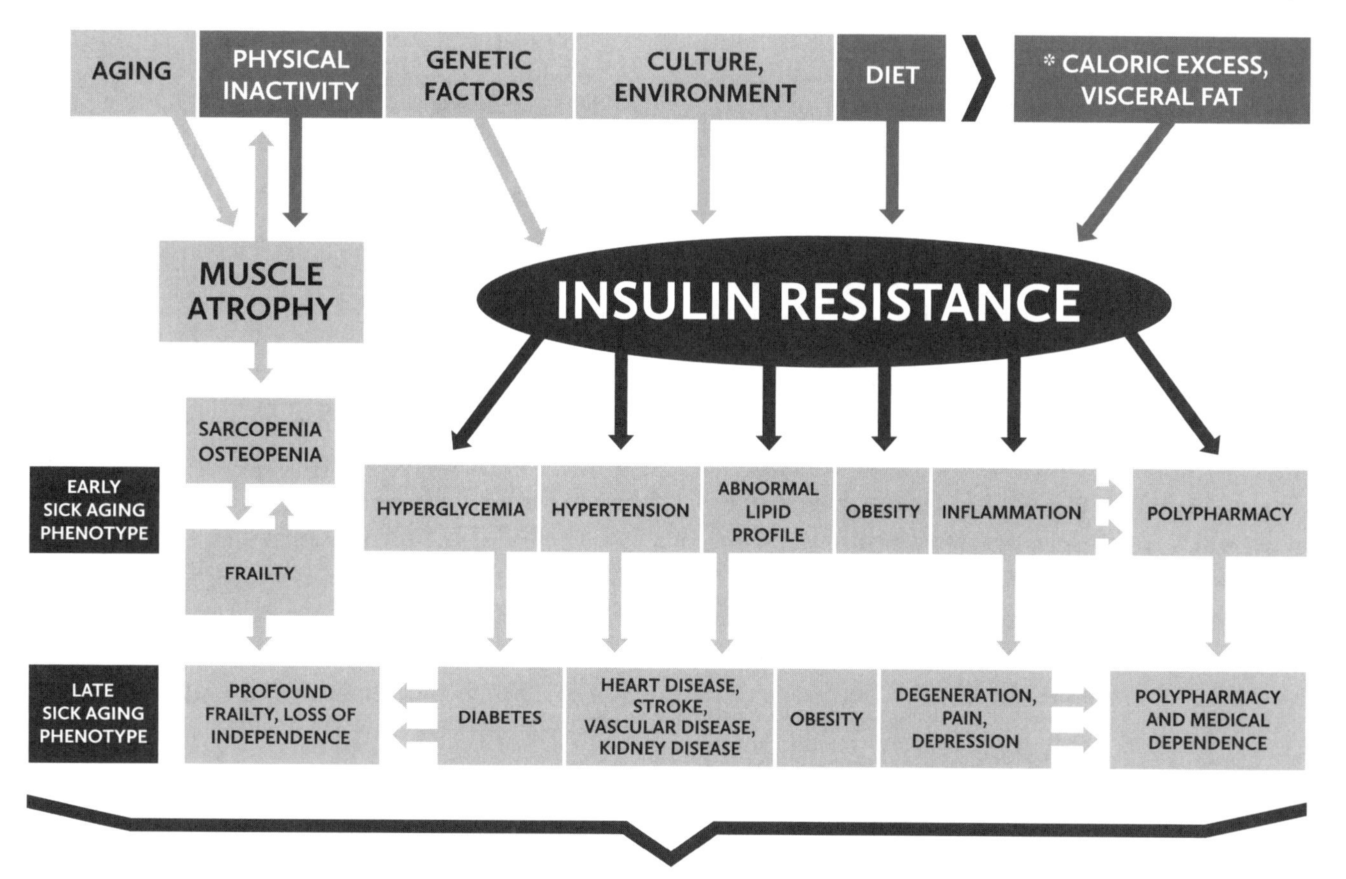


***Figure 1-2.*** Development of the Sick Aging Phenotype. Abnormally high energy balance from diet and lack of exercise, along with genetic and other factors (*top register*), contribute to the development of obesity, "sick fat," insulin resistance and metabolic syndrome. As this aging phenotype progresses (*middle register*), its components become increasingly intertwined and synergistic, culminating in a recalcitrant end stage (*bottom register*) characterized by full-blown diabetes, cardiovascular disease, frailty, and sarcopenia.

That's the metabolic syndrome in a nutshell, and it's bad enough. But the Sick Aging Phenotype gets worse.

### Sarcopenia and osteopenia

The loss of muscle mass (***sarcopenia***) and bone density (***osteopenia***) are not components of the metabolic syndrome, but they are fellow travelers, their clinical impact has long been recognized, and they are central features of the Sick Aging Phenotype, both as cause and effect.

Phil's sedentary lifestyle led to decreased muscle mass even before he developed the metabolic syndrome. Indeed, *loss of muscle tissue was probably his first committed step on the road to the Sick Aging Phenotype*. His declining muscle mass created a parallel decline in muscle glucose utilization and muscle insulin signaling. And, like fat, muscle turns out to be a kind of gland, releasing special signaling molecules called ***myokines***. In Phil's deconditioned state, his myokine profile is likely to be abnormal. The contribution of an abnormal myokine profile to the development of the metabolic syndrome (and hence, to the Sick Aging Phenotype) is not clear. But mounting data suggests that sarcopenic obesity and the metabolic syndrome are partners in crime. You seldom find the latter but in the company of the former.[40]

Because insulin is a growth factor, signaling for anabolic processes, a decrease in insulin sensitivity can be expected to have a disruptive effect on growth and repair. Pertinent examples are ***muscle atrophy***, the loss of muscle mass due to shrinking of muscle cells and connective tissue, and sarcopenia, loss of the muscle cells themselves. Muscle atrophy can be reversed, but once a muscle cell dies, it is difficult or impossible to replace it.

The progression of Phil's sedentary lifestyle to the metabolic syndrome is a perfect scenario for the loss of even more muscle mass – and further decreases in total body insulin sensitivity. Unused, detrained muscle downregulates insulin receptors, turns off protein synthesis, and begins to eat itself to provide calories and amino acids to the rest of the body, which, because of decreased insulin signaling, thinks it's hungry. The result is a progressive loss of muscle tissue and strength. Activity becomes more tiring and more uncomfortable. The organism becomes more inactive.

And so on.

This vicious cycle affects many tissues, not just muscle. Tendons and ligaments lose their stiffness, becoming weaker and more susceptible to strain and injury. Cartilage, a tissue notorious for slow growth and repair, grows thinner and more frail. Even nerve tissue undergoes a progressive deterioration in aging, and declines in growth factor stimulation and insulin sensitivity are at least partly responsible for brain atrophy and dementia.[41]

## Frailty

The Sick Aging Phenotype is coming into focus now. We see how Phil has gone from merely overweight and inactive to a condition in which his insulin signaling is disrupted, his blood pressure is creeping up, his muscles are slowly wasting, his strength is declining, his bones are more brittle, his tissues are more prone to inflammation and degeneration, and his blood is full of fat, giving it the consistency and color of a strawberry milkshake. (That's no exaggeration. I've seen the milkshake many times).

Phil is a wreck, but his nightmare is just beginning.

Hyperglycemia eventually slides into full-blown diabetes, and Phil needs oral hypoglycemic medications like metformin or glyburide to control his blood sugar. These medications are effective for a while, but they don't get at the real root of Phil's disease, and they have significant, occasionally fatal side effects. Eventually, Phil will get his first prescription for insulin, syringes, and needles, and the fun will really begin.

Phil's elevated blood pressure progresses to severe hypertension, and his doctors have him on no less than three blood pressure medicines. These drugs are now absolutely necessary to keep Phil from blowing an O-ring, but they make him a bit dizzy sometimes, which further potentiates his sedentary proclivities.

Phil's sarcopenia continues unabated. His body's muscle mass, which should be a vast landscape of insulin receptors and a major consumer of food energy, is becoming a wasteland of weak, stringy, insulin-resistant, well-marbled, dysfunctional meat. Phil's exercise capacity has gone from poor to pathetic, and his opportunity to turn things around diminishes with every gram of muscle tissue lost. Since Phil never lifts anything heavier than deep-dish pizza, his skeleton doesn't have much to do, and his bone density is dropping fast. Osteopenia is the ever-present sidekick of sarcopenia. Phil is progressing from weakness to full-blown ***frailty***.[42] Illnesses and injuries that would be merely troublesome and painful for a healthy person will shatter him.

Phil is *easy to break.*

Systemic inflammation propels Phil into a twilight realm of *chronic pain*. His joints are creaky and achy. What's left of his muscle mass is sore. His tendons and ligaments are floppy and weak. They injure easily and heal slowly. Phil has knee pain, back pain, neck pain, shoulder pain, headaches, delicate skin, and a chronically upset tummy.

Phil's dyslipidemia prompts his doctor to start him on statins to lower his cholesterol. The available evidence suggests statins will produce a lipid profile (numbers on a lab report) that will make his doctor feel good about himself. But the evidence also suggests that, numbers notwithstanding, Phil is statistically unlikely to reap any meaningful benefit from this therapy.[43] He does turn out, however, to be one of those individuals in whom statins lead to muscle pain,[44] making it even more unlikely that he will begin an exercise program anytime before the Rapture. And the statin doesn't do wonders for his diabetes, either.[45]

Things have gotten out of hand. Hypertension, diabetes, inflammation, and dyslipidemia are inflicting terrible damage on vascular trees and critical tissues throughout Phil's body. His kidneys and retinas are showing signs of damage. Arteries in his heart and brain are riddled with degenerative plaques. He hurts all the time. His strength, exercise tolerance, and mobility are in the toilet, along with his quality of life. He hasn't been laid in years, and couldn't get it up even if the opportunity miraculously presented itself, little blue pill or no. Which brings us to another affliction.

## Polypharmacy

The word ***polypharmacy*** means "lots of drugs." It's a modern epidemic in aging populations, one that harms and even kills people,[46] and it is the final brick in the wall of Phil's Sick Aging Phenotype. When I see patients who display this phenotype in the emergency department, they invariably present with a plastic bag full of powerful medicines, many of which work antagonistically or synergistically in unwholesome ways.

Phil's list of medicines is typical:

- **Insulin** for diabetes – morning and night. Phil injects himself twice a day. He also takes a short-acting insulin throughout the day whenever his sugar is out of control. Which is often.
- **Metformin** for diabetes – morning and night. Has a number of mild side effects. On very rare occasions, will cause a fatal lactic acidosis.
- **Cardizem** for hypertension. A calcium channel blocker. Inhibits Phil's ability to mount a tachycardia (increased heart rate) in response to exercise. If he ever got any.
- **Chlorthalidone** for hypertension. A mild diuretic.
- **Lisinopril** for hypertension. An ACE inhibitor.
- **Vicodin** for chronic pain. "Vitamin V." Phil is addicted.
- **Celebrex** for pain. Not as yummy as Vicodin. May increase the risk of death.
- **Zantac** for chronic dyspepsia. Phil has an extra one whenever he orders a pizza.
- **Senna** for the constipation caused by Phil's inactivity and his Vicodin addiction.
- **Simvastatin** for hypercholesterolemia. Makes Phil's diabetes more difficult to control and makes his muscles hurt. Hasn't made his arteries much healthier though.
- **Fibrate** for hypertriglyceridemia.
- **SSRI-of-the-Month Club** for depression.
- **Quetiapine** for mood disturbances and sleep.
- **Baby aspirin** for coronary artery disease. Anti-platelet therapy.
- **Clopidogrel** for coronary artery disease. Another anti-platelet agent. Phil bruises and bleeds easily.
- **Furosemide** for chronic leg swelling. Another diuretic. Phil has to pee all the time.
- **Albuterol** for chronic obstructive pulmonary disease (COPD, from smoking). Phil has to suck on his "puffer" several times a day. Between Marlboros.
- **Prednisone** for chronic obstructive pulmonary disease. This anti-inflammatory decreases the incidence of Phil's COPD attacks. It also worsens his diabetes, obesity, osteoporosis, and sarcopenia. It's given him a very attractive "buffalo hump" and increased his propensity to a moon-shaped face.

This pharmaceutical stew *seems* to help Phil limp from one day to next. Some of these drugs are actually unnecessary or redundant, and there is a lot of potential for harmful interactions here. For the most part, though, Phil needs these medications now to stay alive and cope with what's left of his existence. *But none of these medicines do anything to correct the underlying pathologies they treat.* The vile potions in his medicine chest keep things under a semblance of control and relieve symptoms, but none of Phil's real problems are being solved.

## End Game

Phil's Sick Aging Phenotype cannot end well. Absent an intervening catastrophe such as a traffic accident, Ebola epidemic, or global war, it can only end with a *Sick Death Phenotype.*

Soon, his pile-driving blood pressure will open a crack in one of the atherosclerotic plaques riddling Phil's left anterior descending coronary artery ("the Widowmaker"). This fissure will cause platelets to gather. On the platelet plug a clot will form and grow, blocking the flow through the artery, starving the heart muscle of oxygen and fuel, leading to a massive heart attack. We've seen how the story ends. With good care, the one-year mortality for this kind of heart attack is on the order of 5–18% for all comers.[47] But Phil isn't all comers. He's a mess, and he has no physiologic reserve to fight back. His 6-week hospitalization is plagued with complications brought on by his obesity, his diabetes, his poor circulation, and his general lack of strength. Phil never has a chance to survive his heart attack, because he has what doctors in polite company call *inadequate physiologic reserve.* Privately we call it the 3Ps: *Piss-Poor Protoplasm.*

All of this was completely preventable. At the very moment Phil's plaque is rupturing, his brother, Will, is playing basketball with his friends on the other end of town. And please remember that *these two guys were identical twins.* They had the same genotype. They grew up in the same house, they went to the same school, they ate the same meatloaf, they shared the same cultural milieu. They're clones. *They have the same DNA.* They were as alike as two people get, but they ended up with vastly different aging and death phenotypes.

Anybody who holds that this doesn't come squarely down to behavior is on the losing side of the argument.[48] Will treated his body like a Ferrari, and never surrendered the keys. Phil treated his body like a rental, and never took ownership of his own flesh. He abdicated his responsibility for Nature's greatest gift to him: the miraculous machine of muscle, bone, blood and brain bestowed upon him at his birth. He abandoned his body, and it abandoned him.

There are a few key points I want you to take away from the foregoing horror story. The first is that Phil's self-destruction wasn't a nice, neat, linear process. It was rather like a slow-motion train wreck. Phil's death was the culmination of a long cascade of interconnected, interdependent processes. It began insidiously, with a little weight gain, a little loss of lean mass, a little decline in exercise capacity, a little elevation in blood sugar and blood pressure. At this stage, Phil looked and felt pretty much the same. He had to buy bigger trousers and his energy wasn't what it once was, but no big deal. Within a decade, these processes had progressed to clinically recognizable disease and moderate functional debility. Within two decades, they had blossomed into full-blown diabetes, severe hypertension, morbid obesity, impotence, chronic pain, disability, frailty, polypharmacy, a miserable quality of life, and the coronary artery disease that would ultimately do him in.

The second point is that Phil's story is an extreme but common one. Depending on multiple factors, including genetics, many people bear the burden of metabolic syndrome and its evil gifts better and longer than Phil. Some will live to be sixty, or seventy. In other words, they get to suffer longer than Phil did.

Many others age without all this extreme pathology. But without intervention, they still face a future of sarcopenia, osteopenia, weakness, and frailty. In other words, as they age, their muscles will atrophy, their bones will become brittle, they will grow progressively weaker, and their resistance to trauma, disease, and even the stresses of everyday life will put them at ever-increasing risk for morbidity and loss of independence. We've all seen this middling phenotype of aging: not Wellness Will, and not Phat Phil. Call it the Scrawny Old Bird phenotype, call it the Bag o' Bones, call it Aunt Helen. Some of us call it "skinny fat." These people don't look fat, but the actual *ratio* of lean mass (bone and muscle) to fat isn't healthy. There is now some evidence to indicate that this *normal weight obesity* phenotype also carries a risk of metabolic deregulation and cardiovascular disease.[49] But even without the burden of hypertension, diabetes, and heart disease, the skinny fat won't live the life they could and should lead: full, vigorous, and healthy.

Now it's time to pause and tip my hat to you, Dear Reader, for wading through all this. It's been a challenging and depressing chapter, full of new and difficult concepts and a picture of aging that might cause us to despair. That's because I've focused heavily on Phil, and what went wrong for him.

*But don't forget Will,* his identical twin, hiking in the Highlands with his girlfriend in his late 80s. There's an alternate future that was always available to Phil, and is still available to most of us. That's what this book is about.

Still, our elaborate picture of what happened to Phil, and what's happening to many of us, is sobering. The Sick Aging Phenotype appears to be self-reinforcing: weakness and decline driving more weakness and decline, circling the drain faster and faster until there's nothing left. The complexity and synergy of the pathologic processes underlying the Sick Aging Phenotype forces us to ask: at what point is it too late to stop the train from leaving the tracks?

Good question, and the short answer is we don't know. It depends on multiple factors, including individual factors, and most particularly upon the determination, will and inner strength of the individual to change course. One thing is certain: the further out of hand things have progressed, *the stronger the medicine* you're going to need to slow the process down. It is just this medicine that we're going to talk about in the chapters ahead.

# 2

# Exercise Medicine

We now take a closer look at what can be done to convert the Sick Aging Phenotype into the Healthy Aging Phenotype, or prevent the Sick Aging Phenotype from developing in the first place. This goal demands the most powerful medicine available: exercise medicine. Exercise has beneficial effects at every stratum of biological organization, from the molecular and cellular levels to the realm of neuropsychiatric health. This chapter illustrates some of the critical distinctions between exercise medicine and standard medical therapies, which are both cause and effect of its unique powers and properties. Exercise is the medicine that actually gets to the root of the Sick Aging Phenotype, instead of just treating its symptoms. These observations will mandate a rational approach to the formulation of an exercise prescription.

## Modern Medicine: How We Traded Syphilis for Heart Failure

One of the problems with modern health care is a deep misunderstanding of what *medicine* is, or at least what it's supposed to be. When I say "medicine," I'm referring to two meanings of the word: Medicine as the *art and science of healing and preserving health*, and medicine as *a specific prescribed treatment or practice*. It goes without saying that Western medicine, after a couple of centuries of extraordinary progress in its understanding and treatment of disease, has entered an era of diminishing returns and reassessment. Germ theory, advances in physiology and cell biology, asepsis, public hygiene, antibiotics, and a revolution in diagnostic imaging have transformed the medical arts. The maturation of surgery from a barber's gig to a scientific discipline permits the correction of many structural diseases, from congenital heart defects to major trauma. Modern pharmacology's manipulation of the organism at every level, from electrophysiology to endocrinology to erections, has given 21st century physicians unprecedented resources in the war against disease and discomfort.

Combined with improvements in public health and nutrition, this awesome medical machinery has contributed to a longer lifespan… and more obesity, cancer, cardiovascular disease, and diabetes than at any other time in human history. We don't die of syphilis and smallpox anymore. Instead, we die of heart failure, stroke, myocardial infarction, or dementia. A particularly tragic manifestation of modern aging is the 65 year-old nursing home pretzel: diapered, demented, immobile limbs twisted like the branches of a dead tree, sore-ridden, tube-fed, chronically dehydrated, kept alive until the insurance stops paying off, finally allowed to die to open up the bed for a more lucrative replacement. This obscenity is perpetuated by modern medicine's ability to keep dead people breathing.

So we live longer, and sometimes in more comfort, but it's not at all clear that we suffer less. Medicine is supposed to preserve life and relieve human misery. It's done very well at the former. The latter seems to be a tougher nut to crack.

## What is a Medicine?

A big part of the problem is that the modern mind conceives of a "medicine" as something you get from a doctor, or the drugstore. "Medicine" has become almost synonymous with "drug," and "health care" has come to mean "going to a doctor to find out what pills to take." The ongoing reassessment of modern medicine is starting to break down this view, thankfully, but it is persistent and pernicious.

It wasn't always so. In traditional societies, "medicine" encompassed a broad range of practices, from the treatment of injury and illness to the maintenance of health, vigor, and integration with the social, natural, and spiritual worlds. A "medicine" could be a tincture, a potion, a poultice or a splint. It could also be a ritual meal, an incantation, a hunt, a tribal dance, a pilgrimage. This all seems very quaint, and indeed much ancient or aboriginal medicine was ineffective or even injurious. But it reflected a different view of medicine and health: *the way we live is, in itself, a kind of medicine*. The screwy idea that health and healing comes in pills, potions and powders is a new one, and serves us no better than the Evil Spirit theory of disease. Unless, of course, you're in the pharmaceutical or supplement business. But those guys have already stopped reading.

*Medicine* is not synonymous with *drug*.

We've already seen this. Phil had medicines for his blood pressure, his diabetes, his arthritis, his messed-up blood lipids, his pain, his depression, his wheezing, his clogged arteries. It made some people a lot of money, but it couldn't stop Phil from descending into a living hell and dying young. These drugs all did what they were designed to do. Each one of them brought about a change in Phil's physiology that made his doctor smile. His blood sugar was tamped down. His blood pressure looked more normal. His lipid profile was closer to what the American College of Cardiology wants to see. His antidepressants tweaked his neurotransmitters exactly as intended. Diuretics made him pee like a race horse, reducing the swelling in his legs. Hydrocodone dulled the physical and existential torment of his slow-motion death.

And not a single one of these drugs made Phil one whit *healthier*. They modulated his physiology, they calmed his symptoms, they may have even helped him live a bit longer. But they didn't decrease his *Suffering*. "Suffering," with a capital S. Phil's *symptoms* (his small-s suffering) may have been moderated, but that didn't remove the simple fact of his misery: prematurely old, frail, fat, impotent, and addicted to a rainbow of pills.

If we think back to our examination of the Sick Aging Phenotype, it's easy to see why this is so. None of Phil's pills could possibly address the multiple factors that lay at the root of his poor health: physical inactivity, epigenetic and environmental factors, diet, aging, obesity, and sarcopenia. Phil's medicines could moderate the effects of his disease, but not the cause.

Let there be no misunderstanding: I am a physician, and I am glad we have these drugs. Patients with hypertension *need* blood pressure medication. Patients with diabetes *need* insulin or oral hypoglycemics to control their glucose. Antidepressants, analgesics, vasopressors, hormonal therapies, anticancer agents, antibiotics – without them, my ability to relieve pain and preserve life and limb would be no better than that of a premodern apothecary peddling leeches and mercury. But I am painfully aware of the limitations of these agents.

Modern drugs don't get to the root of the problem. And they never will.

Because health will never come in a pill.

## Exercise: The Most Powerful Medicine in the World

Back to the twins. You will recall that while Phil was trying to fit all those tablets into his oversized pill organizer, his brother Will was taking his own medicine, in the form of a healthy lifestyle that included vigorous exercise. In fact, because they were twins, with exactly the same genes, our best explanation for why they turned out so differently has to be *the way they lived*, and a big difference in the way they lived was exercise.

Every time Will picked up a dumbbell, went for a walk, hiked a trail, did a bench press, or ran in the park, he was contributing to the phenotypic difference between himself and his brother. In short, Will was taking a medicine that was stronger and more effective than all of Phil's pills combined. And he was having fun doing it.

Doctors have always recommended exercise for health, although the relative emphasis on physical activity and the formulation of an exercise prescription have changed much over the millennia. In the 4th Century BC, Hippocrates said, "eating alone will not keep a man well; he must also take exercise. For food and exercise work together to produce health." In the 3rd Century AD, Galen emphasized the importance of a balanced lifestyle for health, prevention of disease, and correction of certain maladies. The importance of exercise to health continued to be a central feature of the medical model until the late 19th and early 20th centuries, when the emphasis of modern medicine, emboldened by new successes in germ theory, antisepsis, and surgery, began to shift to *treatment of disease* rather than *maintenance of health*, to cure rather than prevention.[1] Since the latter half of the 20th century, we've seen increasing disaffection with the failure of this model, and a growing recognition that regular vigorous exercise has a more profound effect on our health than anything modern medicine has to offer.

*Exercise is the most powerful medicine in the world.* This is not a novel observation,[2] but it is an oft-overlooked one. That's because, as we've seen, the modern concept of a "medicine" is almost synonymous with "drug." Because exercise doesn't make big money for doctors and drug companies. And because, unlike taking pills, exercise involves getting up off your butt and doing something for yourself. There's plenty of blame to go around, but at the end of the day, we each take responsibility for our own health, one way or another.

No drug in the world will ever match the power of exercise medicine. No drug in the world will ever confer so many beneficial effects to so many organ systems, at so little cost, with so few side effects. Let's take a quick survey.

### Musculoskeletal health

The most obvious impact of exercise medicine will be on the fitness of muscle tissue and the skeletal system. Different types of exercise confer different benefit profiles on muscle and bone tissue. But all promote some improvement in muscle metabolism, muscle endurance and, to different degrees, muscle mass, strength and power. Weight-bearing exercise improves bone density,[3] joint function,[4] tendon elasticity and strength,[5] range of motion,[6] and overall physical function.[7] Regular vigorous exercise turns the body's muscle tissue into a vast, insulin-sensitive metabolic sink,[8] an avid consumer of calories and protein. Recently, we have learned that exercise has an impact on the endocrine (hormonal) properties of muscle.[9]

### Cardiovascular health

The effects of regular vigorous exercise on cardiovascular health are well-described and have been known for decades.[10] Exercise improves cardiac stroke volume, decreases resting heart rate, inhibits the development and progression of hypertension, promotes more favorable blood-lipid profiles,[11] and seems to retard the development of peripheral vascular disease, including coronary artery and cerebrovascular disease,[12] with attendant decreases in the risk of heart attack and stroke.

## Metabolic health

Exercise gets to the very root of the metabolic syndrome and the modern aging phenotype. Exercise ramps up energy flux, reduces visceral fat, turns the muscles into calorie-burning ovens, and improves insulin sensitivity. For these reasons, it has gained recognition as a major therapeutic modality for the metabolic syndrome and Type 2 diabetes.[13] This has profound implications for blood sugar, blood pressure, serum lipids, and systemic inflammation. Exercise increases the elaboration of growth factors,[14] which promotes increases in muscle mass and moderates the effects of aging on multiple organ systems, including the central nervous system.[15] Changes in glucocorticoids, thyroid hormone, inflammatory mediators, and sex steroids have all been described.[16] *Exercise transforms the metabolic landscape.*

## Cellular health

Exercise works through multiple pathways to promote cellular health. The anabolic and growth factor responses associated with vigorous exercise retard tissue atrophy, promote healthier energy metabolism, and decrease cellular damage caused by free radicals. *Free radicals* are highly reactive molecules that inflict enormous damage on cellular membranes, cellular organelles, cellular biochemistry and the genetic material itself. The contribution of this free radical *oxidative stress* to a wide variety of disease states, from cancer to cardiovascular disease, is well-established, and a large body of research implicates a progressive decline in the body's ability to neutralize these radicals in many of the degenerative changes associated with the aging process.[17]

There's an interesting paradox here: intense physical activity actually *increases* the production of free radicals, just as an engine running at high RPMs generates more exhaust and heat. Yet regular, vigorous exercise *reduces* actual cellular free radical stress and damage.[18] It appears that exercise-induced oxidative stress promotes healthy biochemical adaptations that increase cellular tolerance to free radicals.[19]

## Neurological health

The depredations of aging and the Sick Aging Phenotype on the body are awful enough, but loss of neurological and cognitive functions are the cruelest cuts of all. This is an area where modern medicine is particularly impotent. It is only recently that we've even begun to *understand* degenerative neurological disease, brain atrophy, dementia, and loss of neurological function in aging. Effective drug therapies for the aging brain are probably still decades away.

Fortunately, exercise medicine has shown itself to be useful even in this difficult area. The effect of exercise on growth factor release,[20] neurotransmitter systems,[21] vascular signaling molecules, antioxidant molecules, the growth of new cellular power plants (***mitochondria***),[22] the growth of new blood vessels, and a beneficial effect on the progression of vascular disease in the brain (as in the heart), have all been cited as mechanisms by which exercise promotes brain health, fights cognitive impairment, and impacts on the development of dementia,[23] including Alzheimer's dementia.[24] Exercise promotes brain plasticity and decreases the loss of brain tissue in aging,[25] and is increasingly prescribed for patients with stroke[26] and Parkinsonism.[27] On the whole, the research literature strongly indicates that exercise is critical for maintaining brain function in aging.[28]

## Psychological health

Psychological and "spiritual" health are the most important realms of all. Here again, when one takes into account risk, cost, and probability of benefit, exercise promises to be the best medicine available, with studies indicating a strong correlation between physical activity and mental health.[29] Sleep, cognitive function, mood, and quality of life have all been reported to respond to exercise.[30] It bears pointing out, however, that of all the spheres of health, this is the one most difficult to assay in a reliable, reproducible fashion. For example, "quality of life" would seem to be a slippery thing to measure. One man's *Paradiso* is another's *Purgatorio*. But on the whole, the preponderance of evidence indicates that exercise, mental health, and a better life all tend to go together, which should surprise exactly nobody.

#### Specific disease states

A rapidly growing body of research has demonstrated the positive effects of physical exercise in patients with a broad range of pathologies: hypertension,[31] heart failure,[32] kidney disease,[33] cancer,[34] diabetes,[35] depression,[36] osteopenia,[37] arthritis,[38] dementia.[39] In some cases, the effect of exercise on an established disease state is primarily palliative. In others, exercise may slow or even reverse the course of existing disease. But the primary power of exercise is its ability to prevent disease. Any disease state, once established, is likely to involve structural, epigenetic, and systemic changes that make reversal difficult or even physically impossible. The best treatment is to not get the disease in the first place. Exercise clearly decreases the risk of developing metabolic syndrome and cardiovascular disease, and there is tantalizing (but not definitive) evidence that it exerts preventative effects against cancer and some forms of dementia.

## Unique Properties of Exercise Medicine

Exercise is indeed a powerful medicine: low cost, excellent side-effect profile, virtually no contraindications (almost everyone can do *some* form of exercise), and completely untouched by the Medicare donut hole. Unlike any other drug, it gets to the root of the modern aging phenotype and the metabolic syndrome. But there are other important differences between exercise medicine and standard medical therapies. It is instructive to examine them.

#### Exercise medicine is self-administered

Yes, I know you take your own pills. Lousy taste and inconvenience notwithstanding, this is nevertheless a straightforward operation: Open the bottle, pop your pill, wash it down. An insulin-dependent diabetic has to be rather more committed, but monitoring your blood sugar and injecting yourself with insulin takes at most a few minutes a day. Other modern medicines and therapies require more invasive or time-consuming processes, of course, and are administered by specialists.

Exercise medicine is quite different. It takes considerably more time and effort than popping a pill or taking your insulin, and you have to do it yourself. This is true whether you work out in your basement alone, go to a commercial franchise gym, or hire a personal trainer. Unless and until you show up and do the work, there's no treatment. *This medicine is on you.* It requires your commitment and involvement in a way no other modern medical therapy even approaches. In fact, this requirement for self-administration is one of the principal benefits of exercise medicine. Exercise demands that the patient engage with his own body in a constructive and therapeutic way, instead of surrendering his flesh to the ministrations of a physician or the effects of a pill or potion. This engagement promotes an entirely healthy sense that the patient has some degree of control over, and responsibility for, his health and physical destiny. And a properly administered exercise medicine requires the patient to assimilate a deeper understanding of his own anatomy, physiology, and adaptive capacities. In short, the requirement of self-administration means that exercise medicine *integrates* the person with his physical being in a way that no pharmaceutical or passive receipt of treatment can ever achieve.

#### Exercise medicine reduces needs for other medicines

This is unusual for modern medicines. The epidemic of polypharmacy described in Chapter 1 is a by-product of the limitations of modern pharmacotherapy. Most drugs treat symptoms, not disease. And those drugs have side effects, leading to still more symptoms. So more drugs to treat the side effects. And so on. Exercise medicine actually reduces the need for other medicines, by preventing or moderating disease processes.

### Lifetime Therapy

In this respect, exercise medicine resembles the *reality* of modern pharmaceuticals, but not the *perception.* It is true that many acute illnesses, primarily infectious diseases, can be resolved with appropriate therapy. But acute conditions like appendicitis, pink eye, a broken arm, or a boil aren't the salient features of the Sick Aging Phenotype. Unhealthy aging is dominated by chronic metabolic, cardiovascular, and degenerative disease. Many patients are under the impression, at least at first, that a course of medical treatment will reverse disease brought on by abuse, neglect, intrinsic aging processes, genetics, or bad luck. Of course, that's usually not the case. Diabetes, hypertension, degenerative diseases, many endocrine conditions, certain genetic conditions – all require a lifetime of medical therapy. Patients ignore this at their peril.

Exercise medicine is powerful, but when the patient stops taking it, the effects wear off. Even when we achieve unusually good results with exercise therapy – for example, the patient is able to reduce or eliminate medication for his diabetes or high blood pressure – the underlying condition isn't "cured." Aging and degeneration are never cured. They're *managed.* Physical inactivity, a principal driver of the Sick Aging Phenotype, can only be treated by regular, vigorous, lifelong exercise. It's a *medicine*. But it's not a *cure*.

### Inverted Dosing

Think about the way we dose most medicines. As the patient gets sicker, we increase the dose or, worse still, add another medicine. If the patient improves, the doctor tries to decrease the dose and number of medications (or should).

Exercise medicine is the exact opposite. When exercise medicine is used properly, *the dose goes up as the patient gets healthier*. We start weak and deconditioned. We begin an exercise regimen. Our strength and fitness improve. So we can work out a little harder, increasing the dose. The increased dose improves our strength and conditioning still further, allowing us to increase the dose again.

This "inverted dosing" of exercise medicine is incredibly important. It illustrates the principle of ***progressive overload***, which is fundamental to the administration of exercise medicine, and it underlies the critical distinction between *exercise* and *training*, which we will explore in great detail in the next chapter.

## Toward an Exercise Prescription

At this point, let's step back and take stock. We've seen that the modern aging phenotype is dominated by the metabolic syndrome, cardiovascular disease, decreased muscle mass, decreased bone density, loss of function, frailty and decline. And we've seen that just one medicine, exercise medicine, is a more powerful preventative and therapy for this phenotype than any drug or intervention offered by modern medical practice.

Of course, our discussion of exercise medicine to this point has been couched in very general terms. Exercise encompasses a vast array of activities: walks in the park, marathons, martial arts, yoga, tennis, volleyball, weightlifting, Pilates, ballroom dancing, Crossfit. What *kind* of physical activity should be the first choice of the aging individual?

This is obviously a complex question, and depends to a large degree on individual factors. Chief among these factors are the individual's preferences, tolerances, abilities, and resources. The "ideal" exercise prescription is useless if one can't or won't do the exercise. But in general, it seems clear that the aging individual will benefit most from an exercise medicine that enhances insulin sensitivity, increases muscle mass, promotes bone density, increases joint integrity and tendon strength, confers all the benefits of exercise medicine to all organ systems, and can be titrated exactly and safely to higher and higher doses as the "patient" gets better and better.

In the following chapters, we're going to look at this question in more detail. By the time we're done, we're not just going to arrive at an exercise prescription for the aging adult. We're going to transform our entire idea of *what modern aging can be.*

# 3

# From Prescription to Program: Safety and Dosing

If exercise is the most powerful medicine, what is its most effective formulation? What is the appropriate exercise prescription for the aging adult? In this chapter, we shall consider the requirements of a rational prescription of exercise medicine for those in their forties, fifties, sixties, and beyond. We will look at the first two of these requirements: safety and therapeutic window. This will compel us to examine the critical distinction between *exercise* and *training*. These considerations lead to the conclusion that the most powerful and rational exercise prescription must take the form of an explicit long-term training *program*. The implications of this approach will confront us with a challenging and transformative picture of the aging adult.

## Requirements for the Exercise Prescription

We've seen how a sedentary lifestyle contributes directly and substantially to the Sick Aging Phenotype and how exercise is a powerful medicine against the development of this slow-motion catastrophe. Of course, *you already know this*. You may not have known about the metabolic syndrome or sarcopenia or phenotypes or insulin sensitivity. But you *know* you need exercise. You know it because friends, family, doctors, and the media constantly tell you so. And you also know it at a biological level, because you weren't made to sit on your ass. You were made to move. Life *is* movement. Exercise is fundamental to our health.

But *exercise* is a broad and fuzzy term, and covers a multitude of sins. At the most fundamental level, exercise is physical activity. Going for a walk is exercise. Yoga is exercise. Cleaning out the garage is exercise. So are jogging, lifting weights, fencing, badminton, and Pilates. All of these are better than being a couch potato. But it should be obvious that not all forms of exercise are created equal. Put another way, exercise medicine comes in different formulations, with different dosing strengths, routes of administration, efficacies, and side-effect profiles. Some exercise medicine is as powerful and specific as the strongest chemotherapy. Other exercise medicine is cough syrup: arguably better than nothing and perhaps a bit soothing, but ultimately ineffective and beside the point.[1] And like any medicine, exercise can be wrongly prescribed or incorrectly administered, and actually become toxic.[2]

So, how do we prescribe an exercise medicine for the aging adult? There are multiple parameters to consider here.

### General Exercise Prescription Criteria

1. **Our exercise medicine must be safe**. I trust I'll get no argument here.

2. **Our exercise medicine must have a wide *therapeutic window***, meaning it should be available in a broad range of effective doses, from low at the beginning of therapy to higher doses as we get healthier.

3. **Our exercise medicine must be comprehensive**. Our exercise prescription should be as integrated and complete as possible.

4. **Our exercise prescription must specifically and effectively combat the Sick Aging Phenotype**: It should attack the metabolic syndrome, reduce visceral fat, arrest or reverse sarcopenia and osteopenia, and fight frailty by retaining or restoring strength, power, endurance, mobility, balance, and function. Ideally, it should also reduce the requirements for additional medication (polypharmacy).

5. **Our exercise prescription should be efficient and as simple as possible.** But no simpler. The prescription must be practical, accessible, and time-efficient. This will promote compliance, enjoyment, and long-term success.

When we look at the foregoing requirements, we begin to see that a prescription to *just get some exercise* is not enough for the aging adult. Yes, going for a walk three times a week is far better than nothing, but it's just not strong or versatile enough a medicine to fully combat and transform the Sick Aging Phenotype. Cage fighting, on the other hand, would be a toxic overdose of "exercise medicine" for most aging adults.

## Safety

This is the first of our requirements. An exercise prescription which increases the risk of injury or illness rather misses the point. Now, if you're in your fifties and you like boxing, that's great. You can follow your bliss, take your licks, and get some exercise at the same time. In general, however, activities that involve blunt force trauma, unexpected twists and turns, high gravitational potential energies (cliff diving) or blood gases boiling out of solution (scuba diving) are poor candidates for a ***General Exercise Prescription***, an exercise program that can be safely recommended for almost all aging adults. I'm *really* not saying that aging adults shouldn't do these activities, although prudence is a beautiful thing. My point is rather that they aren't going to fit the bill *as exercise medicine*, primarily because they can't be considered as safe as other alternatives. There are other reasons, too, and we'll get to those.

So, what makes for a safe exercise medicine?

### Components of Exercise Safety

**Movement patterns.** A primary determinant of exercise safety is the *movement patterns* that make up the activity. An exercise prescription for aging adults should not incorporate extreme, impulsive, or unnatural movement patterns. *T'ai Chi* is a popular exercise prescription for aging adults all over the world,[3] because it takes the practitioner through a complete and natural range of motion without putting undue stress on older joints. The forces involved are moderate and predictable. And it's a classic example of a "low-impact" activity: no jumping, stomping, falling, or striking. Although *T'ai Chi* is lacking in other requirements, it fits the bill for a *safe* exercise prescription.[4] Gymnastics, *Tae Kwon Do,* and figure skating would be less optimal choices.

**Dynamics and Environment.** These factors strongly influence the safety of the activity. Outdoor activities involve exposure to the elements and a virtually limitless array of obstacles and hazards. Hiking, surfing, and mountain biking are terrific exercises, but they involve a certain degree of risk by their very nature. Soccer, martial arts, tennis, and other very dynamic sports demand sudden, explosive movements and unpredictable impacts, twists and turns, with a higher potential for injury. You can see how these factors are related to our first determinant: movement patterns. Blocking a goal in soccer or answering a serve in tennis call for very rapid and dramatic changes in joint moments and force vectors. Such highly dynamic activities intrinsically increase the potential for injury. Again, these are great exercises, and if they bring meaning and joy into your life, you should certainly do them. But they aren't ideal choices for a *General* Exercise Prescription.

Strength training, whether it is done with free weights or machines, is an *extremely* safe exercise modality,[5] as long as the exercises are chosen and performed correctly. Proper strength training is conducted in a controlled (usually indoor) environment. Recent fads involving the use of weights on unstable surfaces have been thoroughly debunked in the scientific literature, and are dying well-deserved deaths.[6] Strength training is traditionally and properly conducted with exercises that describe a natural but complete range of motion on a stable surface, using carefully selected loads that increase over time. So properly designed strength training programs avoid unpredictable forces, impacts, and joint moments. Correct strength training is therefore incredibly safe, and well-tolerated by individuals of any age. This feature alone is enough to bring strength training to our attention as an important candidate for our exercise prescription.

**Dosing range.** Finally, to be safe, the activity should be available in a broad range of doses, from very low to very high. An activity such as judo or sprinting that simply cannot be performed well at low intensity will not be safe enough for the aging adult to be a major component of any General Exercise Prescription. As it happens, the ability to dose an exercise is important for other fundamental reasons, and so we make it one of our major criteria in its own right.

## Dosing: The Therapeutic Window

An ideal exercise medicine should have a wide ***therapeutic window***. That is, it should be available in a broad range of safe and effective doses, and not just to meet the criterion of safety. As we saw in Chapter 2, exercise medicine should incorporate the principle of progressive overload, starting out at low doses and progressing to higher doses as the individual becomes more fit. This criterion eliminates, practically or categorically, a broad range of activities, including many that are commonly used for exercise prescriptions.

For example, how do you dose tennis as an exercise medicine? Or *T'ai Chi*? Or racquetball? From a practical perspective, the short answer is that you really can't. You can practice and enjoy these wonderful activities, partake of their benefits and become more skillful at them, but that's not what we're talking about.

Let's try another example. How do you dose *walking* as exercise medicine? This seems to be a more tractable problem. Two approaches immediately come to mind. The first is to increase the ***intensity*** of our walking. In other words, we increase the speed of our walk, the length of our stride, the swing of our arms. Perhaps we put some weights on our ankles or walk up a steeper grade. Increasing the intensity means that each individual step is harder than it is at a lower intensity.

The other option is to increase the ***volume*** of our walking. Quite simply, this means we walk for longer distances or times, or we walk more often. Instead of walking for a mile at a given intensity, we walk for two miles, doubling our walking volume.

Both of these approaches increase the dose of our walking medicine. And of course, if we wish, we can change both the intensity and the volume simultaneously in some ratio or other. Let's say we walk at a power output (intensity) of 250 watts for a distance (volume) of 4 km, giving us a volume-intensity product – a dose – of 1000 watt-km.[7] We could double the intensity (500 watts) and cut the volume in half (2 km). This would keep our volume-intensity dose product constant at 1000 watt-km. It would, however, change the *quality* of our workout. It would be more of a high-intensity, low-volume routine (and closer to a *run*) than the one we started with. As with a drug, changing the formulation or administration can change the fundamental character and effect of an exercise medicine,[8] even when the dose is the same. Thus, potassium is a vital nutrient, essential for life, but lethal when given as a rapid intravenous infusion.

As it happens, walking as an exercise prescription for the aging adult has a practically limited dosing range. It certainly works as a low-dose exercise prescription. But the intensity can be increased only so far before you're actually into *running*, and the volume can only be increased so far before you die of boredom, your feet start to hurt, or you morph into Forrest Gump and find yourself on a highway in the middle of nowhere. Running has a similar drawback. Its dosing range is broader than for walking, making it a better exercise medicine, but you can only increase the intensity so far before you're *sprinting*, and increasing the volume means mileage, time, and wear-and-tear on shoes, muscles, and joints. There are other problems with running, as we'll see.

For the moment, however, please observe that our examination of exercise dosing has brought us to a very important concept: training variables.

## Training, Exercise, and Practice

***Training variables*** are factors we can manipulate to adjust the dose of exercise medicine and improve our ability to take that medicine productively and in accordance with the principle of progressive overload. We've just seen two such variables, volume and intensity. Other training variables[9] include (but are not necessarily limited to) frequency, work interval, rest interval, set number, repetition number, speed of movement, recovery interval, exercise order, periodization, and specificity. In Part III, Coach Andy Baker and I will show you exactly how the most important training variables are manipulated in long-term programs for enhancement of fitness attributes. The present point is that there's been a subtle shift in our discussion. We're moving from talking about *exercise* to talking about *training*. The difference is critical, as is the difference between *training* and *practice*. In this book we employ these terms as defined by Rippetoe.[10]

***Exercise*** is the more inclusive term, as we've seen. Exercise is just getting up and moving around. It's "getting in a workout." It's a game of tennis. It's washing the car. It's walking the dog. It's working up a sweat. It's far healthier than the sedentary alternative, and to be encouraged under the right circumstances.

***Training***, on the other hand, is a special type of exercise. *Training is exercise that manipulates training variables as part of a long-term program aimed at the improvement of one or more General Fitness Attributes*. The cross-country skier trains to increase endurance. The combat athlete trains to increase power. The gymnast trains to increase flexibility, and the football player trains to increase lean body mass and strength.

Please notice that I don't say the football player *trains* to improve his throwing technique. Similarly, the fencer doesn't train a parry, the boxer a punch, or the dancer a pirouette. These are sport-specific *skills* that are ***practiced*** on the field, on the rink, on the mat. A figure skater doesn't need to practice sword technique, and a fencer doesn't need to practice a breast stroke.

But all these athletes share the need to *train* the ***General Fitness Attributes***. Different authors have presented lists of varying length and detail for the properties of fitness and physical performance. But for the purposes of this text we will define the General Fitness Attributes as ***strength*** (the ability to produce force), ***power*** (the ability to display strength quickly, which includes the property of speed), ***endurance*** (or "stamina," the ability to engage in sustained physical activity), ***balance*** (the ability to statically or dynamically maintain a stable position over the center of gravity), ***mobility*** (flexibility, agility, coordination), and ***body composition*** (most crudely expressed as BMI or the ratio of lean to fat mass).[11] The General Fitness Attributes are common to virtually all athletic or physical performance endeavors – which is why you find the gals from varsity basketball doing the same strength and conditioning exercises as the guys from the wrestling team, or the Marines from Force Recon.

Sport-specific skills are *practiced*. General Fitness Attributes are *trained*.[12]

Now we can see why tennis, *T'ai Chi,* and volleyball, while great exercises, aren't suitable as General Exercise Prescriptions. They aren't *trained*, they're *practiced*. They develop skills, and they each bring some fitness attributes along for the ride, to be sure. Practicing *T'ai Chi* will develop strength, mobility, and balance...up to a point. But such activities aren't effective for the *optimal and progressive* development of an entire range of General Fitness Attributes. Once the athlete has mastered a particular sport through *practice*, the best approach to improving performance is to *train* the General Fitness Attributes. On the flip side, an individual who has trained these fitness attributes is better-prepared to practice a chosen sport more productively and safely.

I'd like you to notice something else. *The requirements for an athletic training program will be identical to those we have enumerated for the General Exercise Prescription.* A coach who wants to train his fencer, football player, or figure skater for strength, power, mobility, and endurance wants the program to be ***safe***. Injuries sustained while perfecting a triple axel, pole vault, or scrimmage in practice, or while using them in competition, constitute risks inherent in the sport. Injuries in *training* are quite another thing. A coach who injures his athletes just to *prepare* them for practice and play deserves last place on the unemployment line.

A good coach wants to be able to titrate or ***dose*** the training for his athlete, focusing on developing General Fitness Attributes early in the training season, then changing the emphasis to maintenance of those attributes as competition draws near so the athlete can focus on skill and competition. Once again, our attention is drawn to strength training. *Strength training fits this requirement beautifully*, because it allows for the very precise loading of human movement patterns.

The coach wants the training program to be ***comprehensive*** and integrated, covering all the fitness attributes necessary for optimizing performance with a program that is as simple as possible. And just as we want a ***specific*** exercise prescription that effectively combats the Sick Aging Phenotype, Coach wants a training program that will produce a fitness attribute profile most appropriate for the sport in question. All athletes need to be strong, powerful, mobile, and conditioned. But cross-country skiers need more endurance than fencers, gymnasts need more power than tennis players, and figure skaters need more mobility than linebackers.

Finally, Coach wants a program that is ***simple*** and efficient, so that his players can develop and maintain their fitness attributes but still focus on skill, practice, and competition.

Does all of this sound familiar?

*Wait a minute,* you say. *Hold on*. This book is about exercise for aging adults. When did we start talking about *training athletes?*

Actually, I've been talking about it from the beginning. I just didn't use those words because, quite frankly, I didn't want to scare you off. But we've arrived at a point where we're ready for a critical transformation in our thinking.

## The Most Extreme Athlete of All

Let's review. We began with an uncomfortable look at the horrors of the Sick Aging Phenotype: Something has to change. The concept of exercise medicine, the most powerful medicine in the world, threw us a lifeline. From there, we began a methodical search for the exercise prescription best suited to prevent, arrest and reverse the Sick Aging Phenotype. That led us to the issue of dosing exercise medicine, and we saw how dosing considerations require us to manipulate training variables. Training variables are used by coaches and trainers all over the world to improve the General Fitness Attributes of athletes, soldiers and other professionals engaged in a wide variety of sporting, combat, law-enforcement, and other activities.

Let's reconsider these General Fitness Attributes: Strength. Power. Mobility. Balance. Endurance. Body composition. These attributes are sought by all athletes who want to win. They are universal. When we improve these attributes, we improve the foundation for the physical performance of *any* athlete, policeman, soldier, or fireman.

Or grandmother.

Or father. Or husband. Caregiver. Mother. Nurse. Contractor. Weekend warrior. Rabbi. Teacher. Grocery clerk.

Because, really, who *doesn't* need to be strong, powerful, flexible, and fit? Who *doesn't* need a healthy body composition, strong bones, mobile joints, and excellent stability and balance? Who *doesn't* need all the General Fitness Attributes?

More to the point: *who needs these things more than you do?* Middle age is upon you, or perhaps it has already passed you by. Time is chipping away at the General Fitness Attributes addressed by training: your strength, your power, your muscle mass, your bone density, your balance. You don't compete for trophies, but you do like to surf, or play with your kids, or keep up with the Young Turks on the job. Fitness isn't just something athletes have. ***Fitness*** is the term that describes the organism's readiness and capacity to meet the physical demands of its life and environment. So you need the General Fitness Attributes, even though you aren't an athlete.

Or *are* you?

The word ***athlete*** comes to us from the Greek ἀθλητής, *athletes,* derived from the word for "prize." The *practical* meaning of this word during the classical Olympic era was something like "contestant" and also something like "combatant."[13] The ancient Olympic games were bound up with profound cultural, political and religious significance – the full slice of life – and the stakes were high. A victor might be housed, clothed and fed for his entire life, and his feats chronicled for the ages. A contestant had to declare an oath before Zeus that he had been *training* for at least 10 months, and competition evoked not so much the niceties of the modern playing field as the dangers of the ancient battlefield: wrestling, boxing, javelin throws, chariot races, and the *hoplitodromos*, a race in full battle armor. Losers (and victors) could be maimed, disfigured, even killed. The games were a reflection of life, and like life, they were brutal.

In our culture, when we think of an "athlete," we think of someone who wins or loses the game and goes home. You, on the other hand, are rather more like the ancient Olympian. You're playing a more high-risk game, and for a much bigger prize. The stakes couldn't be higher. Whether you like it or not, *you are in the arena*, grappling with time, atrophy, decay, and disease. It's a death match.

## From Aging Adult to Masters Athlete

This is the change of viewpoint I've been talking about, and it will transform our language as we move forward. From now on, we're not going to think of you so much as an aging adult who needs to be treated, but as an *Athlete of Aging,* a ***Masters Athlete***, who needs to be *trained*. We get to the same prescription, but the difference in headspace is fundamental and salutary. Exercise medicine isn't the passive receipt of a drug, treatment, operation or gizmo. This medicine you have to seize for yourself, *because that's part of the therapy*.

Exercise medicine must be safe, effective, efficient, quantifiable, and precisely prescribed and administered to achieve specific physiological and performance goals.

That's called *training*.

Training is for *athletes*.

No matter your age, no matter your disabilities, your strength, stamina, mobility, or general situation, you can train. Like any other athlete, you can start where you are and build on that. If you're fat, weak, sick, stiff...*you're still an athlete if you train.* Such miseries and handicaps are your opponents, and they must be dealt with, because they won't just go away. You *must* begin to think of yourself as a Masters Athlete, engaged in the most demanding and brutal sport of all: getting old.

The prize you're competing for isn't cash, honor, fame, trophies, or even a longer lifespan.

No medicine, including exercise medicine, alternative medicine, or any sort of dietary intervention, has ever been demonstrated to lead to significantly longer healthy life spans *in human populations.* Exercise medicine may preserve you from disease that will cut your life short, but it won't extend your *natural* healthy lifespan. The power of any true geriatric medicine, including exercise medicine, is not longevity but *compression of morbidity*: shrinking the sick and dysfunctional part of our dying into a smaller and smaller slice of our lives.[14] The goal line in your sport is to be healthy to the last. That's the *prize* implicit in the word *athlete.*

You're not playing this game for *more* years. You're playing this game for *better* years.

*Aging is an extreme sport*, and you're in the game willy-nilly. You can sit on the benches and pretend it's not real. You can pray for a pill to ease your pain and your fear. You can try to run out the clock. You can surrender to the other team.

Or…you can *play*. But if you want to play, like the Olympian swearing his oath before Zeus, you have to *train*. And the minute you begin to train, you become an *athlete*.

Game on.

# 4

# Enduring Resistance, Resisting Endurance: Comprehensive Training

A rational exercise prescription – or training program – must be comprehensive. This is the third of our prescription criteria, and in this chapter I will make the case that resistance training for strength offers the most biologically and functionally complete training modality available. Strength training promotes favorable adaptations across the spectrum of General Fitness Attributes and biological energy systems to a degree unmatched by any other form of physical training. Moreover, the functional, biochemical, and tissue-level adaptations produced by strength training turn out to be precisely those that are most important for the optimal performance and health of the Masters Athlete. The addition of a low-volume, high-intensity conditioning component to strength training results in a program that addresses all the General Fitness Attributes.

## Comprehensive Training

In the previous chapter, we investigated the first two of our criteria for an exercise prescription. We acknowledged the obvious conclusion that such a prescription should be ***safe***, and we looked at determinants of that safety, including movement pattern, dynamics, and environment.

Safety was also determined, in part, by the second of our criteria: the ability to titrate, or ***dose***, the exercise medicine. Our examination of this criterion brought us to a consideration of training variables, and from there we got to the idea of the Masters Athlete. For the athlete who plays the extreme sport of aging, the proper exercise prescription is a rational manipulation of training variables geared toward the long-term optimization of General Fitness Attributes: strength, power, endurance, and so on.

Exercise is indeed a powerful medicine, but we're well past such a generic observation. Our prescription must *specify* the formulation, administration, and dosing of that medicine, and the goals of treatment, just as an athlete's training program specifies exercise selection, intensity, volume, frequency, and performance goals. For our purposes, *exercise prescription and training program mean the same thing.*

Let's continue fleshing out our prescription/ program, starting with the next of our criteria:

3. **Complete.** ***Our exercise prescription/training program must be comprehensive.***

We need a program that is comprehensive, integrated and complete. That's the focus of this chapter. We're going to look at the different types of training available to the Masters Athlete and how they impact the spectrum of General Fitness Attributes, which will in turn involve an examination of biological energy systems and how they are expressed at the level of muscle tissue. We'll see that muscle tissue is not uniform. It is rather a complex construction of different muscle cell types which use energy and produce force differently. As we age, the loss of muscle is dominated by the loss of fibers which are more critical for strength than for endurance. This will have direct implications for our training prescription. You may find some of this material challenging. I hope you will also find it as fascinating as I do. I promise to make it all digestible.

## Training Modalities and Fitness Attributes

We need a program that hits all the General Fitness Attributes: strength, power, mobility, balance, endurance, and body composition. We have no shortage of options available to us.

### Resistance training

As the name suggests, this form of training uses some form of resistance against which muscles must contract. Up to now, I've used the term more-or-less synonymously with "strength training," as do most exercise scientists and biomedical researchers. I will continue to use the term this way, but resistance training can be used to develop other fitness attributes, including endurance, power, and mobility.[1]

In fact, *all* forms of exercise are based on resistance. There can be no exercise without muscle activity, and for muscles to produce movement or exert force, they have to work *against* something – a resistance. Be all that as it may, let's just agree that, as in most of the published literature on the topic, we will use the terms "resistance training" and "strength training" interchangeably.

Resistance exercise comes in a wide variety of flavors, characterized by the type of resistance, the exercises used, the specific training goals, programming, and other variables. For example, there are cute little "strengthening" bands that you stretch with your arms and legs. You can even do "squats" with them. We find a bewildering variety of machines, Nautilus and the like, which are easy to use and can work practically every muscle and joint of your body. You've all seen the Bowflex, the Soloflex, the Shake Weight, the ThighMaster, and all manner of silly gizmos, most of which probably end up in thrift stores, garage sales, or landfills, without ever having made anybody any stronger. And of course there are free weights. But free weights themselves encompass a wide range of exercises and training goals. Barbells, dumbbells and kettlebells can be used for general strength acquisition, power development, muscle endurance, muscle hypertrophy, or "general conditioning." They can also be used to waste everybody's time and create business for emergency physicians, orthopods, and physical therapists. It's important to know what you're doing.

On the off chance you haven't guessed by now, this book is focused on strength training, so we'll obviously have a lot to say about it later. For now, let's look at some other options.

### Endurance training

Endurance training is focused on aerobic conditioning and the ability to produce relatively low-intensity movements over long intervals. Typical of this type of training is ***LSD***, or ***Long Slow Distance*** exercise, such as running, hiking, cross-country skiing, biking, swimming laps, etc. Such exercises do not produce high levels of strength or power relative to strength training, but they can optimize cardiovascular fitness and tissue oxygen delivery, and condition athletes to produce low or moderate power outputs for extended periods.

### Mobility and balance training

This type of training includes such options as Yoga, *T'ai Chi*, various forms of stretching, balance drills, and the like. They appear to deliver as advertised. For example, *T'ai Chi* has been shown to prevent falls in the elderly,[2] and Yoga practice has profound effects on mobility and balance. These training modalities do not promote progressive development of endurance,[3] strength,[4] or power.

### High-intensity interval training

**HIIT,** or high-intensity interval training, is currently a very popular approach to conditioning, as distinguished from the low-intensity aerobic conditioning promoted by LSD-based endurance training. In this form of training, brief intervals of very high intensity are alternated with short rest periods or low-intensity work. Variants include the Tabata regimen, Fartlek intervals, the Gibala regimen, the Peter Coe method, the Timmons, and, in a loose sense, Crossfit.[5] Regimens differ on the basis of the activity used (sprinting, lifting weights, biking, etc.), target intensities (as measured by subjective markers, heart rate, lactate production, etc) and the number and duration of work and rest intervals. HIIT promotes fat-burning and improvement in body composition, supposedly by inducing a long metabolic "afterburn," although the exact mechanisms remain at issue.[6] HIIT develops aerobic endurance to a similar degree as LSD, but in less training time.[7]

## Interference Effects

At this point, the formulation of our exercise prescription may appear straightforward. The emphasis of each of these types of training seems specific and unambiguous. Strength training builds the attribute of strength, endurance training builds endurance, mobility exercise builds mobility, and so on. What's the problem? Clearly, particular forms of exercise have evolved to address all of the General Fitness Attributes, and if we want to cover all the bases in our training program, we simply combine these modalities in some way. But, like everything else in life, it's actually more complicated than all that.

This becomes apparent as soon as we look at the two fitness attributes that stand out in the minds of most people as being the most important: strength and endurance. When we think of any sort of physical performance, we tend to see these two physical attributes as primary, and all athletes possess them, in varying proportions. So it would seem obvious that the Masters Athlete must train for both.

The problem is that ***concurrent training*** for strength and endurance present us with some fundamental difficulties, both theoretical and practical. In short, serious strength training and LSD endurance training demonstrate ***interference effects***.[8] Strength training and LSD training use different energy systems and demand performance from different populations of muscle fibers. This might seem like a good thing (more comprehensive), but it turns out that concurrent strength and LSD training probably flips a metabolic toggle, the so-called ***AMPK-Akt switch*** (Figure 4-1), in a way that favors aerobic endurance adaptations at the expense of long-term strength adaptations.[9] This has implications for aging muscle at the cellular level. In other words, strength training and LSD training promote the development of different muscle phenotypes. They also promote different athletic phenotypes. "Aerobic" athletes (marathoners, cyclists, cross-country skiers) can perform extraordinary feats of endurance, but they tend to lack strength and power. "Anaerobic" athletes (sprinters, shot-putters, weightlifters, wrestlers, fencers) train to generate high power outputs over short intervals. It is nevertheless interesting to note that power athletes tend to have greater endurance

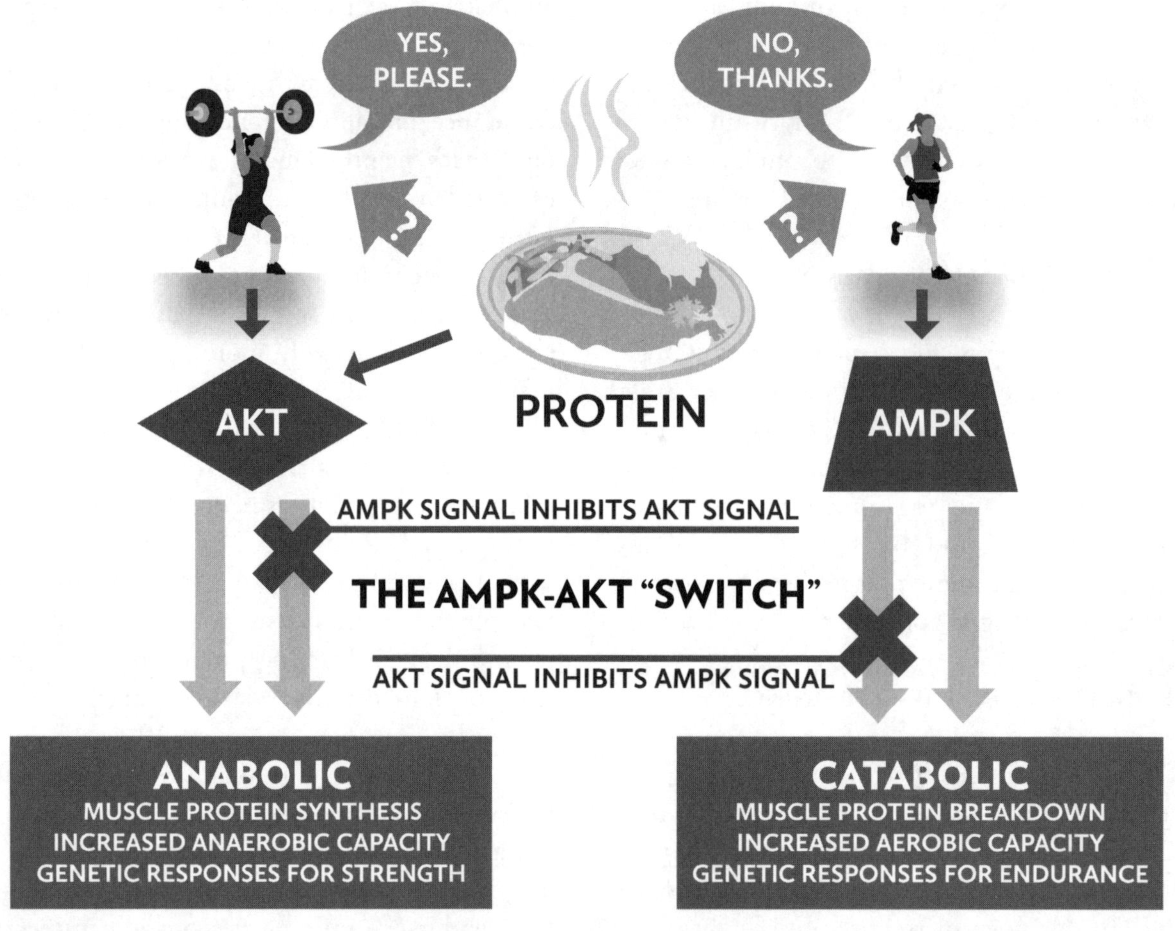


***Figure 4-1.*** The AMPK-Akt switch. Strength training and a corresponding increase in protein intake activate the Akt-mTOR pathway, which signals for anabolic responses that lead to increased muscle mass and strength. Aerobic endurance training activates the AMPK pathway, which signals for decreased muscle protein synthesis, mitochondrial growth, and increased aerobic capacity. The lower caloric and protein intake often associated with this training modality enhances the AMPK signal. Activation of either pathway inhibits the other, hence the comparison to a toggle or "switch." This figure greatly simplifies these complex signaling events, and the mechanisms and practical importance of these processes remain areas of active investigation and vibrant debate.

than untrained individuals, whereas those who train in the LSD-aerobic range do not get stronger or more powerful. This phenomenon will take on greater clarity and significance as we proceed.

The AMPK-Akt switch underlies a classic *biological* interference effect, but concurrent training also confronts us with a *practical* interference effect. Simply put, strength training and endurance training compete with each other for valuable training time. Getting strong requires a substantial investment in both active training and recovery time between training bouts. Building strength and muscle requires a long-term training program, because it requires the addition of new tissue. Strength training is a construction project. Endurance training requires tissue remodeling, but it's more about reprogramming the expression of enzymes for aerobic metabolism, increasing the number of mitochondria, improving circulation to the muscle, and so on. So endurance can be built much more *quickly* than strength, but it takes committed training time to *maintain* endurance, which decays far more quickly than strength.

Our exercise prescription must therefore specify where the emphasis of training should be *vis-à-vis* these two principle attributes, because biological and practical interference would *appear* to dictate that we can't have it both ways. The Masters Athlete can train for strength or endurance, it seems, but not both. Which is it to be?

Even if this weren't a false choice (and it is) the reader might be forgiven for suspecting that my conclusion is foregone. Indeed, as we shall see, emphasizing strength training over endurance for the Masters Athlete is a rational and evidence-based approach. But our analysis will also allow us to bypass the apparent either-or dilemma of strength vs. endurance. *We can, and must, have it both ways.*

To see how this is possible, we need to understand how living systems use and transform energy. We need to have an elementary grasp of ***bioenergetics***.

## Bioenergetics in a Nutshell

Understanding how living systems capture and use energy is fundamental to any understanding of exercise, and nobody who is serious about fitness can make intelligent decisions without it, any more than you can make intelligent decisions about any other aspect of your life without some minimum level of knowledge. I'm going to get you through this in just a few pages. By the time we're done you're going to have a deeper understanding of exactly how your body works during physical activity, and you'll wonder why *bioenergetics* seemed like such an imposing term.

We're going to start where I wish we'd started when I was in med school: the Big Picture. I'm going to show you the whole forest, the most important trails in the forest, and a few trees that mark important turns in the road. But first, I'm going to show you *what we're looking for in the forest*, the Most Important Thing, the thing that bioenergetics is all about: ATP.

### ATP: Energy for life processes

***ATP*** is shorthand for ***adenosine triphosphate,*** the molecule that mediates energy exchange in living systems. Nothing gets done without it. Sugars and fats may be the source of energy for the cell, but that energy has to be in the form of ATP to get used. When a cell needs to do something or make something, it can't just spend a sugar or fat molecule, any more than you can go down to Walgreens and buy aspirin with Krugerrands. The energy in food must be captured in the form of ATP for the energy to be spent.[10] In fact, nobody *ever* talks about ATP for more than a few sentences before they call it "the energy currency of the cell." There – I just did it myself.

As the name indicates, ATP is a molecule of adenosine bound to three phosphate groups. It's not important to know anything in particular about adenosine, or even phosphate. What's important to know is that ATP is just a relatively small molecule, and that the three phosphate groups hang off the adenosine in the form of a chain. For our present purposes, we can think of the adenosine as an inert platform for the chain of phosphates. Figure 4-2 gives us as much detail as we need.

Now, I want you to notice something about that chain of phosphates, which I have represented as little balls. The first two phosphates are attached to the adenosine platform by uninteresting, low-energy bonds. The third phosphate, sticking way out, is attached to the second phosphate by a loose spring, and it wobbles around quite a bit. Looking at ATP in this crude way would make my undergraduate P-Chem professor shriek in dismay, horror, and actual physical pain. But that's okay, because I never liked him anyway. My wriggly-

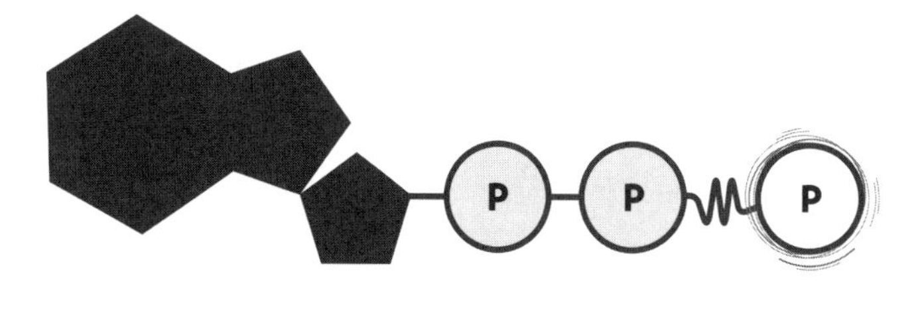


***Figure 4-2.*** ATP – Adenosine triphosphate. The third phosphate is linked to the rest of the molecule by a high-energy bond which contains the energy needed for living processes.

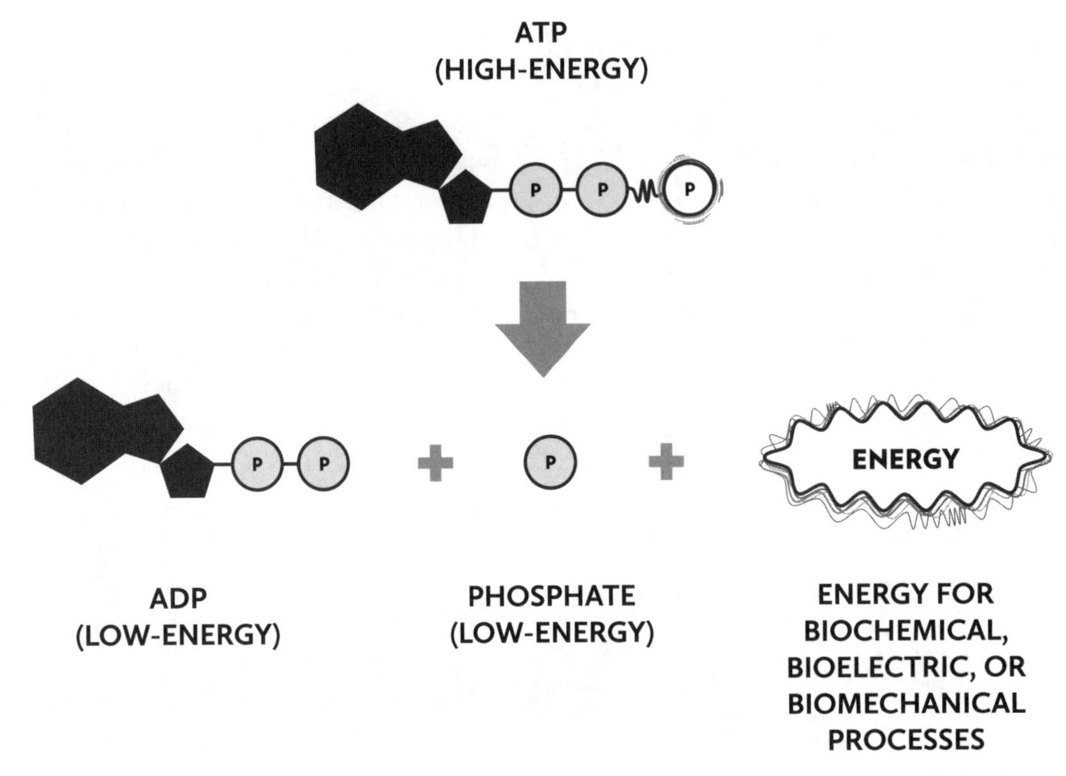


***Figure 4-3.*** Energy transfer by ATP. The third phosphate is released, transferring energy to do biological work, such as charging neurons, conducting biochemical reactions, or contracting muscle tissue.

ball model is perfectly serviceable for our purposes because it underscores that the last phosphate in the chain, the *terminal phosphate*, is just quivering with energy. Chemical energy. Energy that can be used by the cell to *do stuff*.

What kind of stuff? *Biochemical reactions.* All the work of any cell boils down to biochemical work. Cells turn chemicals into other chemicals. And just as Mr. White needs a Bunsen burner to cook up pretty blue meth crystals in a mobile laboratory, you need an energy source to do biochemistry in your cells. That energy is in the form of ATP. The same is true of biological motion. When a muscle cell contracts, it uses ATP to drive biochemical reactions that produce movement.[11]

ATP does this by losing that jittery third phosphate and transferring the energy in its bond to some energy-dependent living process, such as an enzyme reaction, driving the electrical activity of neurons, or powering the movement of muscle fibers. Meditate for a moment on Figure 4-3.

When ATP loses its terminal phosphate (called *ATP hydrolysis* or *dephosphorylation*), the energy in that jittery bond is released in a controlled, specific manner and transferred to another molecule or process. For example, the cell may need to combine a bunch of amino acids to build a protein. This is an energy-consuming process, and uses ATP. In the case of muscle contraction, ATP transfers energy to the filaments that pull on each other and produce motion.[12]

After any such energy-consuming process, the ATP is spent. It is now ***ADP***, or adenosine diphosphate, a much lower-energy molecule. ADP needs to be recharged (*rephosphorylated*), so the cell will have a continuous supply of energy for biochemical reactions and life processes.

*Recharging ADP and keeping ATP levels high is what bioenergetics is all about.* The energy in the food you eat cannot be used for life processes or movement unless and until it is repackaged in the form of ATP. If you keep your eye on the production of ATP, metabolism makes a lot more sense. With that in mind, we can look at the big picture.

Let's start by having a donut.

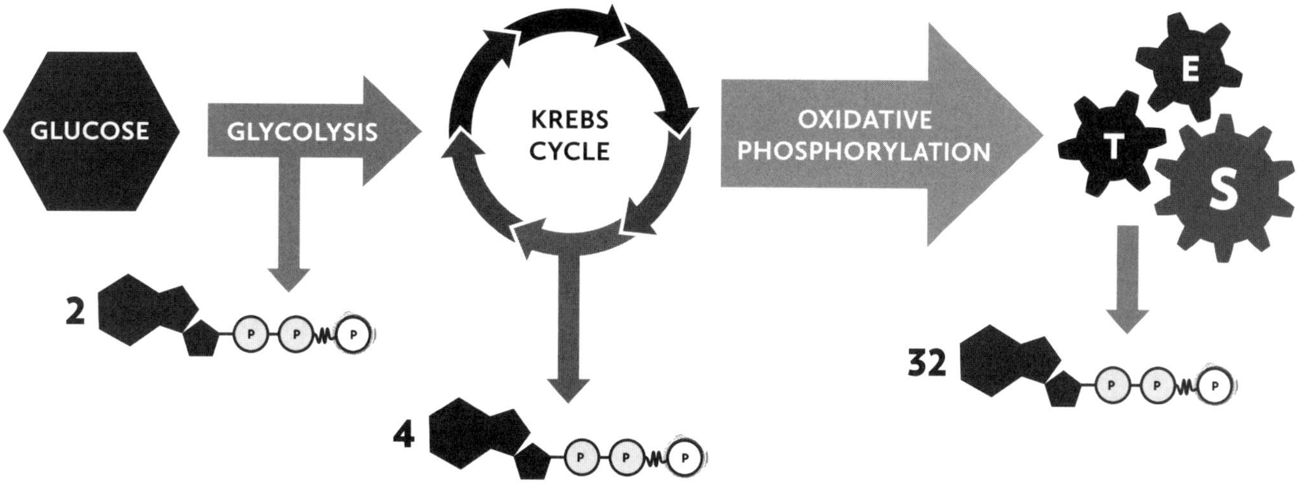

*Figure 4-4.* Overview of energy metabolism of glucose. The energy of glucose is captured in three major steps: glycolysis, the Krebs Cycle, and oxidative phosphorylation. These three steps produce a maximum of 2, 4, and 32 molecules of ATP per glucose molecule, respectively.

## Glucose and fat metabolism: how to turn a donut into ATP

A donut is really an awful thing, if you think about it, which is why most people don't think about it. It's a lump of sugary dough cooked up in a deep fat fryer and then stuffed or painted with more sugar. It's a nutritional junk bond, an abomination, a toxic toroid of carbohydrate and fat. It's so energy-dense that unless you're going to work out immediately, it will put you into a sugar coma at your desk and send fat molecules straight to your spare tire.

But it contains a lot of food energy, *and it sure is tasty*. It will do as an example for our purposes.

When you eat the donut, enzymes from your salivary glands, stomach, and pancreas help break the ghastly thing down into its constituent carbohydrate and fat molecules. Through the action of other enzymes and of insulin, the molecules of the donut circulate in the blood and are ultimately presented to the hungry cells of your body as ***glucose*** and ***triglyceride***. Both glucose (a simple sugar) and triglyceride (fat) will then be converted to ATP. The energy trapped in the chemical bonds of these molecules will be captured to recharge ADP with high-energy terminal phosphates to produce ATP.

Repackaging the energy of glucose into ATP happens in three big steps.

1. **Glycolysis**. The glucose is rapidly split into two fragments, producing a couple of ATPs and some high-energy electrons.

2. **The Krebs Cycle**. The glucose fragments are chemically oxidized ("burned") to form more high-energy electrons and a couple more ATPs.

3. **Oxidative Phosphorylation**: The big payoff step. The cell combines oxygen with all those hot electrons from the first two steps to create a "current" that is used to form *lots* more ATP.

*That's it.* That's the Forest, the big picture of carbohydrate metabolism and bioenergetics. You split the glucose into fragments and high-energy electrons with glycolysis, you burn those fragments down to even more electrons in the Krebs Cycle, and then you use all those hot electrons as "juice" to drive the recharging of ADP to ATP. We're going to unpack these three steps just a little more, to get the very basic level of detail we need to move forward. Stay with me. If you keep Figure 4-4 in mind, you won't lose your way in the woods.

**Glycolysis.** This literally means "breaking glucose," and that's exactly what's happening. At the end of glycolysis, the glucose has been cleaved into two fragments called *pyruvate*, and some of its energy has been captured to produce two molecules of ATP. The rest of the energy is captured in the form of high-energy electrons trapped in *electron carriers* (Figure 4-5). Those electrons will be used in a later step to yield more ATP.

**The Krebs Cycle.** The pyruvate fragments created by the splitting of glucose then go to a special part of the cell called the ***mitochondrion***. The mitochondrion is a little power plant, a sausage-shaped cellular battery. It's where most of the energy from food is converted to ATP. In the mitochondrion, the pyruvate fragments of the glucose are processed further and enter a biochemical roundabout called the Krebs cycle. In the Krebs Cycle, the pyruvate is chemically oxidized ("burned," in a very real chemical sense) to form a couple more ATPs and still more hot electrons (Figure 4-6).

**Oxidative Phosphorylation.** The mitochondrial power plant has compartments, separated by membranes. The many high-energy electrons produced by glycolysis and the Krebs cycle are now used to form a sort of current, driven by the presence of oxygen, which in turn creates an electrical potential across these membranes. In other words, the mitochondrion creates an actual *voltage,*[13] like a little battery. And like any battery, it can do work – specifically, the work of recharging ADP to ATP (Figure 4-7).

**Aerobic vs. Anaerobic.** Now, I want you to notice something about these three steps: The first one is very different from the other two. Glycolysis, unlike the two steps that come after it, does not take place in the mitochondrial battery, but rather in the fluid *cytoplasm* (the common area, if you will) of the cell. The mitochondrion, the cellular powerhouse, is where all the oxygen is consumed and all the actual "burning" gets done.

*Glycolysis does not directly consume oxygen.* Glycolysis is traditionally considered to be ***anaerobic.*** Among other things, this means it is not very efficient, and it generates very little of the ATP ultimately produced by glucose metabolism. One molecule of glucose yields two molecules of ATP by glycolysis. The rest of the energy is still trapped in the pyruvate fragments and the high-energy electrons.

The two big processes that occur in the mitochondrion, the Krebs Cycle and oxidative phosphorylation, *both require oxygen to function,* unlike glycolysis.[14] Thus, mitochondrial energy metabolism is considered ***aerobic***. These processes are more complex than glycolysis, and they yield the vast majority of the ATP produced from metabolizing glucose. Every molecule of glucose ultimately yields (theoretically) about 36 ATP by committing its pyruvate fragments from glycolysis to the mitochondrial furnace. With the 2 ATPs from glycolysis, the total maximum *theoretical* yield for a glucose molecule is about 38 ATPs, almost all of them produced in the mitochondrion.[15]

Now, for a dirty little secret: in reality, none of these three processes are really anaerobic. It is true that bacteria can do glycolysis without oxygen, and so can some of the cells in your body, including muscle. But you're not a bacterium, and in humans glycolysis is intimately connected with oxygen metabolism. Without mitochondrial metabolism to burn off the hot electrons and pyruvate, glycolysis would cease. Talking about glycolysis as "anaerobic" and the processes in the mitochondrion as "aerobic" is a bit misleading. And for our purposes it rather misses the point.

So I'd like to point out another, more relevant difference between these processes. Glycolysis has the potential to be *very fast.* For this reason, and because glycolysis in humans virtually always takes place *alongside* aerobic processes and in the presence of oxygen, it's better to call it *fast glycolysis* rather than *anaerobic glycolysis.* Fast glycolysis doesn't produce very many ATPs, but it produces them rapidly. The mitochondrial processes, on the other hand, are much slower than glycolysis.[16] The oxygen-consuming mitochondrion produces large amounts of ATP, and can do so for much more extended periods than glycolysis. But it cannot deliver energy nearly as rapidly. This will be critical to keep in mind.

So much for the carbohydrate. What about the fat in our donut? The chemical energy in a fat molecule is captured in the mitochondrion in a

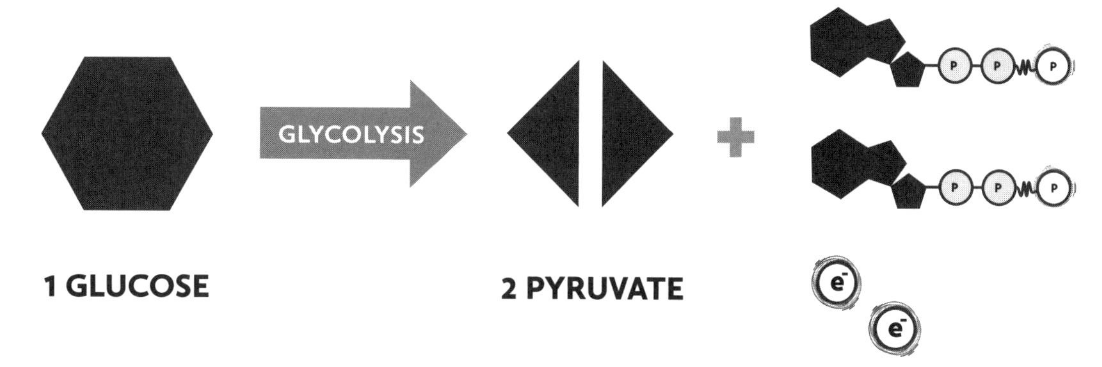


***Figure 4-5.*** Glycolysis. This rapid multi-step process splits glucose into 2 pyruvate molecules, yielding 2 ATP and 2 electron carriers.

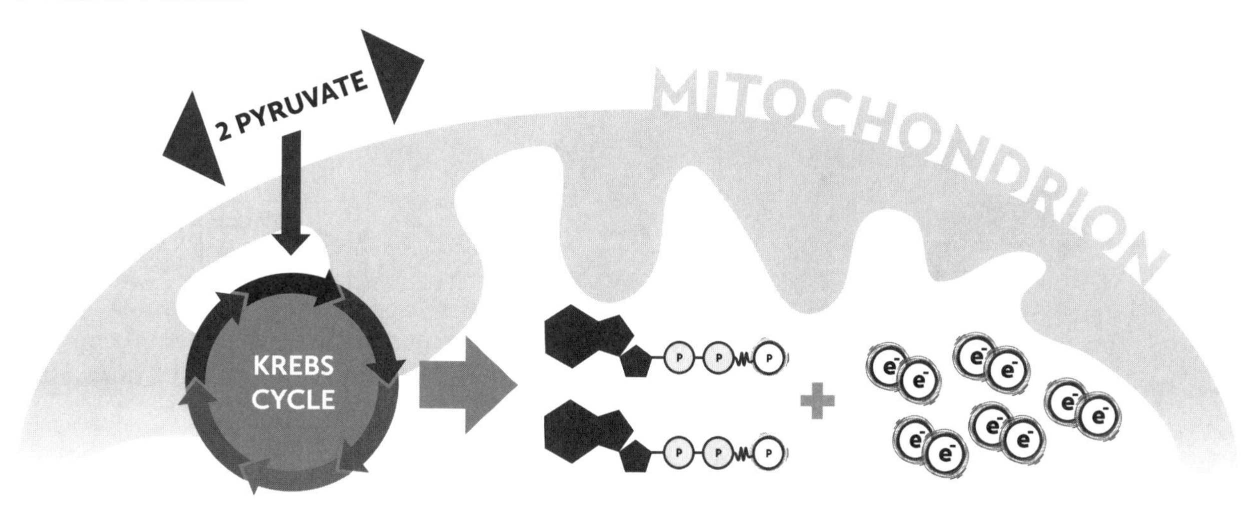


***Figure 4-6.*** The Krebs cycle. Two pyruvate molecules from glycolysis are transferred to the mitochondrial furnace. There, in the Krebs Cycle, the pyruvates are oxidized to produce 2 molecules of ATP, 10 high-energy electron carriers, and carbon dioxide (not shown).

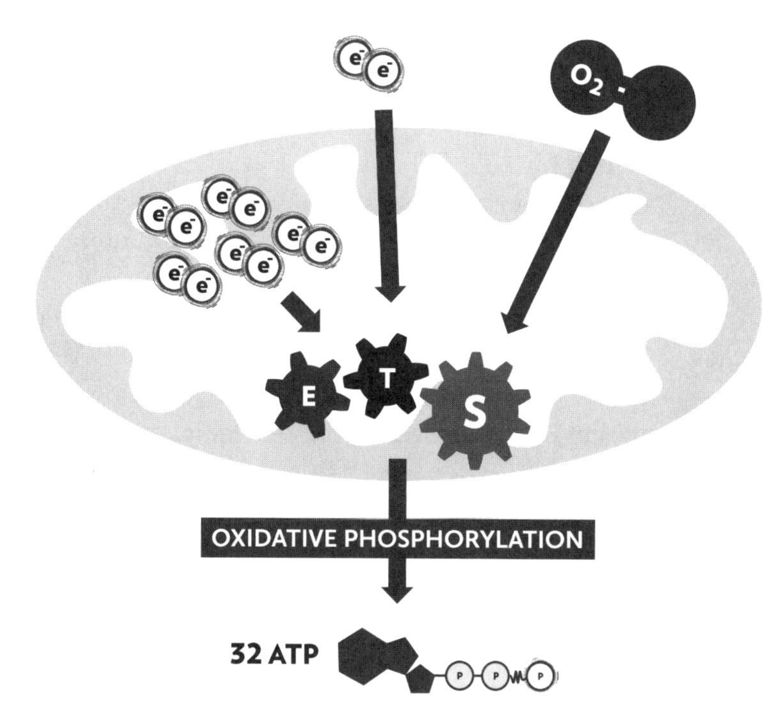


***Figure 4-7.*** Oxidative phosphorylation. High-energy electrons produced by glycolysis and the Krebs Cycle are combined with oxygen to drive a current, or electron transport system (ETS), in the mitochondrion. This current powers the creation of high-energy phosphate bonds and converts ADP to ATP.

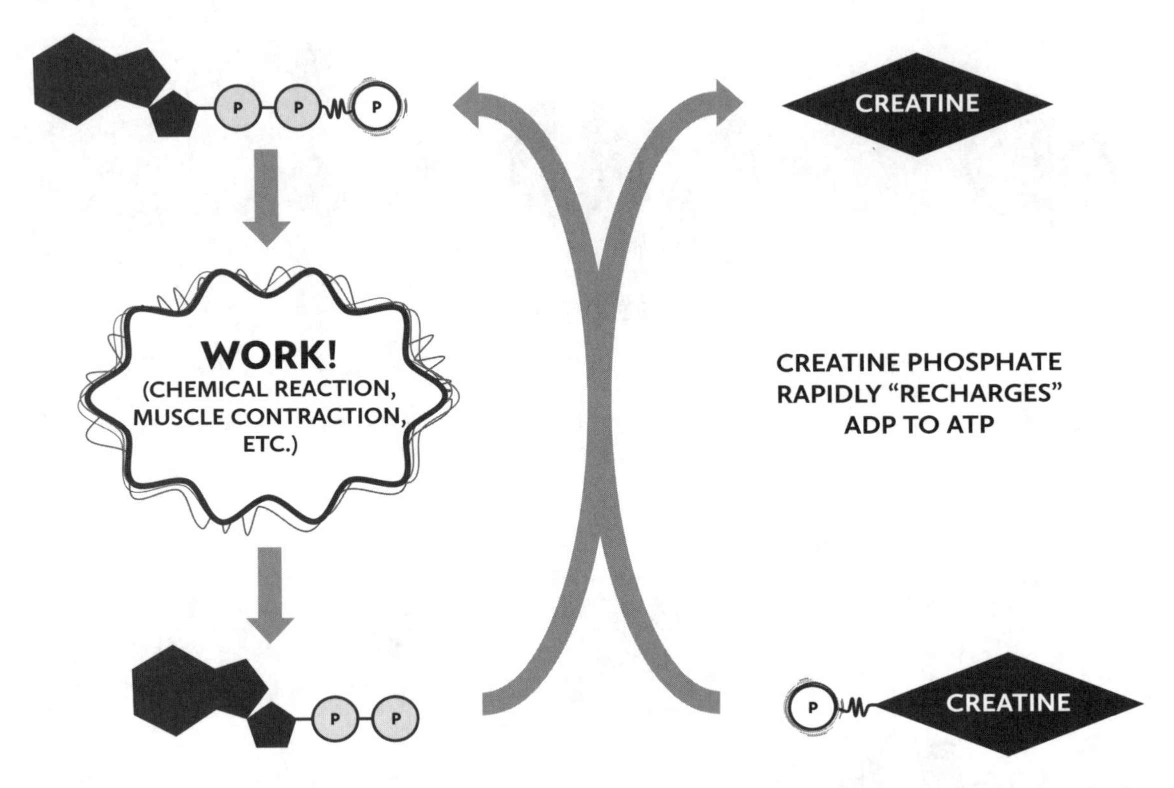


***Figure 4-8.*** The phosphagen energy system. ATP already available in the muscle can be used instantly for very short durations. Creatine stores high-energy phosphate to allow rapid recharge and cycling of ATP during brief periods of high-energy demand.

fashion very analogous to glucose metabolism. It begins with another cyclic process called ***beta oxidation***.[17] This process breaks the fatty acids into short fragments, capturing some of their energy in electron carriers. As with pyruvate from glucose, the fatty acid fragments[18] can be funneled into the Krebs Cycle,[19] producing ATP and more electron carriers. And once again, those high-energy electrons are fed into the oxidative phosphorylation pathway in the mitochondrial battery to drive the production of even more ATP. Like the aerobic metabolism of carbohydrate, the aerobic metabolism of fat is much slower than glycolysis, but much higher yield. For example, a single molecule of palmitate, one of the more abominable fats in our donut, will yield more than a hundred ATPs. Fat is very high in energy.

## THE PHOSPHAGEN SYSTEM: INSTANT ENERGY AND RAPID RECHARGE

We must consider one more important process to fill in our picture of bioenergetics. When the cell needs energy to be delivered extremely rapidly, even more rapidly than glycolysis can deliver, it uses the ATP already available in the cell. This ATP will be depleted quickly, but energy levels are maintained by the ***creatine phosphate*** system. Creatine is found in high concentrations in muscle, kidney and nervous tissues. Creatine can hold on to high-energy phosphate, allowing it to act as a rapid recharging system for ATP. When an ATP is used to do work, such as muscle contraction, it can be recharged almost instantly by a creatine phosphate molecule (Figure 4-8).

This is a one-step process, simpler even than glycolysis, and it doesn't require the ADP to be transported to the mitochondrion for recharging. Moreover, it doesn't require oxygen. It's "anaerobic." Again, the term is a bit artificial, because the energy stored in the phosphocreatine and most of the ATP ultimately comes from mitochondrial ("aerobic") metabolism. As with glycolysis, the salient issue isn't that this system is "anaerobic," but rather that it's *fast*. The use of immediately available

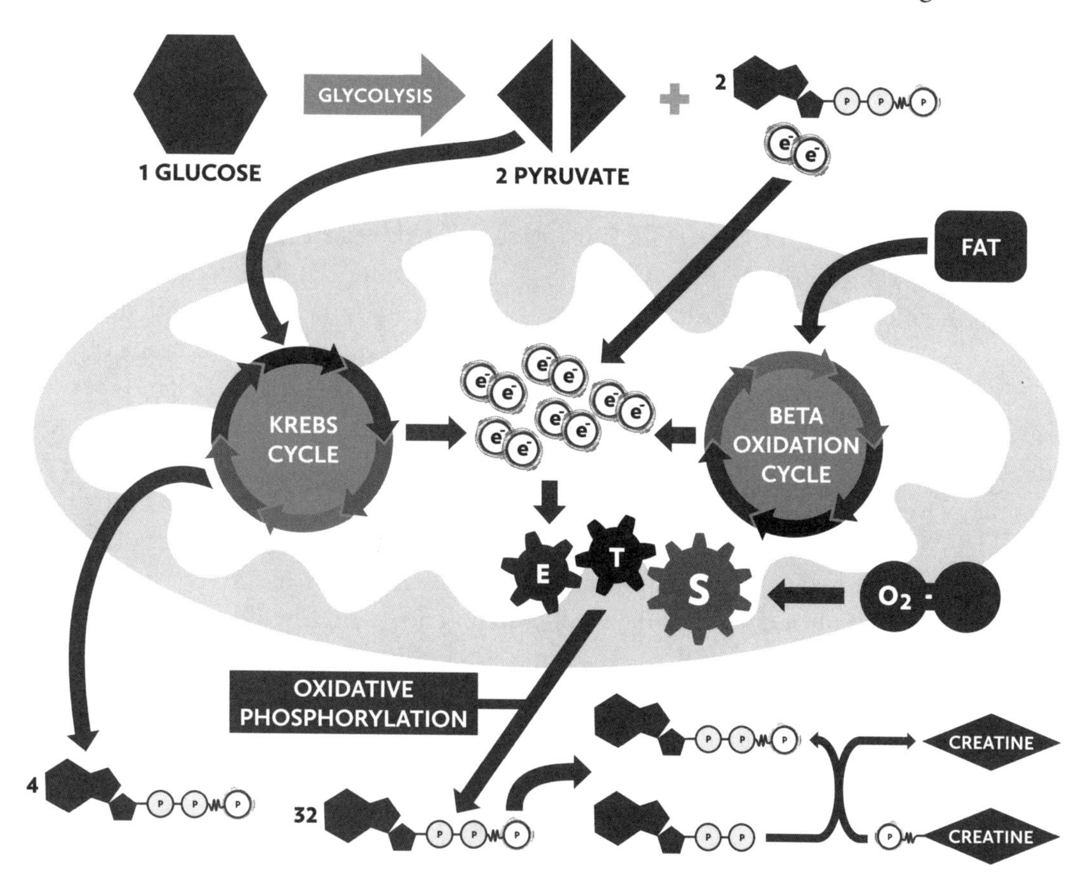


*Figure 4-9.* Overview of energy metabolism. Glycolysis (Step 1) splits glucose to yield ATP, high-energy electrons and pyruvate. Pyruvate, electrons and fat all enter the mitochondrion. Pyruvate is "burned" in the Krebs Cycle (Step 2), producing a little ATP and a lot more hot electrons. Fat is "burned" in the beta oxidation cycle (another Step 2), also producing electrons and fragments for the Krebs Cycle. Electrons from glycolysis, Krebs Cycle, and beta oxidation are funneled into the ETS, where they are used with oxygen for oxidative phosphorylation and the production of a bounty of 32 ATPs (Step 3) from 1 glucose alone. Most of the ATP ends up in the cytoplasm, where it is used to do work. So used, it can be rapidly recharged by the creatine cycle. Please note: everything happening inside the mitochondrion is aerobic. Everything happening outside the mitochondrion is anaerobic. Yet the ATP produced by all these processes fills a common energy pool, and all of these processes work together. You now know more about this than most doctors. Well done.

ATP and creatine phosphate is collectively known as the ***phosphagen energy system***.[20]

Now we have a picture of bioenergetics that, while very generalized and simplified, will allow us to move forward. It is represented in Figure 4-9. It looks daunting! But it's actually far less complicated than, say, your cable remote, your tax return, or your relationship with your spouse. If you just take a deep breath and squint at it for a moment, you'll see that you now recognize and understand all the pieces of the puzzle. Figure 4-9 doesn't introduce anything new. It just shows us how it all fits together.

### A Mixed Energy Policy

From the foregoing, we can see that the cell has three major energy systems to provide ATP for life processes.

The mitochondrial system (composed of the Krebs cycle and oxidative phosphorylation) uses oxygen to burn fragments of carbohydrate and fat in the mitochondrial slow cooker, using oxygen to produce the lion's share of ATP from the food we eat.

The two other energy systems work outside the mitochondrion. *Fast glycolysis* splits glucose rapidly, without *directly* using oxygen, to produce small amounts of ATP at a high rate. Even more rapid is the phosphagen system. The *phosphagen system* is composed of the ATP already present in the cell and the creatine phosphate cycle we examined earlier. The creatine cycle doesn't produce ATP, but rather stores high-energy phosphate so that ADP is rapidly recharged at times of high-intensity energy expenditure.

This is a very effective mixed energy policy, providing the cell with an entire spectrum of power outputs and alternative fuel utilization strategies. But just as an energy infrastructure that uses a bit of solar, a bit of coal, and some nuclear delivers energy to all consumers in the same form – electrical power – so does the mixed energy policy of the cell deliver all its power in the same form, that of ATP.

Now, ATP is ATP, regardless of where it came from. ATP from aerobic metabolism can be used in any biochemical reaction as readily as ATP from glycolysis. It's *energy currency*. The cell can spend it however it likes. And I wish to emphasize that *these energy systems always work together*, in some ratio or another, depending on the needs of the cell and the organism, filling a common ATP pool and keeping the cellular ATP content relatively stable. The functional difference between these energy systems isn't the *type* of energy they produce, but rather *how* they produce it.

There are two vital considerations here: the power output of the energy system and the capacity of the energy system.

***Power*** is the rate at which energy is delivered, and ***capacity*** is the total amount of energy the system can produce, regardless of rate. Consider two batteries, which we call ***C*** and ***P***. Battery C has a high capacity. Plug a motor into it, and it will drive that motor at a moderate rate all afternoon.

Battery P doesn't have even a tenth of the capacity of Battery C. It will run the same motor for just a few minutes, but *much* faster.[21] So even though Battery P's *capacity* is tiny, its *power* far outstrips that of Battery C.

Similarly, the body's energy systems describe a very versatile spectrum of capacity and power, which are inversely related. We spend most of our time in the broad aerobic region of the spectrum. You're soaking in it, right now. Reading, walking, working, running, and sleeping all take place within the low-power, high-capacity aerobic energy system. They don't require high power outputs, so they are supported by a steady stream of ATP pouring out of the mitochondrial slow cooker at a moderate rate. If we decide to walk faster or work harder, we can ramp this system up over a wide range of power outputs, from low to moderately high. Then we'll breathe faster, consume more oxygen, burn more sugar and fat in our mitochondria, and produce more ATP to meet the higher demand. The mitochondrial energy system is efficient over a range of powers, from low to moderate, and has a very high capacity. It's our main energy supply. *We are aerobic creatures.*

There are, however, many activities that require higher power outputs than mitochondrial metabolism can support. Consider, for example, a 200-meter dash, a wrestling match, or a set of push-ups. The power requirements of such activities will quickly consume the ATP and phosphocreatine in your muscles (phosphagen system), and the mitochondria will not be able to churn out new ATP fast enough to keep up. But your muscles can split glucose very rapidly through fast glycolysis. This provides 2 ATPs per glucose instead of 38, but it provides them *right now*, when you need them. You can work at maximum intensity in this high-power system for one to two minutes at most before you exhaust the capacity of glycolysis to deliver energy. It's not efficient, and its capacity is low, but it's damn fast, which means it's powerful.

For even higher power outputs, the muscle can turn to the phosphagen system, and use creatine phosphate to rapidly recharge ATP. When exercise physiologists talk about this system, they're usually focused on the extremes of human power output: wind sprints, high jumps, shot-putting, and weightlifting. Such activities express massive forces over extremely brief intervals. For example, an elite snatch (in which a barbell is lifted from the floor to overhead in one rapid stroke) develops more physical power than virtually any other human movement, because it moves an Olympian weight over a long distance in less than a second. A snatch

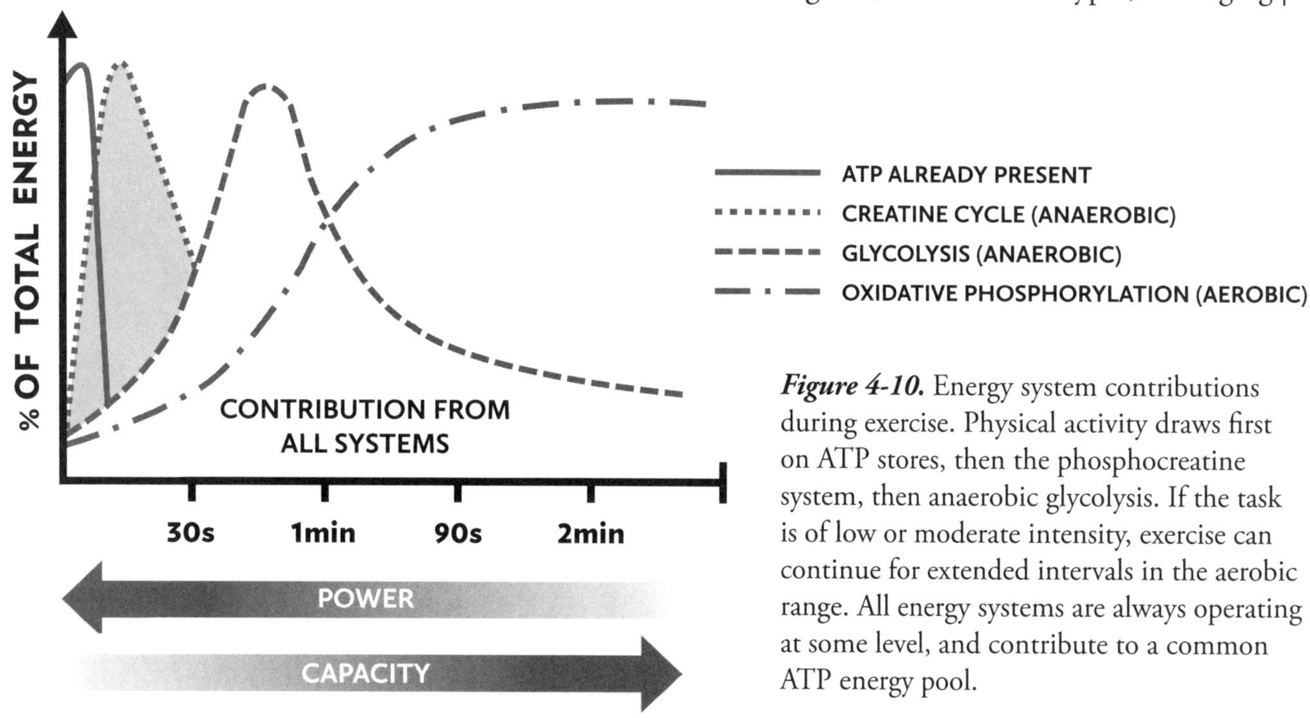


***Figure 4-10.*** Energy system contributions during exercise. Physical activity draws first on ATP stores, then the phosphocreatine system, then anaerobic glycolysis. If the task is of low or moderate intensity, exercise can continue for extended intervals in the aerobic range. All energy systems are always operating at some level, and contribute to a common ATP energy pool.

is performed almost entirely within the phosphagen energy system.

But there are more prosaic, practical power demands that call upon the phosphagen system. Getting out of your car demands power development: heaving a significant fraction of your bodyweight from a seated to a standing position very quickly. It happens primarily within the phosphagen system. Jumping out of the way of danger, throwing a ball for your kid, yanking your dog out of the garbage... all are quick, energetic movements calling for rapid power development and the engagement of the phosphagen system.

Most tissues of the body have both aerobic and anaerobic capacities, with a few important exceptions. Red blood cells do not have mitochondria, and they are strictly anaerobic. Brain tissue is notoriously dependent on aerobic capacity; deprivation of oxygen for only a few minutes results in permanent brain damage. By now it should be clear that muscle tissue uses the entire range of energy systems, but that the power-capacity needs of the task dictate which energy system will predominate (Figure 4-10). This range of energy utilization is expressed not just in the biochemistry of muscle, but also at the level of the tissue organization; specifically, at the level of muscle cells. This is a matter of profound importance for the Athlete of Aging, as we shall now see.

## Bioenergetics, Muscle Fiber Types, and Aging

Skeletal muscle is an incredibly complex and beautiful tissue at every level of organization, although I'm sure you'll be relieved to know that our present purposes do not require an in-depth examination of muscle tissue structure. Muscle tissue may be understood most simply as a "bundle of bundles." The actual contractile elements, the components that produce movement, are the ***myofilaments***, the strands of ***actin*** and ***myosin*** protein that slide across each other to shorten the muscle, consuming ATP in the process. These filaments are bundled into ***myofibrils***, which in turn are bundled together in muscle cells. Muscle cells are unusually long and slender, and are often called fibers. A ***muscle fiber*** is simply a single muscle cell. Muscle fibers are in turn bundled into ***muscle fascicles***, and fascicles are bundled together in a sheath of connective tissue to form a complete muscle (Figure 4-11).

So a muscle is a bundle of fascicles, a fascicle is a bundle of fibers, a fiber is a bundle of myofibrils, and a myofibril is a bundle of filaments. Our attention now shifts to the fibers – the muscle cells.

### Muscle fiber types and energy systems

Now we confront a matter of profound importance for all athletes, and especially the Masters Athlete. It turns out that not all muscle cells are created equal. Just as some athletes and events are "aerobic" and some are more "anaerobic," so it is that muscle fibers are more or less specialized. Skeletal muscles are composed of an *assortment* of muscle fiber types, which differ in their biochemical and biophysical properties. You may have heard of "slow twitch" and "fast twitch" muscle fibers. "Slow twitch" fibers are low-power muscle cells, rich in mitochondria and oxidative (aerobic) enzymes. So they have extremely high capacity, and they'll march all day long. They are, in effect, "endurance fibers." On the other hand, they're small, thin fibers, and they're weak. Because they are "slow twitch," they cannot generate force rapidly, which means they also lack power. Biologists call these ***Type I muscle fibers***.

"Fast twitch" fibers are called ***Type II muscle fibers***, and come in two flavors, the so-called "aerobic fast-twitch" and "anaerobic fast-twitch." For our purposes, these two forms of Type II fibers are more alike than they are different. They both lack the endurance capacity of their Type I brethren, both are capable of performing glycolysis at high rates, both are packed with phosphocreatine, and both are larger, stronger, and more powerful than Type I fibers. Biologists call them ***Type IIa*** ("aerobic fast-twitch") and ***Type IIx*** ("anaerobic fast-twitch"). The attributes of these muscle fiber types are summarized in Table 4-1.

The relative abundance and distribution of fiber types will obviously have implications for performance. It has been said that "sprinters are born, and marathoners are made." Sprinters must perform at the high end of the power spectrum, and muscle biopsy of the most accomplished sprinters reveals a preponderance of Type II fibers.[22] This fiber predominance has a strong genetic component, and it turns out that little can be done to alter it. If you're not born with a large proportion of Type II fibers in your legs, you're not going to be a great sprinter. *Period.*

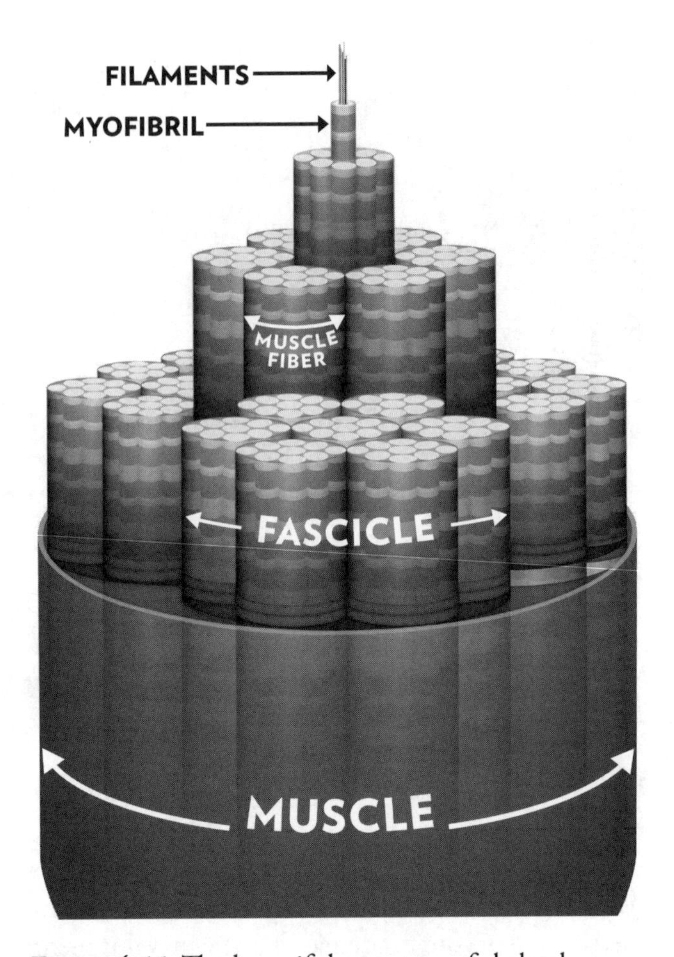


***Figure 4-11.*** The beautiful structure of skeletal muscle. Muscle is a complex tissue we may describe as a hierarchical "bundle of bundles." A complete muscle is a bundle of muscle fascicles, which is a bundle of muscle fibers, which are actually muscle cells. Muscle cells are in turn highly ordered bundles of myofibrils, which are bundles of myofilaments, composed of actin and myosin protein. Muscle cells come in three types, as discussed below, and all three types may be found in a single muscle.

Of course, you can certainly become a *better* sprinter. You can train to increase the size and recruitment of the Type II fibers you have, and with training you can transform some Type IIa fibers into Type IIx fibers, and vice-versa. But *most* exercise physiologists agree that you can't transform Type I into Type II, and you're not going to be able to significantly increase the numerical proportion of fast-twitch to slow-twitch fibers.[23]

The potential of training to increase fiber *size*, however, should not be dismissed, because while we probably cannot change the *numerical* proportion of fiber types, we can increase the *cross-sectional* proportion of a fiber type. In other words, we can increase the amount of muscle area and muscle mass contributed by one fiber type or another, by engaging in training that focuses on that particular muscle fiber type. So if we engage in LSD endurance training, focused on our low-power Type I fibers, those fibers will become somewhat larger, richer in mitochondria, and coated with more capillaries, while the high-power Type II fibers will tend to become smaller. This is the muscle phenotype of the endurance athlete.[24] Similarly, the sprinter, weightlifter, or wrestler will increase the size of his Type IIa and Type IIx fibers, and express a more high-power muscle phenotype, which will be larger and stronger than the endurance muscle phenotype.

## Aging and Type II Muscle Fiber Atrophy

All of this is critically important to the formulation of our Exercise Prescription/Training Program. Aging is characterized by a progressive decline in muscle mass, but that loss of muscle is not uniform across fiber types.[25] *The loss of muscle mass in aging is dominated by the atrophy of Type II fibers*, the largest, strongest, and most powerful fibers, which are more specialized toward anaerobic metabolism. In this limited sense, *aging and endurance training have a similar impact on muscle tissue*. They both decrease the relative mass, or even the number, of Type II fibers.

## MUSCLE FIBER TYPES

| Type / Subtype | Type I | Type IIa | Type IIx |
|---|---|---|---|
| Brospeak | "Aerobic Slow Twitch" | "Aerobic Fast Twitch" | "Anaerobic Fast Twitch" |
| Fiber Size | Small | Medium | Large |
| Mitochondrial Density | Very High | High | Low |
| Capillary Density | High | Intermediate | Low |
| Endurance | High | Intermediate | Low |
| Strength/Power | Low | High | Very High |
| Phosphocreatine | Low | High | Very High |
| Glycolytic Capacity | Low | High | Very High |
| Aerobic Capacity | High | Intermediate | Very Low |
| Anaerobic Capacity | Very Low | High | Very High |
| Atrophy in Aging | Moderate | High | High |
| **Good for** | **Long, Slow, Boring:** Distance running, cross-country pogo-stick races, Yoga marathons, Disneyland with grandchildren, etc. | **Short and Intense:** Tennis, soccer, wrestling, climbing the stairs, fleeing from danger, chasing grandchildren, etc. | **Exciting Explosions:** Shot put, high jump, leaping for joy, weightlifting, Olympic Sneezing, tossing grandchildren, etc. |

***Table 4-1.*** Muscle fiber types. The power-capacity spectrum of bioenergetics is reflected at the tissue level in Type I (low-power aerobic), Type IIa (high power-aerobic/anaerobic) and Type IIx (very high-power anaerobic) fibers.

This is a very troubling observation. Type I fibers are there to be trained, even in very aged and atrophic muscle, and the potential for increasing our aerobic capacity and endurance is *relatively* well-preserved as we get older. But a preferential loss of Type II fibers would indicate a corresponding loss of potential for strength and power, or even the ability to meaningfully train these attributes. This would be particularly devastating, because these are the most important General Fitness Attributes for the older athlete[26] (and indeed, for all competitive athletes) – the domain of Type II fibers.

But all is not lost. More precisely, *Type II fibers are not lost*, even in aged muscle. Consider the important study by Nilwik et al.[27] published in 2012 showing that the decline in muscle mass with aging is almost entirely due to a reduction in Type II muscle fiber size – *but not number*. Nilwik's group took 25 healthy young men and 25 healthy older men and performed muscle biopsies for fiber typing. They found that the muscles of older subjects were, unsurprisingly, smaller than those of younger subjects, and that the difference in size could be attributed almost entirely to the smaller size of Type II fibers in the older group. The older subjects then underwent a six month strength-training program. Their muscles got larger, naturally, and the investigators found that the concomitant increase in Type II fiber size completely accounted for this change. Related studies by Verdijk[28] and Frontera[29] found similar results.

In short, aging muscle is characterized by the preferential *atrophy* of high-power Type II fibers, and the atrophy of these fibers is disproportionately responsible for the loss of muscle mass and strength in aging. Fortunately, it would appear a population of shriveled-up Type II fibers lingers in aged muscle, like so many ghosts. These fibers remain responsive to training stimuli. Training in the high-intensity, high-power, "anaerobic" range, and in particular strength training, allows the Masters Athlete to hang on to this vulnerable population of fibers, or, if they have atrophied, to return them to the land of the living, and to make them bigger and stronger. This means that high-intensity training, and in particular strength training, will have a powerful effect on the maintenance of muscle mass and strength in the athlete of aging, in a way that aerobic endurance training simply cannot begin to approach.

## Beyond Strength: The Other Fitness Attributes

Let's take stock. We began this chapter by turning to the third of our criteria for an exercise prescription: a training program that was ***comprehensive*** with respect to the fitness attributes. This immediately confronted us with a biological and practical competition for emphasis between strength and endurance. As we have seen, this tension is the manifestation of deeper structures, at the levels of muscle tissue organization and biological energy systems.

At this juncture, it would appear the unfortunate biological realities of aging indicate training for strength should take precedence over training for aerobic endurance. Training for strength puts us at the high-intensity end of the energy spectrum, and promotes the salvage, retention, and development of the precious high-power Type II muscle fibers that are disproportionately lost as we grow older, maximizing our ability to hold on to muscle mass and function.

That's great. *But is training for strength really the most comprehensive approach to an exercise prescription?* After all, there are other fitness attributes to be considered besides strength and endurance: power, mobility, balance, and body composition.

The Masters Athlete needs them all. And, yes, all of these attributes are addressed more substantively and appropriately by training for strength than by training for endurance.

***Strength,*** after all, is the ability to exert a force against a resistance. It's the ability to pick up something heavy, push it away from you, or press it overhead. ***Power*** is the first derivative of strength, the ability to express strength *quickly* – to snatch a heavy object up from the floor, to heave, to leap, to throw, to strike, to lunge. You may have the *strength* to get off the toilet, but if it takes you all afternoon because you don't have the *power*, you're in deep, deep trouble. Strength and power are fitness attributes, the *most fundamental* fitness attributes, and neither of them can be rationally trained or improved without using programmed resistance exercise.

But the payoff of strength training goes beyond the obvious. Properly performed and programmed, resistance training increases ***mobility***, our ability to perform within the full and natural range of motion with agility and coordination, by strengthening normal human movement patterns throughout that full range of motion. The idea that strength training reduces mobility and makes us "muscle-bound" is a discredited artifact of fitness mythology and improper exercise prescription.[30] Correct strength training doesn't just increase mobility, it actually *demands* and therefore *trains* mobility, in a way that running, cycling or even swimming can't even approach. We shall have more to say about this in Chapter 6.

Further still: properly performed and programmed, resistance exercise trains the General Fitness Attribute of ***balance***,[31] our ability to express normal human movement patterns not just with power, but with stability, safety, and confidence. *Correct* strength training through the entire range of motion *demands* and therefore *trains* our so-called "kinesthetic" perception,[32] which tells us where our body, our body parts, and our center of mass are located relative to the gravitational field and the horizontal reference (the floor). And it *demands* and therefore *trains* the contribution of neuromuscular and skeletal components that maintain our center of mass over a stable balance point. More on this in Chapter 6 as well.

And even further: strength training optimizes ***body composition***.[33] Properly performed and programmed, it reduces visceral fat and promotes the retention of lean tissue: strong muscle, hard bone, and resilient tendons and ligaments. The importance of these changes for any athlete, but especially the Masters Athlete, are obvious.[34]

The prevailing caveat in the foregoing discussion is "*properly performed and programmed.*" Strength training that is improperly performed or programmed, or that is directed at the achievement of purely short-term or cosmetic results, will not reap these benefits, and isn't really *training* at all. Recall that the difference between *training* and *exercise* has to do with the manipulation of training variables, or the *dosing* of our exercise prescription. It turns out that strength training, properly programmed and performed, offers us the opportunity to manipulate training variables with an exquisite precision not found in any other training modality. Fortunately, as Andy Baker and I will show you in Parts II and III, proper performance and programming are ultimately guided by a few basic, easy-to-understand principles, although a lot of people will try to convince you otherwise, usually while picking your pocket.

## Enduring Resistance; Resisting Endurance

For the Masters Athlete, the tension between LSD training for endurance and resistance training for strength resolves with a decided preference for strength training, which allows us to work on the high-intensity end of the energy spectrum, build strength and power, retain our Type II fibers, and simultaneously train the other fitness attributes.

Even so, *endurance is no more to be dismissed than any of the other attributes.* Every athlete needs all the attributes in some proportion or other, even highly specialized athletes working at the extremes of the power-endurance energy spectrum, such as Olympic weightlifters (high power/low endurance) and cross-country skiers (low power/ high endurance). And the athlete of aging is most certainly not such a specialist. Even granting that strength should take center stage in our training prescription, endurance is still important. Isn't it possible to build endurance *and* strength?

Here's the good news: if we focus our training on strength and the high-power end of the energy spectrum, it's not only possible, it's virtually *inevitable.*

The conventional wisdom in exercise physiology holds that strength training does not make an impact on biomarkers of aerobic capacity, such as maximal oxygen uptake and aerobic enzyme activity. Recent research, including investigations focused on older subjects, has begun to challenge this view[35] and much of the research that contributes to the conventional wisdom is highly flawed, consisting primarily of small, short studies using what I call "low-dose" resistance training, poorly programmed and administered. But even studies that do not find increases in *biomarkers* of aerobic *capacity* nevertheless find that strength training improves *practical measures* of aerobic endurance *performance*,[36] such as treadmill time to exhaustion or overall exercise tolerance.

An illustration is in order. My friend and teacher, the noted strength coach and author Mark Rippetoe, has frequently cited the following example of a distance cyclist. The cyclist is an endurance athlete, and he believes with an almost religious conviction that strength training is not only useless, it's actually *poison* for competitive cycling. We snatch this guy off his bike on a deserted trail, kidnap him, and bring him to Rippetoe's gym, far away from civilization, in Wichita Falls, Texas. Using a dynamometer and a cattle prod, we measure the strength in his legs and come up with a number – call it $x$. His execution of an average pedal stroke while cycling requires him to exert some fraction of his maximal leg strength, say $\frac{1}{4}x$. We keep this guy locked up and compel him, through bribery, trickery, or threats of violence, to engage in strength training for 6–8 weeks. We force him to consume adequate protein and fluids, make him go to bed early, and let him call his Mom on weekends. At the end of his captivity, we find little change in his maximal oxygen uptake, his aerobic enzymes, or other commonly-assayed biomarkers of aerobic capacity. And yet we find that his endurance *performance* has improved. How?

When we measure his post-training strength, we find that it has doubled to $2x$. This means that his execution of an average pedal stroke while cycling now requires only $\frac{1}{8}x$, half as much of his maximal leg strength as before. In other words, *each pedal stroke is now easier than it used to be,* because it requires a smaller fraction of his maximal leg strength. We may also find, if we do the necessary testing, that strength training has improved his economy of motion and efficiency.[37] In short, *by making him stronger we have increased his endurance performance, and made him a better endurance athlete.* Our data collected, our point made, we release him back into the wild, possibly with some sort of radio tag so we can monitor his future training and mating habits.

There are multiple factors at play in this phenomenon. High-intensity exercise like strength training and HIIT demand a higher level of muscle fiber recruitment than low-intensity LSD work. Intensity modulates a protein called PGC-1α, which in turn promotes the development of mitochondria.[38] And perhaps most importantly, training at the high-power, "anaerobic" end of the energy spectrum demands support from mitochondrial (aerobic) metabolism.

Consider the athlete who performs a heavy bout of high-intensity exercise, say a set of heavy deadlifts or a wind sprint. This bout will demand a higher power output than mitochondrial metabolism can support, and will take place almost entirely in the phosphagen system, with some input from fast glycolysis. Remember that these are low-capacity energy systems. So by the time the athlete has completed his set or his sprint, they will be more-or-less depleted. And yet, after a few minutes of rest, he will do another set or sprint. How can this be? Because the high-power ("anaerobic") energy systems will be restored by the mitochondrial ("aerobic") system. During the rest interval between bouts, oxygen consumption is elevated, and the energy is used to replenish muscle energy stores. *But this support does not go both ways.* Training at low or moderate intensity does not produce significant improvements in anaerobic capacity[39] (Figure 4-12).

And so, here's the take-home point at last: *Low-intensity endurance exercise increases low-intensity endurance performance, but not strength or power.*[40] This mode of training interferes with strength development, and consumes valuable training time while progressively developing only two fitness attributes: endurance and body composition. In fact, the "improvement" in body composition induced by aerobic LSD training is characterized by the loss of fat (good) but also the atrophy of Type II

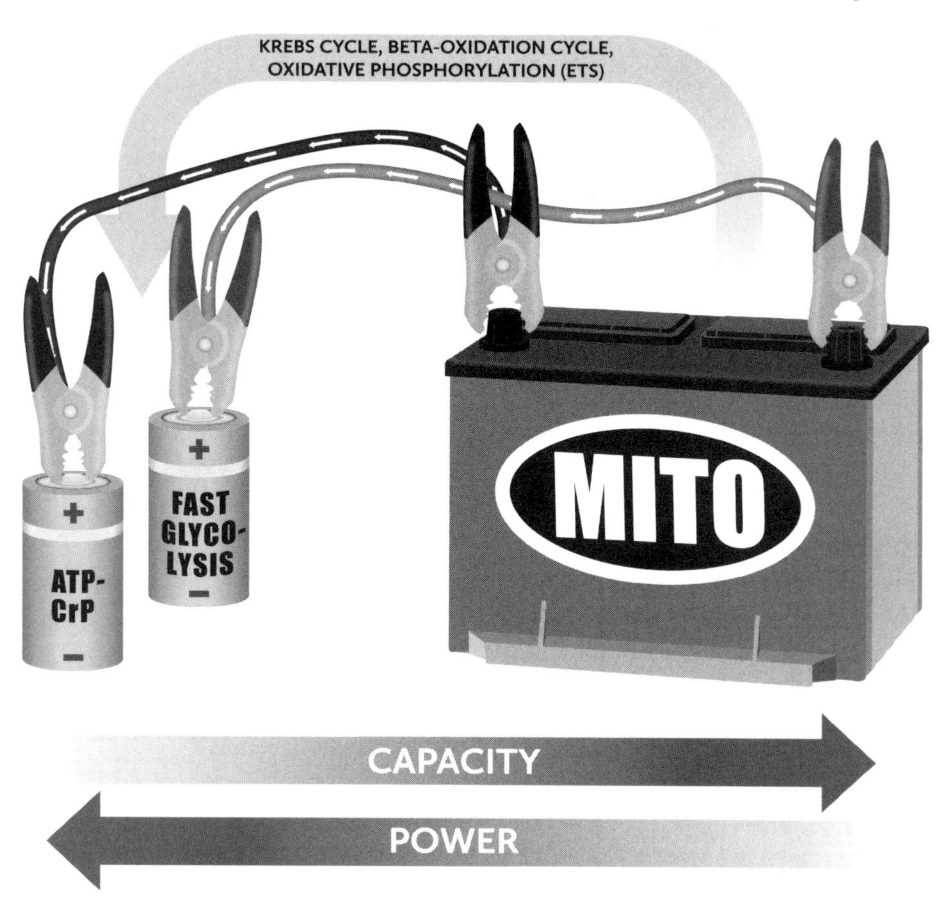


***Figure 4-12.*** The mitochondrial energy system supports cytosolic energy systems. Cytosolic or "anaerobic" energy systems have high power and low capacity, and consist of the phosphagen system and fast glycolysis. Mitochondrial or "aerobic" energy systems have low power and high capacity, and consist of the Krebs cycle and oxidative phosphorylation. During recovery from high-intensity work, the mitochondrial system works to "recharge" the cytosolic system.

fibers (very bad) and is arguably *contraindicated* for the Masters Athlete.

*Strength training increases both strength and low-intensity endurance performance*, and also trains the attributes of power, mobility, balance, and body composition. The addition of a complementary program of *high-intensity* conditioning (Chapter 26) develops both high-power performance and low-power endurance in less time than LSD, while avoiding any practical or biological interference effects of concurrent strength and LSD training.[41]

## Strength for the Extreme Sport of Aging

*All athletes need strength training*, even endurance athletes.[42] Strength is the most fundamental fitness attribute and pays dividends in any sport, with the possible exception of chess. Extreme athletes, such as those involved in the brutal sport we call aging, need strength the most. This is because the athlete of aging must perform a myriad array of activities in the game of life, even while time continues to pound away at him.

We're talking about what the gerontologists call *functioning*: the ability to carry out activities of daily life, including the activities that bring us joy and give our lives meaning. The Masters Athlete would more properly call it *performance* in the Arena of Life. Whatever we call it, we're talking about the ability to get out of bed, snatch a child from danger, lift a box overhead into a cupboard, pick up a heavy bag of groceries, leap for joy, play Frisbee with the dog, remodel the bathroom, row a boat across the fishing pond, or make love to our spouse.

I'd like you to notice something about those activities – activities that play out in the Arena of Life. *None of them involve running, biking, swimming or skiing for hours.* None of them are feats of aerobic endurance. Instead, they all involve expressions of strength, power, mobility, and balance. Let's face it: If you find you *have* to run 10 miles tomorrow, you have quite probably just lost the game of

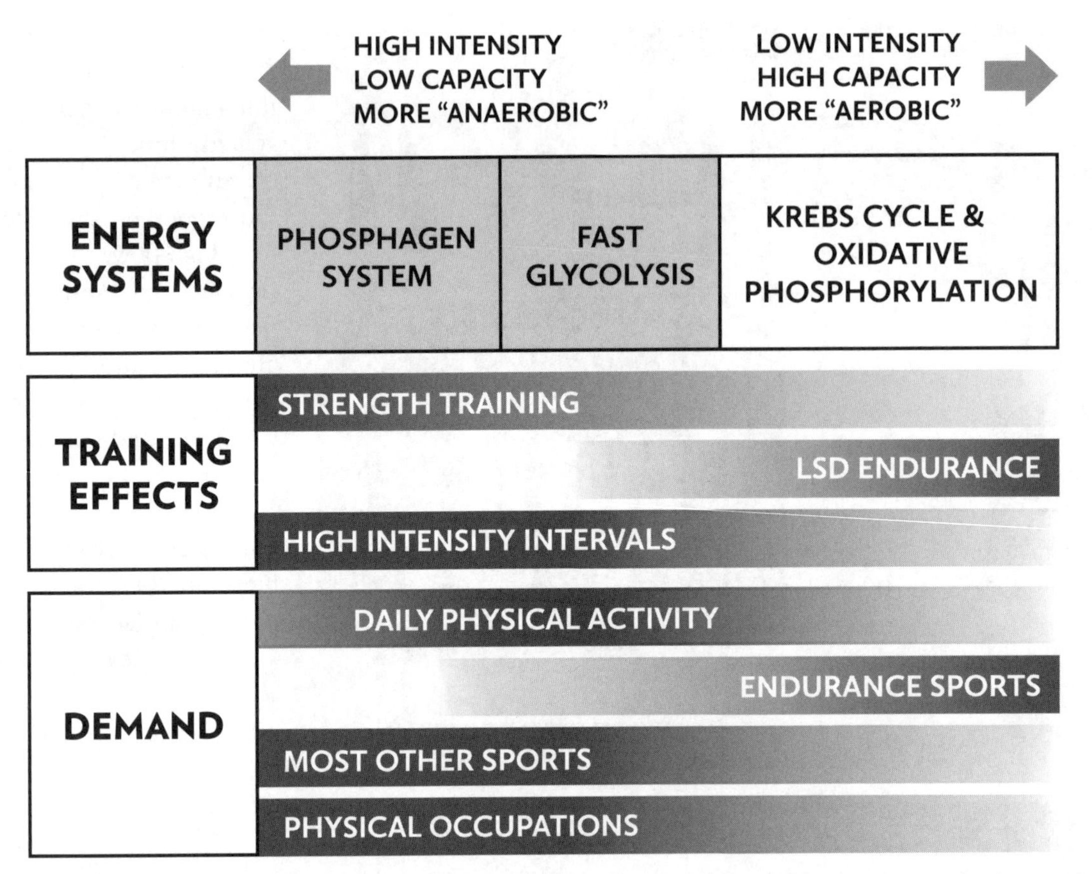


***Figure 4-13.*** Impact of different training modalities on energy systems. All forms of exercise draw ATP from all three energy sources (see Figure 4-10), but this figure emphasizes the extent to which different forms of exercise train and induce adaptations in those energy systems, and the demands of various physical activities on these systems. Strength training is conducted within the high-intensity anaerobic range and produces robust adaptations in the phosphagen and glycolytic energy systems, with some training effects on the aerobic energy system (depending on how the training is conducted). High-intensity interval training (HIIT) consists of short bursts of intense effort in the anaerobic system, but produces adaptations across the entire energy spectrum. LSD endurance training (running, distance biking, etc.) trains the aerobic energy system almost exclusively, and does not produce meaningful increases in anaerobic capacity. Most daily, occupational and sport activities do not demand the sort of aerobic endurance developed by LSD aerobic training.

life. Something Extraordinary And Very Bad has happened. Sure, you *could* train for this exigency, just as a fencer *could* train for the unexpected need to run a marathon. But it's not a particularly productive use of training time for either of you. The fencer will need power and balance on the practice floor tomorrow, not extreme aerobic endurance, and you'll have to pull a trunk out of the attic or heave your granddaughter up onto your shoulders (Figure 4-13).

The Masters Athlete needs endurance, to be sure, and many studies show that the health benefits of strength training in older individuals are increased when combined with a conditioning program. But strength, power, mobility, and balance are more important for the extreme sport of aging than the ability to huff and puff down a road for an hour. Moreover, in agreement with everything we've learned about energy systems, fiber types, and interference, evidence indicates that older individuals who train exclusively in the aerobic endurance ranges with LSD actually get *weaker* with time.[43]

*Only strength training covers so many fitness attributes.* Only a strength training prescription fits the bill for the athlete committed to performance

| | ENERGY SYSTEMS | | | ATHLETIC ATTRIBUTES | | |
|---|---|---|---|---|---|---|
| | Aerobic Endurance *Biomarkers* | Aerobic Endurance *Performance* | Anaerobic Capacity | Strength and Power | Mobility and Balance | Body Composition |
| LOW-INTENSITY LSD | **YES** | **YES** | NO | NO | +/- | ↓ fat, no muscle ↑ |
| HIGH-INTENSITY CONDITIONING | **YES** | **YES** | **YES** | +/- | +/- | ↓ fat, +/- muscle |
| STRENGTH TRAINING | NO* | **YES** | **YES** | **YES** | **YES**** | ↓ fat, ↑ muscle |

***Table 4-2.*** Summary of the effect of different training approaches on energy systems and athletic attributes. *Although some recent data suggests that strength training improves biomarkers of aerobic performance, we have acceded to conventional wisdom, which holds that it does not. **Mobility and balance are improved by strength training only when exercises demand mobility and balance; this has obvious implications for exercise selection and will be addressed in Chapter 6.

in the extreme sport of aging. If you enjoy tennis, hiking, swimming, skiing, or ballroom dancing, that's fine. Really. They're good for you. *Please* do them. But you'll do them better, longer, and more safely if you *train* for them in addition to *practicing* them. You just can't have a comprehensive exercise prescription without training all the fitness attributes. Strength training comes closer (Table 4-2) to filling a comprehensive prescription for the Master than any other exercise modality, by a long shot.

The winning athlete trains for strength. This applies doubly to the Masters Athlete, as we shall see in the next chapter.

# 5

# Specificity and Effectiveness: Your Physiological 401k

A correct prescription must specify a therapy with specific biological targets in order to produce a desired treatment outcome. A rational training program for any athlete will aim at the attainment of specific improvements in fitness attributes to optimize performance in practice and play. In this chapter, we will see that programmed strength training effectively combats the components of the Sick Aging Phenotype, while allowing the Masters Athlete to optimize the General Fitness Attributes and retain muscle, bone, strength, power, and function.

## Phat Phil Rises Again: Strength Training and the Sick Aging Phenotype

We've seen that a proper exercise prescription for the aging adult will take on the form of a training program for the Masters Athlete, because only a *program* that modulates training variables can be precisely administered over a broad range of doses. We've also explored the General Fitness Attributes that must be addressed by the training program of any athlete, including the Masters Athlete. In the previous chapter, we considered the various exercise modalities available to us through the prism of the fitness attributes and biological energy systems.

These investigations have now reached a point where strength training is the leading contender to be the linchpin of any training prescription. Strength training is a ***safe*** exercise if properly prescribed – that is, if it employs normal human movement patterns and manipulates training variables to achieve appropriate ***dosing***. And a properly designed program of strength training and conditioning is ***comprehensive***, driving improvements in all the General Fitness Attributes and imposing a productive training stimulus on all three energy systems.

Nevertheless, other considerations remain. In this chapter, we will look at the 4$^{th}$ of our criteria:

4. **Our exercise prescription/training program must specifically and effectively combat the Sick Aging Phenotype: metabolic syndrome, cardiovascular disease, sarcopenia, osteopenia, and loss of strength, function and mobility.**

After all, we've decided that the "event" we're training for is the brutal contest we call aging. It's all well and good if our training addresses the General Fitness Attributes and spans the three energy systems. But will that improve our game?

For most sports, this is not necessarily an open-and-shut question. Sports scientists and exercise physiologists are very good at showing that a particular training program will affect mobility, power, strength, or some obscure biophysical or laboratory value. But they've had a devil of a time showing that any particular approach to training delivers *better performance on the field*. This is an admittedly difficult task, hindered in part by the complexity of evaluating how the manipulation of any single exercise variable affects competitive outcomes, and partly by the lack of generally-accepted, practical, and relevant sport-specific metrics. Many people *think* that practicing explosion through Olympic lifting variants like the power clean will make you a better linebacker, or that a strong press will make you a better pitcher, and there are very compelling reasons to think so.[1] *Proving* it, on the other hand, seems a tall order. This is why most coaching practice is based on experience rather than "peer-reviewed research."

But we're in luck, because assessing the impact of training on the extreme sport of aging turns out to be a rather more tractable proposition. That's because, for this one very important game, we *do* have a set of readily assayed and relevant "sport-specific" metrics, and a comprehensive and ever-deepening knowledge of the opponent. We've already seen these metrics and our principal adversaries, when we examined the aging phenotypes. Our training prescription must address the Sick Aging Phenotype and its components if it is to be a winning strategy for the Athlete of Aging. Strength training is our leading candidate to be the cornerstone of such a prescription, so in this chapter we'll investigate whether it combats the Sick Aging Phenotype.

Let's briefly review the components of maladaptive aging that we saw exemplified in Phil's miserable decline and early demise. Phil's inactivity, lousy diet and deplorable habits led to the development of a deranged energy balance (too many calories for not enough work) and the accumulation of unhealthy fat. His condition progressed to insulin resistance, which ultimately blossomed into metabolic syndrome and finally full-blown diabetes. Metabolic syndrome produced chronic inflammation, dyslipidemia and vascular changes that resulted in high blood pressure, atherosclerotic heart disease, and generally poor circulation. Phil's muscles got progressively smaller and weaker (sarcopenia and dynapenia), his bones got progressively more brittle (osteopenia), and his tendons got floppier, weaker, and more easily injured. Phil developed frailty, chronic pain, depression, polypharmacy and loss of functioning. His Sick Aging Phenotype ultimately killed him through coronary artery disease and a massive heart attack, but it could just as easily have done him in with congestive heart failure, an arrhythmia, venous thromboembolism, a stroke, a nasty skin infection, an unanticipated drug interaction, suicide, or a broken hip. Or instead of killing him quickly, the syndrome could have simmered on for another couple of decades, culminating in an interminable purgatory in a nursing home as a diapered, demented meat pretzel, waiting for the final bout of pneumonia or sepsis. (The great physician William Osler said that pneumonia is "the old man's friend." Some old men might beg to differ.)

That's the opponent we confront as Masters Athletes in the Arena of Life: the Sick Aging Phenotype. Does strength training prepare us to grapple with this monster? The answer is a resounding *yes*. This is not a mere assertion, but a conclusion based on the best evidence we have accumulated over the last twenty or thirty years, and especially since the dawn of the 21st century, when we've seen an explosion of research literature on the topic. In this pivotal chapter, we'll survey some of that evidence.

This is as good a time as any to point out an inconvenient truth about published scientific research: Like all other human endeavors, it's about 90% shit by weight. This has always been true, and if anything it's even more true now, as research effort is heavily impacted by publication bias, the pressures of academic life, and the corruption of science by industry, which has a decidedly non-scientific axe to grind.[2] This sad fact of life does not exempt the biomedical literature,[3] whether we're talking about exercise medicine,[4] cancer chemotherapy, diagnostic imaging, or even basic cell biology.

So I want to be perfectly up front with you: Just as you can easily find studies showing that generally accepted and widely used medical therapies do not actually produce the desired results, so are there contrary findings in the literature on strength training for various disease states and their markers.[5] This overview of the literature focuses on the *overwhelming preponderance of the evidence,* draws heavily on physiological reasoning and experience, and would of necessity involve my own very human biases, whether I admitted it or not. I choose to admit it. Like any scientific or medical analysis, mine must be considered provisional. I invite you, I encourage you, I *implore* you to evaluate views contrary to those in this book and reach your own conclusions.

Sorry, but if you were looking for Timeless Truths, you came to the wrong place. I believe the conclusions offered here represent our best *current* understanding of the impact of resistance training on the Sick Aging Phenotype. But a career in medicine rapidly teaches one that there are no capital-T Truths. The biomedical literature on exercise medicine, which until recently ignored strength training and gave primacy to aerobic exercise, is itself a perfect example of this.

With all the caveats out of the way, let's take a look at the evidence, bearing in mind the structure and development of the Sick Aging Phenotype as discussed in Chapter 2 (Figure 5-1).

## Strength Training, Sick Fat, and Inflammation

An abnormally positive energy balance is a principal cause of the metabolic syndrome. Any form of exercise, in conjunction with fewer Twinkies, Doritos and Big Gulps, is going to move energy flux in a more negative direction, with a concomitant reduction in bodyfat. Although fat loss is associated in the public and medical minds with aerobic exercise, there is growing recognition that resistance training can increase fat loss and decrease fat gains by maximizing muscle mass and muscle energy expenditure. Moreover, strength training contributes to the loss of *visceral* fat, which is more closely associated with the development of metabolic syndrome than total bodyfat.[6]

This is important, because visceral fat is actively involved in systemic inflammatory processes.[7] I use the term ***sick fat*** to describe this situation. In sedentary individuals with excess energy flux and insulin resistance, *visceral fat becomes a pro-inflammatory tissue.*[8] Inflammation promotes degenerative changes in blood vessels and other tissues that drive the development of cardiovascular disease and other elements of the Sick Aging Phenotype.

Strength training has been studied in this context, and demonstrates the power to reduce the burden of sick fat and decrease systemic inflammation.[9] This is partly through the ability of exercise to increase energy expenditure and reduce the amount of fat in the body. But a more important effect may be the *reprogramming of fat tissue* by high-intensity exercise, transforming sick fat into healthy fat, a tissue with a signaling profile that actually promotes health, regulates appetite, and works in harmony with muscle and other tissues. This has implications for blood pressure, coronary artery health, insulin sensitivity, chronic pain, and possibly even long-term neurologic health.

In short, strength training has the power to fight the accumulation of sick fat, a major player in the development of metabolic syndrome and the Sick Aging Phenotype.[10]

## Strength Training, Metabolic Syndrome, and Diabetes

*Any* form of regular, vigorous exercise combats the development and progression of the metabolic syndrome, and this most definitely includes resistance training.[11] Vigorous exercise creates a

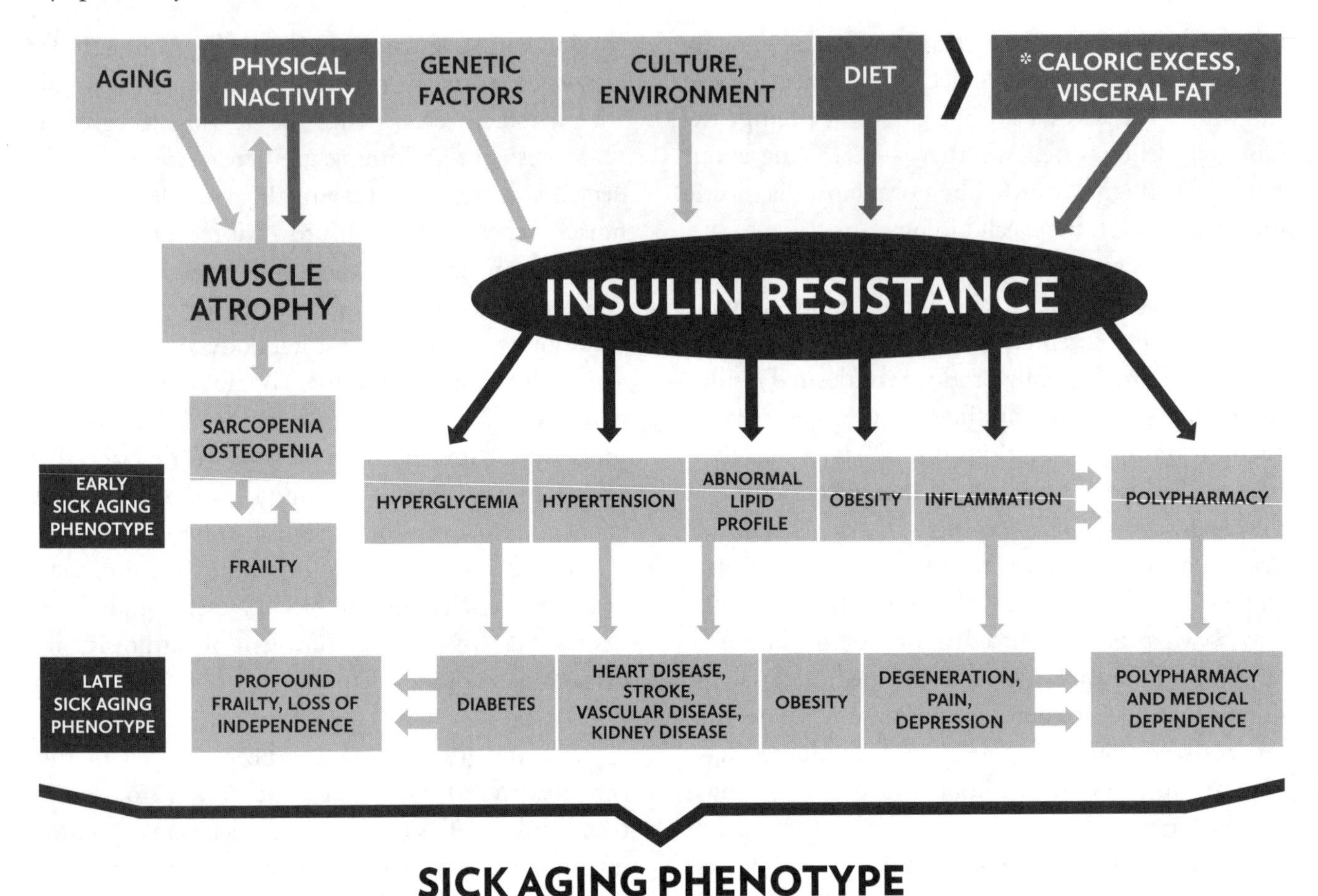


***Figure 5-1.*** The Sick Aging Phenotype (Reprise). An abnormally high energy balance from excess caloric intake and low physical inactivity, combined with aging and genetic and environmental factors, precipitates the development of obesity, visceral fat, muscle atrophy, and insulin resistance. The development of the metabolic syndrome promotes ongoing physiological imbalances, inflammation, and damage to tissue, especially vascular tissues. These processes culminate in the full-blown Sick Aging Phenotype: diabetes, atherosclerosis and vascular disease, heart disease, stroke, sarcopenia, weakness, frailty, chronic pain, and tissue atrophy. As the meta-syndrome develops, its component processes become more interlinked and reinforce each other, so the Sick Aging Phenotype becomes progressively more established and difficult to treat.

demand for energy by working muscles, and it's *usually* through the action of insulin that hungry cells suck calories out of the bloodstream for work.[12] So it makes sense that muscles roused from their torpor and forced into a training program will increase their insulin sensitivity, thereby increasing total body insulin sensitivity. Strength training, however, doesn't just increase the *activity* of muscle. It increases the *mass* of muscle tissue as well, which has a profound multiplier effect on the impact of exercise on metabolism, and increases energy expenditure even at rest.

At this juncture we should take note of an interesting physiological wrinkle. Glucose entry into muscle cells does not require insulin signaling *during exercise*. It does, however, require an increased availability of muscle *glucose transporters.*[13] Trained muscle produces more of these transporter proteins to adapt to training stress, promoting the ability of muscle to sop up food energy during exercise even in the absence of insulin, an important effect for those with insulin insensitivity or diabetes. After exercise, muscle energy demands remain elevated, and during this period glucose uptake by the muscle

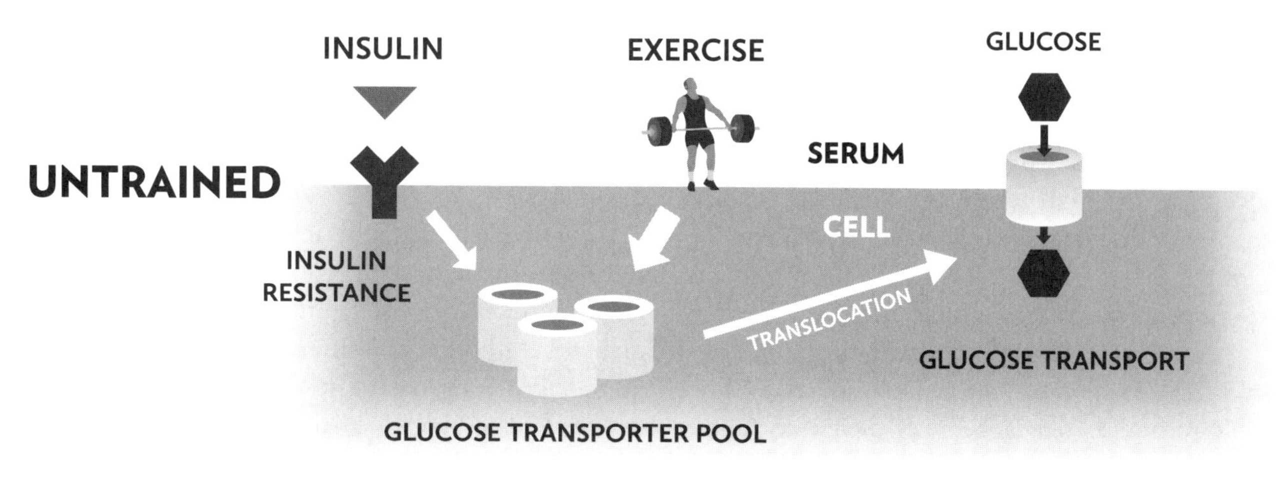


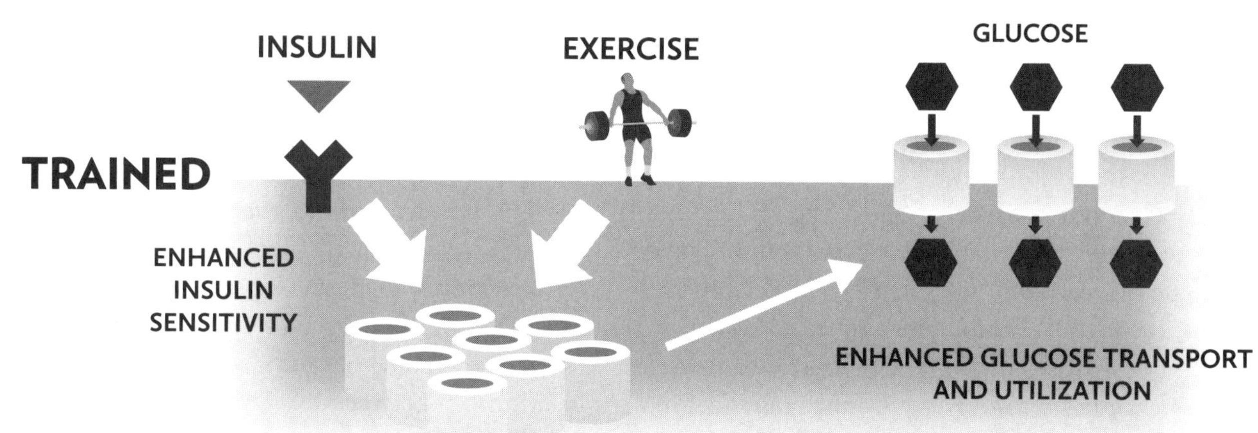


***Figure 5-2.*** Training increases both insulin-independent and insulin-dependent glucose flux in skeletal muscle. At rest, insulin is required to recruit glucose transporters to the muscle membrane, but this process is impeded by insulin resistance. During exercise, the recruitment of glucose transporters is independent of insulin. In the trained state, increased expression of glucose transporters enhances both insulin-dependent and exercise-induced, insulin-independent glucose transport.

is dependent on insulin to activate the glucose transporters (Figure 5-2).

Think of the implications of this physiology for the patient with insulin resistance or diabetes. Normally, this individual will have elevated serum glucose levels because his insulin signaling systems aren't working properly, meaning that glucose can't be efficiently removed from the bloodstream. But this blockade to glucose flux is bypassed during exercise.[14] Exercising muscle is a huge volume of tissue that will rapidly take up glucose in an insulin-independent manner. What's more, this exercise forces an important adaptation: the production of more glucose transporters to prepare the tissue for the next bout of exercise.[15] This increased availability of glucose transporters is one reason why exercise increases muscle insulin sensitivity,[16] and is in fact very similar to one of the putative mechanisms of metformin, a widely-prescribed anti-diabetic drug.[17] As training progresses, the tissue will become more insulin-sensitive, to allow for increased glucose disposal during the post-exercise, insulin-dependent period.[18] In other words, *exercise promotes both insulin-independent and insulin-dependent glucose disposal,*[19] with profound effects on an insulin-resistant phenotype.

The sheer volume of research data indicating that strength training combats insulin resistance and the metabolic syndrome has become overwhelming. Study after study shows that resistance training increases skeletal muscle insulin sensitivity, increases muscle glucose uptake, promotes glucose tolerance, and decreases the high serum insulin levels found in patients with metabolic syndrome and Type 2 diabetes.[20]

Resistance training also decreases levels of *HbA1c* or *glycated hemoglobin.*[21] Hemoglobin, as you will recall from your high school biology, is the molecule that gives red blood cells their color and allows them to carry oxygen to the tissues of your body. You can think of HbA1c as hemoglobin that has marinated in sugary blood so long that glucose molecules have become chemically bonded to it. This abnormal form of hemoglobin can still carry oxygen, but its accumulation in the blood is a marker for the metabolic syndrome, the onset of Type 2 diabetes, and cardiovascular disease. I suspect HbA1c may also exert direct pathological effects, although this is not known for certain. An important systematic analysis of the data on *progressive* resistance exercise (that is, actual *training*) by Irvine and Taylor,[22] encompassing 9 randomized controlled trials and 372 experimental subjects, found that strength training led to reductions in HbA1c in patients with Type 2 diabetes.

Data on the beneficial effect of resistance training on insulin sensitivity and metabolic syndrome goes back decades,[23] although its implications have been slow to percolate up into the consciousness of the public, or even the modern medical mind. Multiple studies demonstrate that muscular strength is inversely associated with the incidence of the metabolic syndrome.[24] In other words, the stronger you are, the less likely you are to display the hellish constellation of visceral obesity, insulin resistance, hypertension, dyslipidemia, and systemic inflammation that points the way to the Sick Aging Phenotype. Accumulating evidence of the effect of resistance training on the metabolic syndrome was analyzed in depth by Strasser, Siebert, and Schobersberger in a study published in the journal *Sports Medicine* in 2010.[25] They identified 13 randomized trials of resistance training, and found that, when pooled and analyzed, the data from these studies indicated beneficial effects on obesity, HbA1c levels, and blood pressure. They recommended resistance training as a therapy in the management of metabolic syndrome and related disorders.

If unchecked, the insulin resistance that is central to the development of metabolic syndrome may ultimately blossom into full-blown Type 2 diabetes. Although conditioning with aerobic LSD exercise has long been known to decrease the risk of *developing* Type 2 diabetes, there was scarce evidence in the literature of a similar effect of weight training, primarily because it hadn't been studied as much. While a great deal of research on the effect of strength training in patients who already have Type 2 diabetes is in print, very few studies have looked at prevention. A 2012 investigation by Grontved et al.,[26] however, found that strength training was indeed associated with a profound decrease in the risk of developing diabetes, especially when combined with a conditioning program. Given everything we know about physical activity in general, the relationship between exercise intensity and the risk of developing diabetes, and the well-established effects of strength training on muscle metabolism and glucose flux, these results are hardly surprising. And they comport well with everyday coaching and clinical experience: People who remain active, stay strong and eat wisely don't become diabetic.

For many, however, the horse is out of the barn. What if you *already* have Type 2 diabetes? Although there is no shortage of anecdotal reports that lifestyle changes, including strength training, can normalize blood sugar levels and eliminate the need for medication, there is no good randomized prospective data that any form of exercise or diet will *cure* diabetes once established. But there is an *enormous* amount of evidence that exercise, and in particular resistance exercise, has profound beneficial effects on the disease.[27] In the last 10–15 years, strength training has garnered increased recognition for its ability to manage Type 2 diabetes by increasing muscle mass, improving total body insulin sensitivity, enhancing glucose oxidation, decreasing HbA1c levels, and improving serum glucose control.

In summary, strength training combats insulin resistance across the entire spectrum of severity, up to and including the development and management of Type 2 diabetes. Because of the centrality of insulin resistance to the development of the metabolic syndrome and the Sick Aging Phenotype, it is difficult to exaggerate the importance to the Masters Athlete of training for strength.

# Cardiovascular Health

Because insulin resistance and the metabolic syndrome promote the development of cardiovascular disease, and because strength training combats insulin resistance and metabolic syndrome, we might expect strength training to have a beneficial impact on the cardiovascular system in health and disease.

## Strength training & cardiovascular fitness

For a long time the conventional wisdom held that, while resistance training could certainly make for stronger muscles and bones, it didn't really train the heart or promote cardiovascular health. This was a classic case of physiological reasoning, and it was based in part on a misunderstanding of the interplay between the energy systems. It went like this: aerobic conditioning (particularly LSD work) clearly has profound beneficial effects on cardiovascular health. Strength training, on the other hand, operates within the anaerobic energy system, meaning it isn't aerobic, and it uses short bouts of intense effort rather than long, extended, incredibly boring ordeals of low-intensity work. Therefore, strength training should not confer the benefits of LSD and other endurance training modalities.

This view is beginning to erode as researchers look more closely at the impact of resistance training on cardiovascular fitness and reassess old assumptions. For example, conventional wisdom has long held that structural adaptations of the heart muscle are fundamentally different in resistance-trained and endurance-trained athletes. On this view, weightlifters demonstrate *concentric hypertrophy*, with increased cardiac wall thickness and little increase in chamber size, while endurance athletes display *eccentric hypertrophy*, with balanced increases in chamber size and wall thickness. But a systematic analysis of the available scientific literature on this point, published by Utomi et al. in 2013,[28] found that *both endurance training and strength training produced similar structural cardiac adaptations.* Strength athletes and endurance athletes both displayed increased wall thickness and changes in chamber size compared to sedentary controls. There were some differences in functional parameters, but not anatomy. Of particular interest were the findings on *ejection fraction*, a measure of how hard the heart can pump, and arguably the most important variable studied. There was no difference in ejection fraction between the resistance- and endurance-trained groups.

In the world of exercise physiology, cardiovascular fitness is closely associated with the athlete's ***$VO_2$max*** (pronounced vee-oh-two-max). This quantity represents the maximal rate at which an individual can deliver oxygen to tissues during exercise, and is sometimes referred to as *maximal aerobic capacity*. $VO_2$max is heavily dependent on cardiovascular function, and the highest values for $VO_2$max have been recorded in endurance-trained athletes. However, athletes who work in mixed aerobic-anaerobic sports, and anaerobic athletes like sprinters and weightlifters, also have higher $VO_2$max than sedentary individuals.[29] Although the values for $VO_2$max displayed by such athletes are not as high as those of marathoners and cross-country skiers, they nevertheless indicate significantly higher levels of cardiopulmonary fitness than those seen in sedentary populations (Table 5-1).[30] On the other hand, many investigators find that a program of strength training produces only very small increases in $VO_2$max, or no changes at all. These findings underscore the importance of including a conditioning component in our exercise program. As we saw in Chapter 4 and as Andy Baker and I will describe in Part III, this component of our training prescription can be satisfied in a very simple and time-efficient manner.

## Strength training & cardiovascular disease

Cardiovascular disease is an inclusive term, encompassing hypertension, peripheral vascular disease (particularly coronary artery disease and cerebral vascular disease), heart attack, heart failure and stroke. Accumulating data indicates that resistance training has a beneficial impact on risk factors for cardiovascular disease, even when its impacts on total bodyfat and $VO_2$max are minimal.[31] Hypertension, coronary artery disease, and congestive heart failure have all been studied in the context of strength training, and all have been found to respond favorably.

**Hypertension.** No form of exercise that I am aware of is able to *cure* established hypertension, but it now appears that both aerobic and strength training exert positive influences on this condition. Early studies of the effect of strength training on blood pressure were mixed,[32] primarily because of differences in study design. The most recent work in this area tends to be of somewhat higher quality, and a growing body of literature indicates a beneficial effect of resistance training on blood pressure.[33] In men with hypertension, there is an inverse relationship between strength and all-cause mortality.[34] Contrary to what your grandma may have told you, there is no good evidence that strength training causes high blood pressure. In fact, it appears that the opposite is true.[35]

**Dyslipidemia.** Resistance training improves a number of risk factors for cardiovascular disease, including serum lipid profiles[36] although the data on this point is decidedly mixed. A recent paper by Braith[37] concluded that resistance training has *manifold beneficial impacts on cardiovascular disease risk factors*, although limitations of the research conducted so far make estimation of risk reductions difficult. For example, the evidence that resistance training impacts serum lipid and cholesterol profiles is equivocal, and most of this research has been done in individuals who already have total cholesterol levels <200 mg/dL at study entry. People whose cholesterol is already reasonably well-controlled are unlikely to manifest further improvements with any exercise intervention, especially the low-dose, poorly programmed resistance training interventions studied in most research. In Braith's view, the primary mechanism by which strength training decreases cardiovascular disease risk is by increasing insulin sensitivity, decreasing systemic inflammation, decreasing visceral fat, and moderating blood pressure.

**Heart Failure.** The use of strength training in patients with heart failure is a new and very exciting area of investigation. ***Heart failure*** is a chronic condition arising from accumulated damage to the heart, either from repeated heart attacks (ischemic events) or from longstanding uncorrected hypertension. The heart muscle becomes progressively incompetent to meet the demands of the circulation. It's an unspeakably miserable disease, its five-year survival rate is in the toilet, and in developed countries this monster has become an epidemic and a gigantic sink for health care resources. It is now apparent that strength training in patients with heart failure is safe and improves exercise tolerance, function, and quality of life.[38] Moreover, a study by Smart et al.[39] suggests that strength training, characterized by bouts of intense effort interspersed with lighter activity or rest, may be more appropriate for this population than endurance-based aerobic training.

**Coronary artery disease** is characterized by the accumulation of fatty plaques in the arteries that serve the cardiac muscle. Similar plaques are found in the arteries of the brain, and this is known as ***cerebrovascular disease***. Rupture of these plaques can lead to the formation of a clot, which blocks the blood vessel, leading to heart attack or stroke. I am aware of no noninvasive therapy, including exercise, that has been conclusively shown to result in significant regression of established vascular plaques with associated decreases in cardiac events and stroke. However, strength training is generally safe in patients with coronary artery disease[40] and other forms of cardiovascular disease, and is in fact recognized as an important component of the

**$VO_2$max (ml/kg/min)**

| | |
|---|---|
| Sedentary (Couch Potato) | 30 |
| Active but untrained | 40 |
| Wrestlers | 55 |
| Weightlifters | 55 |
| Cyclists | 75 |
| Runners | 70-80 |
| Cross-Country Skiers | 82+ |
| HIIT-trained | 55-70 |

***Table 5-1.*** Maximal oxygen uptake ($VO_2$max) in various training states. $VO_2$max is a measure of aerobic capacity and is generally taken as an indirect metric of cardiopulmonary fitness. Aerobic endurance athletes at elite levels of training have very high $VO_2$max values. However, even anaerobic athletes, such as weightlifters, wrestlers and HIIT-trained athletes, who condition at high intensity and do little or no LSD endurance work, have much higher $VO_2$max values than sedentary and untrained individuals.

exercise prescription for these patients and for the rehabilitation of patients after heart attack and stroke.

On balance, it must be said that the preponderance of available scientific evidence *to date* indicates that endurance training is *probably* superior to strength training for the optimization of cardiopulmonary fitness and health. There has been some significant erosion in this view, but let's take that conclusion at face value for now. If cardiovascular health were our only consideration, endurance training would be hands-down our exercise modality of choice. But of course, it is *not* our only consideration, and in any event the data also makes it clear that the addition of a conditioning component to a strength program improves cardiovascular fitness more than either training modality alone. This most emphatically does *not* mean that we are stuck with LSD training after all, as we'll see in Part III.

## Sarcopenia, Osteopenia, and Other Atrophic Components of the Sick Aging Phenotype

From 1995 to 2013, I was involved in cerebral ischemia research. This means that I investigated what happens to the brain when blood flow is interrupted, as happens in stroke or during cardiac arrest.[41] My focus was on molecular mechanisms that lead to brain cell death or survival. To make progress in this research, I had to learn a lot about how cells decide to die.

That's right. Cells can *decide* to die. It's not a passive process, but rather the culmination of an elaborate biomolecular self-destruct program called ***apoptosis*** or ***programmed cell death***.[42] Apoptosis is critical to advanced, multicellular life forms like you. Without it, embryonic development would be a disaster. Viral infections would spread like wildfire if cells weren't programmed to sacrifice themselves for the greater good when compromised. And apoptosis is one of the body's primary defenses against malignant transformation and the development of cancer.[43]

Apoptosis is horribly complex in the particulars, but the big picture isn't hard to sketch out. There are two basic pathways: *extrinsic apoptosis* and *intrinsic apoptosis*. In extrinsic apoptosis, another cell or tissue sends a death signal, which is picked up by the target cell and tells it to die. In the intrinsic process, some stressor causes the cell's mitochondria (the power plants we saw in Chapter 4), to spill certain proteins into the cytoplasm. Think of a leaky nuclear reactor. Bad news. These leaked proteins don't kill the cell outright, but rather trigger a complex series of events that lead to cell suicide. In both intrinsic and extrinsic patterns, the terminal phase of apoptosis is carried out by enzymes that cut up cellular components and DNA. These enzymes take the cell apart in an orderly fashion and clean up the mess.

At some point during apoptosis, the cell will become unrecoverable. It will be, in a word, *dead.* When the nucleus, mitochondria, and other cellular structures start to shrink up and disappear, there is little hope for the cell. And once a cell has cut up its DNA, it has blown its own brains out. Game over. However, because apoptosis is not a passive falling-apart, but a molecular *program*, one that has to be signaled, triggered, activated, and executed, it can be modulated. Up to a point, apoptosis can be inhibited or reversed, and the most effective way to do so is through *growth factor signaling.*[44]

***Growth factors*** are hormones like human growth hormone (HGH), insulin, insulin-like growth factors (IGFs), endothelial-derived growth factor (EDGF), and nerve growth factor (NGF), among many others. As the name implies, they signal for cells to grow and multiply. But growth factors don't just promote growth – they promote *cellular survival.*

For example, you can subject cultured cells to any number of noxious stimuli that will cause them to snuff themselves. Such stimuli include lack of oxygen, radiation, poisons, certain types of viral infection, or toxic levels of calcium or free radicals. The cells will promptly activate their self-destruct programs, shrivel up, and die. However, you can slow down or arrest the cell suicide program by administering a growth factor, such as insulin or IGF-1, to the culture. As a result of observations like these, growth factors are under intense scrutiny for their potential to treat any number of devastating diseases, including stroke.[45]

But that's not all. If you take cultured cells, which are growing in blood serum, and you remove that serum, they will die, *without any other insult.* Why? Because the serum contains growth factors. Removal of growth factor signaling is sufficient to trigger apoptosis in many types of metazoan cells.[46]

One (somewhat contentious) way of looking at this is that *the default mode of these cells is not to live, but to die.* If you remove growth factor stimulation, they will kill themselves. The death machinery is there, just waiting to be activated. The teleological, evolutionary, developmental, and philosophical implications of this view are staggering, but beyond the scope of this book.

### Apoptosis and aging: the molecular perspective

Apoptosis seems to be a key player in the biology of aging. At the time of this writing, there is abundant evidence that apoptosis, *autophagy* and other programmed cell death processes are important mechanisms underlying the neural degeneration, muscle atrophy, sarcopenia, and osteopenia that descend on us like vultures in the second half of our lives. And there's increasing interest in the use of growth factors and other anti-apoptotic strategies to retard the loss of these critical tissues.[47]

Let's take muscle atrophy (loss of muscle mass) and sarcopenia (loss of muscle cells) as examples. Muscle loss is endemic in older individuals, and it predicts frailty, illness, loss of independence, injury, and all-cause mortality.[48] This makes perfect sense, because muscle is what allows us to move and function in the physical world. Healthy muscle is also a deep biological sink for carbohydrate and fat disposal, bristling with receptors sensitive to insulin signaling, and the most abundant secretory tissue, pound-for-pound, in the human body – your most massive "gland."

So the atrophy and loss of muscle tissue in aging is not just a matter of getting weaker and skinnier, which is bad enough. *Muscle tissue loss is nothing short of a catastrophe.* The impact of muscle atrophy and sarcopenia on health care costs is astronomical,[49] and the impact on quality of life and human suffering is simply incalculable.

Muscle cell apoptosis, autophagy, and other programmed cell suicide processes are key contributors to the muscle atrophy and sarcopenia seen in geriatric and sedentary populations.[50] High levels of suicide proteins, including proteolytic enzymes, have been found in the atrophic skeletal muscles of aging rats, and the fibers in these muscles demonstrate apoptotic changes, including DNA fragmentation. The data in humans, while limited, also implicates apoptosis in muscle tissue loss.[51] For example, older human subjects demonstrate large numbers of apoptotic muscle cell nuclei compared to controls.[52] Adults who do not engage in regular strength training lose up to 1 pound of muscle per year after 40.[53] The dominant factor in this process is loss of Type II fibers. By age 80, untrained adults have lost up to 50% of Type II fibers.[54] This is particularly devastating, because these are the largest, strongest, and most powerful type of muscle fibers.

The age-related loss of muscle tissue tracks a corresponding decline in growth factors and anabolic sex hormones. For example, levels of IGF-1 fall with advancing age, and lower IGF-1 levels are associated with the loss of strength and muscle mass that progresses as we grow older. Conversely, growth factors such as IGF-1 induce skeletal muscle accumulation, or ***hypertrophy***.[55]

Observations like these led to a burst of studies investigating the administration of growth factors to older individuals.[56] The results trend toward improvement in lean body mass, decreased bodyfat, some improvement in serum lipids, increased strength – and an increase in adverse events, including insulin resistance, diabetes, gynecomastia (man-boobs), joint pain, and swelling.[57] The take-home message here is that, while it may be tempting to take trophic factor supplements to retard the aging process, a far better approach is to *make our own*, in our own bodies, for as long as we can, so the responses are physiologic, regulated, and healthy.

When we engage in strength training and eat correctly, we are sending a signal to our body that an ***anabolic*** state, a physiological environment favoring growth, repair and survival, is called for. An anabolic environment means growth factors. Growth factors suppress apoptosis and atrophy. And apoptosis and atrophy are fundamental components of aging.

## Apoptosis, atrophy and aging: the clinical evidence

**Resistance Training and Muscle Atrophy.** The clinical evidence from human studies comprises a virtual mountain of data showing that strength training prevents and reverses age-related declines in skeletal muscle mass and function.[58] The disproportionate loss of high-powered Type II fibers in aging is primarily due to muscle atrophy rather than actual loss, and can be significantly reversed if not too advanced.[59] Strength training not only restores muscle mass, but also muscle function, resulting in increases in mobility, power, strength, *and* muscle secretory function. Muscle isn't just the biggest gland in your body, it's also the one that you can most directly influence with your behavior.

**Osteopenia and Osteoporosis**. The effect of strength training on atrophic aging doesn't end with muscle. Strength training also sends a strong message to bone tissue. Just as muscle must adapt to increasing resistance in a progressive exercise program, so too must bone be remodeled to accommodate the increasing stress on skeletal components. *Any* sort of sufficiently intense resistance exercise stimulates increased bone mineral density at muscle attachments and other points of mechanical stress. For example, if you do curls with heavier and heavier weights, you will increase bone mineral density where the biceps muscle attaches to the bones. That's terrific, but the real payoff comes with structural exercise.

***Structural exercises*** are those that place a significant *axial* (compressive) stress on the spine, and almost always on the pelvis and hips as well. In the absence of adequate and regular loading of the axial skeleton and the hips, aging and atrophy lead to decreased bone mineral density (osteopenia) loss of bone structure (osteoporosis) and ultimately pathologic bone failure. The result: vertebral collapse, spinal deformation, chronic pain, hip fracture (which can still be a death sentence), and the miserable and disfiguring curse of the Dowager's hump. Exercises like squats, deadlifts, and standing presses place significant training loads on the axial skeleton, pelvis, and hips, and force increases in bone mineral density where the Masters Athlete needs them most.

## Fighting Frailty: Strength, Mobility, Balance and Function

Here we're getting beyond what some would narrowly consider to be the health benefits of resistance training and moving into the realm of performance. Of course, by now it should be clear that performance is a critical component of our health.

It would seem obvious that *strength training should increase strength*, and the first derivative of strength, which we call power. Of course, as with everything else in life, creative people can find a way to thoroughly screw this up. Some of the most perversely gifted of these individuals become personal trainers, many of whom have *absolutely no idea* how to exploit the human body's miraculous capacity for adaptation to drive the development of increasing strength. We shall have more to say about how this is *properly* done in Part III. For now, suffice to say that resistance training, properly administered, performed, and programmed, can indeed produce remarkable and continuous improvements in strength and power, even in extremely old individuals, as demonstrated in hundreds of studies published over the last half-century or so.[60] As we have already discussed at length, this has profound implications for the Sick Aging Phenotype.

Picking up a heavy box and putting it in the cupboard requires not just strength, but also the ability to move throughout the required range of motion, to maintain truncal and spinal stability while doing so, and to keep one's balance while moving a heavy weight from the floor to overhead. Thus, mobility and balance are, along with strength and power, essential components of physical functioning, and they tend to decline with age. The power of strength training to positively impact these factors depends entirely on the manner in which it is administered. As General Fitness Attributes, these qualities can be trained, but only if training stress is properly applied in a way that forces the organism to adapt and improve these attributes.

If strength training is performed sitting down in fancy machines, or by performing truncated, artificial movement patterns with your butt supported by a bench (picture a seated dumbbell curl), you can expect little in the way of improvement in these parameters.

If, on the other hand, strength training is constituted by structural (standing) exercises with free weights over a full range of motion, it will stress the trainee's ability to move through that range of motion, to maintain spine and joint stability, and to keep the center of mass of the lifter-load system balanced over the middle of the foot. This training stress will force corresponding muscular, skeletal, tendon, ligament, neuromuscular, perceptual, and cognitive adaptations that preserve and increase flexibility, mobility, balance[61] and, above all, *function* in the aging adult.[62] Strength training is a powerful tool for promoting the ability of the Masters Athlete to *perform* in the Arena of Life.

### Frailty

The end stage of the Sick Aging Phenotype is characterized by frailty, which means exactly what you think it means: an inability to withstand the rough-and-tumble encountered in the Arena of Life without breaking. Wasted muscles, brittle bones, a sick and torpid metabolism, poor mobility and balance, and a diseased cardiovascular system render us more susceptible to injury and illness, and less capable of coping with them when they occur. In the setting of frailty, tripping on the sidewalk, a case of the flu, or a "minor" bout of pneumonia can be a death sentence. Phat Phil was an example of this. His heart attack was a bad one, but he might well have survived if he'd had the physiological reserve to fight back. He didn't.

Muscles and ligaments made strong by training are less likely to sprain or snap. Bones made hard and dense by programmed structural exercise are more resistance to fracture and collapse. Minds made tough by struggling under the bar, and awake to possibilities of ongoing physical accomplishment offered by training, are less likely to succumb to despair and depression. As Mark Rippetoe is fond of saying, *strong people are harder to kill.* The wise athlete engages in training, in part, to make himself resistant to injury. It is no different for the Masters Athlete. Strength training is a powerful tool against age-related frailty.

## Psychosocial and Spiritual Dimensions: Human Apoptosis

Earlier, we explored the role of cell suicide in the atrophy of aging. Biomolecular self-destruct programs are triggered and executed at the microscopic and biochemical levels of the organism, but they can be modulated or even aborted by growth factor stimulation. We've seen how strength training fits into such a picture of aging and atrophy.

That's the *molecular* perspective. But I think the macro perspective is even more illuminating. I maintain that apoptosis doesn't just occur on the cellular or biochemical level. A similar process of self-destruction takes place *at the level of the human being*, and like cellular apoptosis it is accelerated by aging and aggravated by the withdrawal of growth and survival stimulation.

Call it *human apoptosis*.

Aging is characterized by a loss of strength, flexibility, and adaptive physiologic reserve. These losses go with the senescence of growth and repair systems, blunting of hormonal responses, and atrophy of muscle, nerve, tendon, ligament, and bone. This physical atrophy is accompanied by an equally deadly psychological decline. Too often, the aging individual sees that he is getting weaker, and so lowers his expectations and his efforts – and thereby grows weaker still. This is analogous to the cell cutting up its own DNA. Once the psyche has surrendered to decline and death, it's all over but the suffering.

Like cellular self-destruction, I think human apoptosis also comes in both intrinsic and extrinsic flavors. Fortunately, in the last few decades we have seen a decrease in extrinsic "death signaling" to older people, with the growing acknowledgment that it is possible to remain fit and active well into our extended life spans. Still, aging individuals are told by cultural stereotypes, TV, family, doctors and other "experts" that they need to slow down, eat less meat, and for God's sake act their age.

But the intrinsic signals are even worse: "I'm fat. I'm weak. I'm worthless. My joints ache. *And I'm too old to do anything about it.* Where are the Cheetos?"

I believe that intrinsic human apoptosis is a powerful contributor to the Sick Aging Phenotype: a living hell of progressive weakness, obesity, inactivity, shrinking horizons, sexual impotence, decreased expectations, mounting despair, a growing list of expensive drugs, learned helplessness, sickness, and pain. It's being *all over* at sixty…or fifty. It's a life of waiting to die from a skin infection or a broken hip or a blot clot, of needing a stupid little go-cart to get from here to there, of not being able to reach your own ass to wipe it, of narcotizing yourself with alcohol, cigarettes, *American Idol* and Doritos so you don't have to face your own grim existence as a slowly rotting Jabba The Hut.

I see it every day. Some doctors call it "old-itis." A grim joke, I guess, an attempt to dissipate the impact of an obscenity that offends the eye, the mind, and the spirit. This gruesome avatar of aging cries out for compassion and correction.

*Strength training is a macroscopic growth factor,* countersignaling *all* of this horror. It negates the extrinsic form of human apoptotic signaling: Every octogenarian who strides into a gym and trains for strength is a vivid refutation of the stereotype of the frail senior, and a living example of what aging can and should be. More importantly, training blocks the intrinsic form of human apoptotic signaling. It's a way for the Masters Athlete to send a survival signal to the gray goo in his own skull: "I'm still getting stronger. I'm still living. *I'm not done yet.*"

This is not my wishful extrapolation of cellular phenomena to the human sphere. It's a medical fact, supported by study after study. Strength training has been extensively studied in the context of what I call intrinsic human apoptosis, where the data indicates that it fights depression, improves outlook and quality of life, increases independent functioning, and can even retard or reverse cognitive decline.[63]

## Strength Training is the Weapon of Choice Against the Sick Aging Phenotype

We've covered a lot of ground, which I have summarized in Table 5-2. When we evaluate strength training's suitability as a General Exercise Prescription for the aging adult (first tier of the table), as a training program directed at the required performance attributes of the Masters Athlete (second tier), and its specificity for the Sick Aging Phenotype (third tier), we find that it is indispensable for health and performance as we age. No other single approach comes close. Aerobic LSD exercise fails to address a number of fitness attributes, because it is comprised of repeated movements describing a limited range of motion, does not drive improvements in strength and power, and does not span biological energy systems. High-intensity interval training (HIIT), which we examine in detail in Part III, fares better, depending on the movement patterns used, but still falls short in a number of areas.

Strength training is by far the most comprehensive modality available, and must therefore be the dominant component of our exercise prescription. Nevertheless, strength training alone is not entirely sufficient, especially if we accede to conventional wisdom and take a critical view of its ability to address cardiovascular health. (This critical evaluation is reflected in Table 5-2, where I deliberately handicapped strength training and gave the benefit of the doubt to LSD endurance exercise in those areas where the literature was particularly mixed.)

However, when we combine strength training with a conditioning component, we have a comprehensive and powerful training prescription for the Masters Athlete. The question then becomes which of these strength + conditioning combinations we will use: strength + LSD or strength + HIIT. This decision will hinge to a considerable degree on the preferences of the individual. If you love cross-country skiing, biking, running, or some other form of LSD training, then your choice is clear. Performance of a sport or vigorous physical occupation will *usually* provide a suitable conditioning stimulus, both for that activity and for health (Chapter 26). For those who are not active outside of training, or who wish to maximize their physical capacities, the combination of strength training and HIIT offers the most comprehensive and efficient approach.

I want to point out one more thing before we sum up. I told you at the beginning of this very long, very dense chapter (well done, Dear Reader) that the biomedical literature suffers from any number of significant methodological problems. When it comes to exercise in health and disease, a particularly common problem is the ***dosing*** of exercise medicine. When one looks at this literature, one finds that the overwhelming majority of studies utilize "low-dose" resistance training and inappropriate exercise selection (non-structural exercises that do not exert optimal loading stresses on the organism for long-term adaptation). Moreover, this literature is characterized by short training periods. Few studies go beyond 10 weeks and most are far shorter. This means that most studies of exercise medicine are terminated before the patient even has a chance to mount serious increases in muscle mass, because most strength accumulation during the early phases of training is mediated by neuromuscular adaptations and muscle fiber recruitment, not by the addition of muscle mass, which contributes proportionally more later.[64]

In short, most of the literature inadvertently but systematically handicaps resistance training, using exercise medicine that is poorly dosed, poorly administered, poorly programmed, and discontinued far too early.

*And yet,* even with these pervasive shortcomings in the exercise medicine literature, an overwhelming amount of data clearly indicates that resistance training has profound and beneficial impacts on the Sick Aging Phenotype. *How much more effective can we expect it to be when the medicine is prescribed and administered correctly?*

| TIER 1: EXERCISE RX PARAMETERS | STRENGTH | LSD AEROBIC | HIIT | STRENGTH + LSD | STRENGTH + HIIT |
|---|---|---|---|---|---|
| SAFETY | ✓✓✓ | ✓✓✓ | ✓✓✓ | ✓✓✓ | ✓✓✓ |
| DOSING | ✓✓✓ | ✓ | ✓✓ | ✓✓✓ | ✓✓✓ |
| COMPREHENSIVE | ✓✓ | No | No | ✓✓✓ | ✓✓✓ |
| SPECIFIC TO SAP | ✓✓✓ | No | No | ✓✓ | ✓✓✓ |
| SIMPLE AND TIME-EFFICIENT | ✓✓✓ | No | ✓✓✓ | No | ✓✓✓ |

| TIER 2: PERFORMANCE ATTRIBUTES | STRENGTH | LSD AEROBIC | HIIT | STRENGTH + LSD | STRENGTH + HIIT |
|---|---|---|---|---|---|
| Endurance | ✓ | ✓✓✓ | ✓✓ | ✓✓✓ | ✓✓✓ |
| Mobility and Balance | ✓✓✓ | No | ✓ | ✓✓✓ | ✓✓✓ |
| Strength | ✓✓✓ | No | No | ✓✓✓ | ✓✓✓ |
| Power | ✓✓✓ | No | ✓ | ✓✓✓ | ✓✓✓ |
| Body Composition | ✓✓ | ✓✓ | ✓✓ | ✓✓✓ | ✓✓✓ |

| TIER 3: SICK AGING PHENOTYPE | STRENGTH | LSD AEROBIC | HIIT | STRENGTH + LSD | STRENGTH + HIIT |
|---|---|---|---|---|---|
| Physical inactivity and positive energy balance | ✓✓✓ | ✓✓✓ | ✓✓✓ | ✓✓✓ | ✓✓✓ |
| Obesity and visceral fat | ✓✓ | ✓✓✓ | ✓✓✓ | ✓✓✓ | ✓✓✓ |
| Insulin Resistance | ✓✓ | ✓✓✓ | ✓✓✓ | ✓✓✓ | ✓✓✓ |
| Cardiovascular Disease | ✓ | ✓✓✓ | ✓✓✓ | ✓✓✓ | ✓✓✓ |
| Sarcopenia | ✓✓✓ | No | ✓ | ✓✓ | ✓✓✓ |
| Osteopenia | ✓✓✓ | ✓ | No | ✓✓ | ✓✓✓ |
| Weakness and Frailty | ✓✓✓ | No | ✓ | ✓✓✓ | ✓✓✓ |

| SUMMARY: EXERCISE RX SUITABILITY | STRENGTH | LSD AEROBIC | HIIT | STRENGTH + LSD | STRENGTH + HIIT |
|---|---|---|---|---|---|
| A complete, efficient, and effective Exercise Rx for the Master's Athlete? | YES | NO | NO | NO | YES |

***Table 5-2.*** Summary of the suitability of various exercise modalities and their combinations as exercise prescriptions and training programs for the Masters Athlete. The assignment of scores for each category was made by the author in an entirely implicit fashion, based on his evaluation of the literature, his interpretation of the preponderance of the available evidence as expounded in the foregoing text, and his own experiences and biases as an athlete, coach, and rapidly aging dude. Readers are invited to examine the relevant literature on all the parameters tabulated here and to draw their own conclusions.

## Your Physiological 401k

When you're sixty or seventy, you're *not* going to need to be able to run 20 miles, or 10, or even 3. You're going to need muscle, bone, strength, power, mobility, balance, and yes, some endurance. But will they be there for you? When you enter your golden years (if you haven't already) will you be strong, resilient, supple, healthy, functional, and useful?

If you're reading this book and have made it this far, my guess would be that you're mature, intelligent, probably well-educated, of middling socioeconomic status or higher and, well, a bit of a nerd. Like most people in this demographic, you probably obsess over your 401k or other retirement plan. How much money will you need in retirement? Are you socking away enough to have a secure nest egg in good times and bad? Is that nest egg growing at a healthy rate? Are your investments diversified?

I would suggest that your physical being is *at least* as important a part of your retirement plans as your Vanguard account or your pension plan, because otherwise you risk a future in which you retire as an affluent physical wreck, if you make it that far. When you think about saving for retirement, you can't just think about money. You need to think about muscle, bone, tendon, power, strength, mobility, and function.

You need to make regular, rational deposits into your physiological 401k. You need to bank tissue for retirement. Resistance training for strength, more than any other exercise modality, allows you to offset the inexorable decline of musculoskeletal tissue with aging, and all the suffering that goes along with it.

Strength training is a powerful medicine for the prevention and treatment of the Sick Aging Phenotype. Strength training is ***safe***. It has a ***wide therapeutic window*** and can be applied in a broad range of ***doses***. It is ***comprehensive***, hitting all the General Fitness Attributes and energy systems. And as we have just seen it is ***specific and effective***, combating all the components of the Sick Aging Phenotype. So it should come as no surprise that inclusion of strength training in an exercise program is endorsed by the American Heart Association,[65] the American College of Sports Medicine,[66] and the American Diabetes Association.[67]

All that's needed now is the prescription itself. How, *exactly*, is our strength training medicine to be administered, dosed, and programmed? This leads us to the last of our criteria: ***simplicity and efficiency***. This requirement is critical whether we look at exercise from the perspective of a prescription or a training program. The training program of an athlete must develop the General Fitness Attributes (that is its function), but it must also prepare and free up the athlete for play and practice without injuring him or taking up too much valuable practice time. So, too, must the Master's exercise prescription prepare him, safely and efficiently, for the Game of Life. We don't live to train. We train to live.

As we shall see in the next chapter, this is why all savvy athletes end up in the same place: a gym equipped for serious barbell training.

# 6

# Simplicity and Efficiency: From Black Iron to Grey Steel

The biology of aging, the Sick Aging Phenotype, and the effect of various exercise interventions on the physiology of aging populations indicate that strength training is the correct focus of a General Exercise Prescription for the Masters Athlete. It remains to determine precisely how this type of exercise medicine is to be formulated and administered for maximal benefit and safety. Barbells optimize the suitability of strength training for older adults. Barbells maximize muscle recruitment and range of motion, permit training within the widest therapeutic window, demand concomitant training for balance, load the axial skeleton, and train the broadest range of fitness attributes with the least number of exercises and a minimum of complexity and training time.

## Simplicity and Efficiency

In the previous chapters, I have laid out the case that when an exercise *prescription* for aging adults takes on the form of a training *program* for Masters Athletes, it conforms beautifully to our criteria. Resistance training for strength is safe, can be dosed precisely over a broad range, encompasses the majority of physical performance attributes, and spans all three energy systems. And as we saw in the last chapter, a strength and conditioning program specifically addresses the Sick Aging Phenotype, combating insulin resistance, cardiovascular disease, sarcopenia, osteopenia, loss of mobility and function, frailty, depression, and the whole sick spiral of human apoptosis.

Strength training has long been thought of as the domain of burly young men. We have seen that it is a powerful tonic for the depredations of aging. A 22-year-old Gym Bro can certainly train harder than a 66-year old grandmother, and he might even look better with his shirt off. But Grandma *needs* to train in a way that Gym Bro cannot begin to fathom. Gym Bro is pumping iron to look good on the beach at Ft. Lauderdale. Grandma is engaged in an existential death match, fighting to hang on to tissue, mobility, function, independence, and years of quality living.

It remains for us to finally determine exactly how we will prescribe, deliver, dose, and exploit our exercise medicine. We now turn to the last criterion of our prescription:

5. **Our exercise medicine should be as simple and efficient as possible.**

There's no shortage of complicated exercise "programs" out there. In recent years, the concept of "muscle confusion" (a principle not employed by elite athletes, who know better) has made training complexity – or, rather, chaos – into a virtue. Programs like P90X and Crossfit, not to mention most personal trainers, are keen to keep changing things up from session to session, so that every workout is different, new, and exciting. This keeps muscles "confused" (whatever that means – I'm trained in physiology and I sure as hell don't know). It keeps the program "fresh" and "interesting," and most importantly it keeps the client coming back. After all, when the workouts change constantly, the "program" must be so complex as to be beyond the ken of the trainee. Only the trainer, with his deep understanding of the principles of muscle confusion, extended domains, and facilitated neuromuscular quantum interdimensional myosin phase activation (or whatever) has the competence to decide what unique combination of stability board, dumbbell, battling rope, and kettlebell exercises the client must do today to get sweaty, sore, pumped, and not bored. When this guy's finished with you, you're going to *know* you got your money's worth.

This is all very silly. If your doctor changed your blood pressure or diabetes prescription three times a week, wouldn't you begin to suspect that something just wasn't quite right? I should hope so. So why is it that when our personal trainers or the oh-so-buff guys on the training DVD shuffle exercises around like so many Tarot cards, we're somehow willing to believe they have anything like an exercise prescription with long-term goals in mind?

Thinking of *exercise as a medicine* clarifies the picture dramatically. When we think of exercise as a medicine prescribed to achieve long-term goals, we begin to see that such "programs" aren't exercise medicine at all. They're just random admonitions to thrash about.

This is not to say that random thrashing about isn't better than sitting on your ass with a remote in one hand and a bag of chips in the other. We know that such regular, unprogrammed thrashabouts can improve body composition and aerobic fitness.[1] Exercise is *usually* better than no exercise (unless the thrashabout gets you hurt). But we decided several chapters back that the Masters Athlete needs more than just a prescription to "get some exercise." He needs rational, effective *training*, directed at long-term goals, to prepare him for the arena of the most brutal sport of all.

More to the point, he needs to get his training done in the most effective, efficient, and simple way possible, so that he can actually get into the arena and *play*. Grandkids wait for no program. We don't live to take medicine. We take medicine to help us live. So it is with training. Training is not the game; it *prepares* us for the game. The Athlete of Aging doesn't live to train, he trains to live.

Now, just as training complexity can be taken to an extreme (a different workout for every day of the year!) simplification can also get out of hand. No single exercise or type of exercise will ever fill our training prescription. We can see this simple truth at work with the example of running, which many people still see as the exercise *par excellence*. Running, like other LSD aerobic exercises, clearly decreases bodyfat, increases endurance, modifies cardiovascular risk factors, and has a beneficial impact on metabolic parameters, including insulin resistance. But it doesn't increase muscle mass, it has relatively minor effects on axial skeletal bone mineral density, it does not exploit or train the full musculoskeletal range of motion, and it doesn't build strength or power.

Moreover, once the runner has trained for a relatively short period of time, running does not deliver the exercise intensity needed to drive *progressive* improvements in performance or health. Beyond a certain intensity (a certain percentage of the athlete's $VO_2$max), the only dosing parameter practically available to the LSD runner is to increase volume, that is, the length and frequency of runs. To be clear, running can be a salutary exercise, but it just doesn't cover all the bases for a Masters Athlete. It's a single movement pattern with a small range of motion, practiced at low intensity, almost entirely within a single energy system. Running four miles three times a week is a very simple exercise prescription, and far, *far* healthier than being sedentary. It is also completely inadequate to the demands of the General Exercise Prescription.

So we want our training program to be as simple as possible. But no simpler.

These considerations confront us with a fairly obvious set of parameters. We can unpack the last of our criteria as follows:

5. **Our exercise medicine should be as simple and efficient as possible.**

    a. The number of exercises should be kept to a minimum.

    b. The complexity of programming (the formula for progress in the program) should be kept to a minimum.

    c. The program should permit significant progress with 2–3 days/week of training, and total weekly training time should be kept to a minimum.

    d. Despite its simplicity, the program should be comprehensive with regard to the musculoskeletal and energy systems, and should apply training stresses sufficient to drive progressive, long-term improvements in the maximal number of fitness attributes (strength, power, endurance, mobility, balance, and body composition).

We have seen that strength training offers us a comprehensive training stimulus that drives improvement in virtually all performance attributes, even endurance. When we combine strength training with focused and efficient conditioning in a rational program, we can cover all the bases, but only if we select the correct exercises.

## Strength Training Modalities

As discussed in Chapter 4, we have a vast array of resistance exercise options open to us, most of which are not to be taken seriously. Rubber bands, silly little spring-loaded dumbbells you shake until your arms get sore, and that ridiculous doodad you squeeze open and shut with your thighs...anything advertised on TV that arrives in a box and weighs less than several hundred pounds will not get you stronger. These contraptions aren't for strength training. They're gadgets, gizmos, gimmicks, and rip-offs. As a great man once said, there's one born every minute. We shall speak no more of these things.

***Bodyweight training*** utilizes one's own mass as the "load" to be lifted. Depending on the movements prescribed, it can be safe, and it will produce improvements in strength, up to a point. That point is sharply delimited, as you might imagine, by the weight of the individual. Beyond this point, only volume can be manipulated, not intensity. The dosing range for this modality is far too constrained to be suitable as a formulation for our exercise prescription.

What's left? Free weights and machines.

***Machine systems*** were popularized by Arthur Jones in the 70s. Over the ensuing decades, they transformed the fitness industry, and even people who should have known better jumped on the bandwagon. A new training paradigm emerged: jumping from one machine to the next to combine strength training with aerobic conditioning. This ***circuit training*** with Nautilus machines and other products became the industry standard. Machines don't require special skills to use or teach or coach, they're non-threatening, and they appeal to the innate and often unreasoning technophilia of human primates. And with a machine for just about every single muscle in the body, this technology seems to offer a comprehensive approach to training. On one machine, you can flex your elbow against a load and work your biceps. On the next, you can extend your knees under a load and work your quads. Across the room you can flex your abs against resistance, and then go blast your hamstrings on the leg curl machine. Let there be no doubt: such machine-based exercises will, if programmed correctly, improve strength over the range of the movement trained by the machine, add mass to the selected muscles, and improve the ability of the tissue to dispose of glucose and fat and respond to insulin stimulation. That's all good.

So what's wrong with machines? Actually, a great deal, but we're going to focus on just a few issues relevant to our purposes. To that end, I'm going to tell you a story.

Not long ago, I was away from home attending a research conference. When our work was done for the day I got a one-time pass at a national franchise gym ("Something Fitness" or "Fitness Something") near the hotel. During my workout, I observed a gentleman in his mid-fifties who had procured the services of a personal trainer. This corpulent fellow had all the clinical features of a recalcitrant couch potato who had, to his credit, finally decided his body had declined quite far enough. Phat Phil in an alternate reality, as it were. His trainer was a perky and oh-so-supportive young lady with 8% bodyfat in a very fetching black leotard, with the inevitable clipboard perched on her hip. She was employing a classic machine circuit approach, driving Phil to work in the muscular endurance range.

First, she put him on the pectoral fly machine. He *sat down*, settled in, and pulled his straight arms together in front of him against a resistance, working those all-important pecs. Twenty reps! With only enough rest time to steal a swig of bottled Norwegian spring water, Phil was then herded onto the leg extension machine. He *sat down*, put his shins under the padded armatures, and straightened his legs out against resistance, slamming the old quads. Twenty reps! *Good job*, chirped his adorable trainer. But no rest for the weary: She then ordered Phil over to the leg curl machine. He *lay down on his belly*, put his heels under the padded bar, and flexed his knees against resistance to bring his ankles up to his butt. Toning up those hamstrings. Twenty reps!

Phil was beginning to look a little gray by now, but clearly this young lady could have asked him to walk naked over hot coals with a pair of dumbbells in his hands and gasoline on his toes and he would have dutifully complied. On to the ab machine, where Phil again *sat down*, strapped in, and flexed at the waist against resistance. Move over, Leonidas. Phil's gettin' a washboard belly. Twenty reps!

No rest: next he *sat down* in the curl machine (biceps!) then he *sat down* in the shoulder press machine (delts!) and then he did *seated* lat pulls (back!). Another quick swig from the *fjord*, and it was back to the pectoral fly machine for another circuit.

Round and round Phil went with his beautiful young *Dominatrix*, giving his all to satisfy her, getting sweaty and exhausted, going nowhere fast.

It was like...*Love*.

Phil got the workout of his life that night. When he was done, he was dripping, trembling, pale, excited, and by all appearances just this side of needing a bypass. There could be no doubt in Phil's mind that he'd had his money's worth, and more. But I knew he was wasting both his money and his time. First of all, Phil's trainer was working him in the twenty-rep range. This is excellent for muscular endurance, but a lousy programming approach for strength. So even if Phil weren't too crippled with soreness to come back for another fling with his trainer later in the week, this program wouldn't produce *long-term increases* in strength in the muscles being worked. It would increase the endurance of the muscles, and Phil's overall endurance. That's not a bad thing, but it's not what Phil needs to combat his aging phenotype.

Even if Phil's trainer had worked him in the strength-rep range for these exercises, they would have both missed the boat, because this approach focuses on muscles and muscle groups. We shouldn't be too hard on this young lady. This focus reflects how she was programmed at the Personal Trainer Factory. And her clients are programmed by the culture and the media to crave firm, "toned," attractive muscles. They want to beef up their arms, calves, buttocks, biceps, or whatever. The machine-based approach to resistance training is perfectly suited to this muscle-centric, cosmetic, superficial view of fitness: a machine for every muscle.

We can get an idea of just how completely bankrupt this muscle-centric view is if we think of Phil not as an aging adult, but as a Masters Athlete who needs to train for the merciless game of getting older. What does Phil need as an athlete? He needs to function in the physical arena of his daily life. He would like to be able to push a lawn mower, pick a box up off the floor, jump out of the path of a wayward driver, lift his daughter up onto his shoulders, support his wife when they Tango, and stand up off the toilet without hurting himself. Phil needs to be able to *move* over his entire natural range of motion – confidently, smoothly, powerfully, safely.

In the Arena of Life, Phil does *not* need to lie on his belly and flex his hamstrings against resistance, or do an isolated knee extension, or (for heaven's sake!) a pectoral fly. No normal human being *ever* performs these movements against a significant resistance outside a gym. They are not in the repertoire of normal human movement patterns. People at home, at work and at play *do not do hamstring curls.*

What aging adults do in the Arena of Life is *sit down, stand up, push things away, pull things in, lift stuff up off the floor, and heave stuff over their heads.* These simple, natural movement patterns are the building blocks of our lives as physical beings, and taken together they encompass the functional range of motion of the human organism.

The problem with machines is not that they don't strengthen muscles. The problem with machines is that they *strengthen muscles instead of movements.*

Individual muscles, no matter how big, beautiful, or "ripped," are absolutely useless outside a normal human movement pattern. In fact, training a muscle in isolation on a machine, outside its normal movement patterns, is liable to unbalance and distort those patterns, and actually increase the potential for those patterns to become dysfunctional or even injurious. Big strong pecs combined with weak shoulder or back muscles unbalance the forces across the shoulder and make the movement patterns involving the shoulder *less* functional. Or consider the big-chested, chicken-legged Gym Bro, for whom every day is upper body day. His arms and chest are huge, but he's liable to injure himself picking up a heavy box. He's devoted his life to training the muscles he can see in the mirror with his shirt off, *but he's never trained the basic movement pattern of lifting an object off the floor.*

The inappropriateness of machine-based training for the Masters Athlete comes into even sharper relief when we realize that Phil performed his entire circuit either sitting or laying down. The only time I saw the poor bastard stand up was to follow his trainer's perky little butt to the next station. None of this work encompassed a full human movement pattern, and none of it applied a training stress to his axial skeleton, his gait, his balance, or his total body strength.

## Training Movement Patterns with Barbells

When we focus on natural human movement patterns instead of individual muscles, joints, or muscle groups, an entire new perspective on training opens up to us. We no longer have to wonder whether we're training the correct muscles in the correct way to the correct, balanced level of strength, because instead of training the muscles, we're training *the movement that uses the muscles,* and all the other tissues and systems that support the movement. Each muscle, bone, joint, tendon, ligament, and nerve will contribute its natural and correct share of work or support to the movement, because we are using all of these components to do what nature designed them to do.

The advantages of focusing on movements instead of muscles goes much deeper. There are about 640 muscles in the human body. But just a few basic movement patterns capture input from the vast majority of this muscle mass. If we take the basic patterns of squatting down and standing up, pushing something away, lifting something overhead, and lifting something heavy off the floor, we will strengthen and condition the entire musculoskeletal system, and make all of those movements stronger throughout the natural range of motion, increasing both strength *and* mobility. Loading the movement will also demand improvements in proprioception and balance, something that sitting down in the leg press machine can never do.

In short, when we focus our resistance training on movement patterns instead of muscles, we open up the opportunity to train the entire musculoskeletal system with just a few exercises in a way that improves strength, mobility, and balance, while exploiting the potential of resistance training to drive adaptation across the entire energy spectrum, enhance insulin sensitivity, reverse the atrophy of muscle and bone, and combat the Sick Aging Phenotype. Focusing on *movements* instead of *muscles* gets us one step closer to our exercise prescription.

Only one form of strength training allows us to do this: *Barbells*.

Unlike machines, barbells are not designed to train isolated muscles or muscle groups. The primitive, humble, venerable barbell is the best technology yet developed for the safe, ergonomic loading of natural human movement patterns. With a barbell, we can apply a load to any of the major movement patterns, and thereby *train* those movements. Exercises with barbells call for the trainee to perform each exercise according to his own anatomical dimensions (***anthropometry***), rather than forcing the trainee to conform to the geometry of a machine. Barbell exercises demand balance and the contribution of all the muscles of the trunk and back, not just the extremities, to stabilize and support the load.

Finally, barbells can be loaded with as little or as much weight as we like. Very weak trainees can start out performing the movements with bars weighing as little as a few pounds, or even a broomstick. Barbells permit us to dose exercise medicine in precise increments according to the needs of each trainee. Because of this unparalleled range of dosing and the whole-body nature of the exercises, a precise training stress can be delivered to the Masters Athlete in a manner that drives steady increases in strength in just two or three sessions a week. Barbell training offers the Master a training system that is safe, doseable, comprehensive, simple, efficient, and effective against the Sick Aging Phenotype.

Such is the program we will describe in Parts II and III: Four simple exercises performed over the course of a 2- or 3-day/week program, combined if necessary with intense conditioning drills, will drive profound and dramatic improvements in strength, power, endurance, mobility, balance, body composition, and health.

The ***squat*** is the cornerstone of this program. In this exercise, you simply squat down and stand up again. Loading this normal human movement pattern recruits a *vast* volume of muscle tissue over a complete range of motion, forcing major improvements in overall strength, muscle mass, joint integrity, back strength, conditioning, and overall athleticism.

The ***deadlift*** is nothing more than lifting a heavy barbell off the floor – another fundamental movement pattern. It is complementary to the squat and allows trainees to lift more weight than any other exercise, more weight than they ever thought possible. It strengthens the back, legs, trunk, hips, shoulders, and grip. It is particularly accessible to older trainees with limitations in their range of motion, and it produces transformative changes in confidence, self-image, and outlook. Something about knowing you can bend over and pick up something damn heavy just makes us feel more alive.

The ***press*** trains the fundamental movement pattern of lifting something overhead. But it's far more than an arm and shoulder exercise. Because it is performed standing, it demands balance, and recruits muscle mass from the entire body, including the legs, thighs, hips, back, abdomen, and chest.

The ***bench press*** trains the basic human movement pattern of pushing something away from you. It is complementary to the overhead press and promotes massive increases in upper body strength.

Although they are not essential to our exercise prescription, the ***Olympic lift variants***, the ***power clean*** and the ***power snatch***, may be used by a few select Masters with the necessary aptitude and desire.

After the initial stage of training, which is devoted entirely to the rapid accumulation of strength, a conditioning component will be added. This may simply be the athlete's sport of choice:

tennis, swimming, biking, hiking, martial arts, etc. But the General Exercise Prescription fills this requirement through the addition of a high-intensity interval conditioning (HIIT) component, which can be pursued using a number of modalities, including a stationary bike, kettlebells, rowers, or sleds (our preferred option). Like resistance training with barbells, HIIT can be dosed precisely according to the needs of the athlete, allowing safe, steady progress. HIIT optimizes anaerobic and aerobic conditioning, endurance, cardiovascular fitness, and body composition, while being far more time-efficient and comprehensive than LSD training. We will discuss this approach to conditioning in Chapter 26.

There it is at last: an exercise prescription for the aging adult.

## Conclusions: Grey Steel from Black Iron

We've come a long way. We began with an unflinching look at the misery of the Sick Aging Phenotype. This hellish and pervasive form of aging is driven not just by the unavoidable vagaries of time and biology, but also by an excessive positive energy balance (too many calories), a sedentary existence (not enough exercise), sarcopenia, and insulin resistance. The Sick Aging Phenotype progresses into metabolic syndrome: hypertension, worsening insulin resistance, truncal and visceral obesity, abnormal serum lipid profiles, and a global inflammatory state. The Sick Aging Phenotype comes to full bloom with Type 2 diabetes, cardiovascular disease, severe hypertension, some degree of heart failure, brittle bones, threadbare muscles, a shopping bag full of prescription medicines, exercise intolerance, frailty, and loss of function. The phenotype comes to lethal harvest with stroke, heart attack, congestive heart failure, hip fracture, vertebral collapse, end-stage kidney disease, retinal hemorrhage or degeneration, toxic polypharmacy, dementia, depression, despair, and loss of independence. A Sick Death Phenotype is not far behind.

This is unacceptable. And we don't *have* to accept it, because, as we saw in Chapter 2, exercise medicine, the most powerful medicine in the world, combats the Sick Aging Phenotype in a way that no standard medical therapy can even approach. We seized on this lifeline, and determined to formulate an exercise prescription for the aging adult that was safe, could be dosed precisely according to the needs of the individual and in a way that permitted ongoing improvements, was comprehensive and integrated, specifically and effectively addressed the components of the Sick Aging Phenotype, and was as simple and efficient as possible.

***Safety*** was our first consideration, and led us to narrow our field of candidate exercises to repeated motor activities with predictable movement patterns describing the normal range of motion, with a minimum potential for unexpected forces or trauma. This ruled out scuba diving, combat judo, *parkour*, tennis, pole-vaulting, and any number of other activities that, fun and life-affirming though they may be, are nevertheless unsuitable as a General Exercise Prescription.

The consideration of ***therapeutic window*** narrowed the field further, and introduced us to the concept of training variables, such as intensity, volume, recovery, frequency, etc. In fact, it led us to the very concept of *training* itself: a long-term program manipulating training variables to achieve improvements in General Fitness Attributes. This discussion brought us to the distinction between *training* and *practice*, and it helped us to identify resistance training for strength as a prime candidate to be the keystone of our exercise prescription. Most importantly, this phase of our investigation transformed our pursuit of an exercise prescription for the aging adult into the formulation of a training program for the Masters Athlete.

When we advanced this search to the criterion of a program that was ***comprehensive*** and integrated, we found that training for strength put us deep in the anaerobic energy system. Unlike LSD training in the aerobic range, this kind of training promotes adaptation across the biological energy spectrum, applying training stress to the phosphagen, glycolytic, *and* mitochondrial energy regimes, all while improving strength, power, and body composition. We saw how this sort of training – repeated bursts of effort requiring high power outputs – more closely matched the demands we face in the Arena of Life than the interminable ordeals of LSD aerobic training. People don't need to run twenty miles in their daily lives. They need to stand up, push, pull, lift, and leap.

With strength training now a prime candidate for the foundation of our exercise prescription, we investigated whether or not such a program could prepare us to compete against our archrival. In other words, we wanted our training to ***specifically and effectively attack the Sick Aging Phenotype***. This led us to a mountain of evidence, a rapidly-growing body of biomedical data indicating the power of strength training to improve insulin sensitivity, decrease abdominal and visceral fat, improve glucose regulation, fight the metabolic syndrome, improve cardiovascular fitness and health, restore muscle mass, improve bone mineral density in the axial skeleton, decrease inflammation, fight depression, maintain function and independence, and improve quality of life. We found that most of these benefits were magnified when strength training was combined with some sort of metabolic conditioning.

Finally, in the present chapter, we concluded our investigation by considering the last of our criteria: a training program that was ***simple and efficient***. A program consisting of just a few barbell exercises, combined with some limited conditioning work, offers the most powerful and direct approach. Instead of training individual muscles or muscle groups with elaborate machines, we can simply apply training loads to a small but complete repertoire of normal human movement patterns that we all use in our daily lives, increasing total body strength and power while reaping all the other health benefits of resistance training with a minimum of time and fuss.

I have laid out this case as clearly and explicitly as my poor abilities will permit, and perhaps I have persuaded you that a barbell-based strength and conditioning program is an ideal exercise prescription for the Masters Athlete. Is there another approach, one that is just as good or even better?

There certainly *could* be, but if there is I haven't found it.

It's not for lack of looking. Like many of you, I've been searching for the best approach to fitness for my entire life, and I've tried it all. In recent years, my search has become increasingly systematic, evidence-based, focused…and urgent. You see, I am a physician, and a physiologist, but most importantly, *I am a Masters Athlete*. The material in the last six chapters isn't just a nerdish or professional abstraction to me. It's *personal*. I have no intention of going quietly. I am committed to growing old with as much strength, vigor, and function as I possibly can. I aim to cling to every muscle cell, every bit of bone tissue, every inch of my range of motion, every iota of functional independence…*for dear life*. I have no intention of showing up in some other guy's ER as a dwindling, depressed, defeated lump of weak, wheezing, miserable fat. Anything can happen, of course, and in the end time will defeat me. But I will go down fighting. The Sick Aging Phenotype is not for me.

Perhaps you feel the same way, and perhaps I have persuaded you that *resistance is not futile*. But not every patient is a candidate for therapy. Some patients are too sick, too complex, or too unreliable to be candidates for tricky drugs, organ transplants, or intensive therapy. In the same way, not everybody can take the medicine I'm talking about. That's not warm and fuzzy, that's not nice, and that's not fair. But it is true, nonetheless. The patients who take this medicine don't have to be strong, talented, rich, fit, or even healthy. But they must be compliant, intelligent, patient, hardworking, consistent, courageous and, above all, ferociously committed. At the risk of sounding enigmatic, I would say they don't have to be *athletic* – but they must be *athletes*.

Does that describe you? If so, and if you're willing to put in the limited time and extraordinary effort to play the extreme sport of aging well, Andy Baker and I have some very strong medicine to prescribe for you. We'll take a closer look at your treatment, and training, in Parts II and III.

# Part II: WHAT

## An Introduction to the Exercises

# 7

# Elementary Iron

This chapter gives the reader a brief introduction to the practical requirements of barbell training. Although some Masters will be able to learn adequate performance of the exercises from text and video resources, it is by far preferable to obtain proper instruction from a qualified coach. The necessary equipment, facilities, and gear are minimal, but are absolutely mandatory for safe and effective training. The pros and cons of home gyms and "black iron" gyms are described. Commercial franchise gyms will usually prove to be less than optimal or even completely unsuitable. Observation of a few simple, common-sense rules will make barbell training the exceptionally safe activity it should be. We discuss the role of the Valsalva maneuver, in which the breath is held against a closed glottis to increase thoracic and abdominal pressure and provide support for the axial skeleton, and we affirm the safety and utility of this oft-maligned practice.

## Learning to Lift

In this Part II of this book, we'll introduce the basic exercises used in our barbell prescription. The idea is to familiarize the reader with these exercises, provide a rationale for their inclusion in a training program, illustrate their suitability and safety for aging populations, and give you an *idea* of how they are performed.

*This book is not intended to instruct the reader in the performance of barbell exercises.* Instruction in these exercises is beyond the scope of this work. Moreover, Rippetoe's indispensable and definitive book, *Starting Strength: Basic Barbell Training, 3rd edition,* deals with the proper performance of the barbell movements in superb detail. Any individual who decides to pursue a barbell training program should acquire *Starting Strength* and find a coach, or a least a lifting partner or two.

Although some particularly motivated, intelligent, and talented individuals will be able to make considerable progress in the exercises with an appropriate text, instruction in the barbell lifts, especially for those who are trying to claw their way back to fitness after a long decline, will ideally be under the direction of an experienced and qualified strength and conditioning coach in a suitable facility.

Let's expand on this a bit more. There are three approaches to adequate learning of the barbell exercises.

### Self-instruction with book and video

There are many materials available for instruction in barbell training. Rippetoe's text and videos (available on StartingStrength.com), are far superior to any other instructional materials available *anywhere*. Period. No other text comes close in terms of detail, anatomic and biophysical rational, clarity, and efficiency of approach to *Starting Strength*. The videos are invaluable ancillary tools that will provide the student with examples of the correct movement and common problems and their corrections.

Individuals who elect to engage in self-instruction with the book and videos would be well-advised to read the entire book and view the videos prior to commencing training, and to make liberal use of video recording to check their form and to solicit feedback. This feedback may be readily obtained from Starting Strength coaches on the forum at StartingStrength.com.

Although practicable for some individuals, this option will likely result in a much longer learning curve and slower progress, with false starts and resets for form. For older, weaker, and more detrained individuals, it may be positively unsafe.

### Learn from the book and videos with a dedicated partner(s)

This is much like the first option, except in this case you have a training partner to critique form in real time, to give you somebody to watch and evaluate (this is invaluable), to engage with in regular reviews of the material, to help you change plates, to spot you, to encourage you and share in your victories, and to keep you company. A good training partner is a treasure. Of particular importance for this option is that you and your partner(s) pay careful attention to the ***cues*** noted for every exercise, and listen and look for the cues used in the videos. *Cueing is a critical component in the Starting Strength model,* and trainees ignore it at their peril. This option also benefits from "video coaching."

### Learn from the book and videos and a qualified strength coach

This is *by far* the most desirable option. The approach we recommend is to read the book and watch the videos, and then get qualified coaching (preferably by a certified Starting Strength Coach). This includes all the advantages of the other two while promoting quicker learning of the correct movements, avoidance of form errors during learning that can lead to bad habits (some of which can be extremely difficult to break), and the institution of modifications (stance, grip width, exercise inclusion/exclusion) demanded by the lifter's anthropometry and unique physical circumstances.

## Equipment and Facilities

The physical requirements for barbell training are minimal but they are *requirements*, nevertheless. Without good equipment in a good facility and proper gear and clothing, barbell training simply cannot be done safely or effectively. The good news is that the equipment itself is virtually unbreakable if used properly, and will last a lifetime after an initial minimal investment.

### The gym

Our first consideration must be the gym itself. By ***gym*** we mean a facility with adequate space, equipment, flooring, ventilation, shelter from the elements, and so on. For a single person to train safely and effectively requires *a bare minimum* of about 550 cubic feet of space: 8' x 8' of floor space and 8 or 9 feet of overhead clearance, depending on the individual's height, with a little additional space for plates, equipment, and safe margins. This is the amount of space required to accommodate a decent squat rack and small platform. The facility should ideally be on a slab, and exotic hardwood or marble flooring would be poor choices.

We tell you all this because most commercial gyms, while they may have adequate space for training, lack many of the other requirements for proper performance of barbell exercises. For this and other reasons, we believe that a well-appointed home gym is one of the best investments the Masters Athlete can possibly make, once he has learned the basics of barbell training. If the space is available, an investment of about $3000–$5000 will result in a home facility far superior to what is available in the community. No waiting, no commute, no curl-bros doing ridiculous stunts in the squat rack, no stupid rules, and you can listen to whatever music you like. Please consider it.

This option may not be available or appealing to you, in which case you would be wise to investigate any facility thoroughly and do some comparison shopping before you join. The best option would be an actual "black iron" gym catering to people who are serious about getting strong. These are few and far between, although they are growing in popularity. The very best option would be one of the Starting Strength gyms scattered throughout the country. These facilities offer coaching by certified Starting Strength Coaches in a facility with approved space and equipment.

Some older athletes may find black iron gyms intimidating at first, especially if their experience with "gyms" has been limited to hotel exercise closets and Planet Fitness. Serious strength gyms are usually located in warehouses or other light industrial properties, are less antiseptic in appearance, more crowded, full of chalk- and rust-covered equipment instead of gleaming white machines, occupied by bigger, earthier creatures, and *loud*. Try to look past all that. The rates are probably competitive with the shiny-but-useless commercial franchise gyms in your area, the equipment is *far* more likely to be exactly what you need, the atmosphere is more conducive to the kind of work you'll be doing, and most of the inhabitants will turn out to be gentle giants who *love* to help others, including you, get stronger.

The music is just the music. You'll get used to it.

If such a facility is available to you, we strongly urge you to consider membership. It is a decision you'll likely be glad you made.

If, on the other hand, your options are limited to commercial franchise facilities, then comparison shopping becomes even more critical. Cost considerations aside, you will want to evaluate such facilities against the following checklist:

1. **Is the facility reputable?** Talk to current and former members, investigate via Angie's List, your local chamber of commerce, and other resources.

2. **Is there at least one squat rack?** If not, you're done. A gym without a squat rack is not a gym. No squat racks, no squattage. No squattage, no training. *Period.* Two squat racks would be better. Three even more so. This is because squat racks will often be occupied by people doing ridiculous things like curls, or rows, or something bizarre that they just made up. This can sometimes be entertaining, but watching silly people perform antics in the squat rack is not the best use of your training time. At best, when it's time to squat you may find the single squat rack occupied by a bunch of bros doing squats incorrectly. And later, when *you're* doing squats, they'll be happy to give you uninformed and unsolicited advice about how you're doing it wrong, or how your method of performing squats will disable, disfigure, or kill you.

3. **Is there at least one pressing bench?** If not, you're done. This is not a gym.

4. **Does the facility have polygonal plates?** Red flag. Whoever came up with this idea needs to be taken out back and maimed with his own creation. The *polygonal plate* is an invention akin to the *salad shooter*, *fenestrated condom,* or *triangular wheel.* The ostensible purpose is to prevent plates from rolling around. The *real* purpose is to discourage pulls from the floor (deadlifts and cleans), which are loud, require appropriate flooring, encourage the use of chalk, and are disturbing to the *decent*

people who are trying to work out on the Stairmasters and yoga mats while listening to Bon Jovi blaring from the speakers. From the perspective of the management of a commercial gym franchise, deadlifts and other pulls from the floor are *evil.* Hence the polygonal plates. It is in fact possible to do deadlifts in a facility with polygonal plates, if you can ignore the glowering looks of disapproval and disbelief from the management and other patrons, and if you are willing to endure the endless devastation to your shins from the bar bumping back into your legs.

5. **Are they, in fact, playing Bon Jovi?** Red flag. You can still join, but it will *suck*.

6. **Does the facility forbid the use of chalk?** Another red flag. Chalk is essential for proper and safe performance of the barbell lifts. It ensures a positive grip on the bar and controls callus formation. A gym that forbids the use of chalk isn't serious about helping its clients get stronger. If you have no other options, it is possible to keep a little chalk ball in your gym bag and use it surreptitiously, at least until you are caught, convicted and jailed. Smuggling of white powders is, after all, a serious offense in most countries.

7. **Does the facility forbid grunting and sweating**? Seriously. Some places do. In fact, at least one very successful gym franchise marketed itself on the basis of considering such behavior worthy of public reprimand and shaming. Be very afraid.

## The equipment

The minimum equipment needed for lifting is a squat rack or power rack, a pressing bench, a barbell, and a complete set of plates. This ground is covered definitively in *Starting Strength*, so we'll simply emphasize that *barbells are not the place to save on money.* This goes for any gym you join and especially for trainees outfitting their home gyms. Bars range in price from less than a hundred dollars to over a thousand, and here is where the old maxim that you get what you pay for really applies. Any new bar selling for less than about $300 is bound to be a poor investment. Cheap bars are poorly milled, have sloppy tolerances, poor elastic characteristics, and lousy spin. Worst of all, they can bend or even break, usually at exactly the wrong moment. A good bar is a thing of beauty, growing more attractive as it ages. With proper care it will be there to help your great-grandkids get strong for *their* retirement. Do your homework and invest in a good bar.

## The clothing

You'll need cotton t-shirts, stretchy shorts or pants, long socks, and lifting shoes. That's it, *but you need it all.* Synthetic fabrics are usually poor choices for upper body wear during lifting, because they tend to be slippery and/or stretchy, which can transform a routine set of heavy squats into a real *adventure.* Lower body wear, on the other hand, needs to be flexible and unrestrictive. It shouldn't bind anywhere in the range of motion, from the bottom of a low squat to a fully erect posture. Long socks will prevent the bar from scraping your shins during pulls from the floor.

Proper shoes are absolutely essential. Once you commit to strength training, you have to make an investment in weight lifting shoes. Running shoes, crosstrainers, and other athletic shoes available in stores are unsuitable for lifting weights, because they are designed to minimize impulsive shocks to the foot from repeated ground strikes. The soft soles and squishy heels of such shoes make for an unstable surface while lifting, as if one were trying to hoist a heavy weight while standing on the surface of a warm marshmallow. Weight lifting shoes have rigid, incompressible soles to provide a firm foundation for moving heavy loads. They are generally only available from web-based suppliers.

## The gear

We sometimes get the impression that novice lifters suffer from gear envy. Unlike many other forms of exercise, lifting does not offer the athlete many opportunities to adorn his body with sexy, shiny, cool-looking doodads. Most lifters will wear a belt at some point…and that's about it. Wraps and warmers can help support old or injured joints, and sometimes you'll see a lifter with lifting straps hanging on his wrists. Usually this will be under circumstances that are not appropriate for straps.

**Belts.** If you had to buy one piece of gear, a belt would be it. The belt assists the lifter by optimizing the effect of the Valsalva (see below), and thereby helps to stabilize the spine, which helps you lift more weight, which helps you get stronger. The belt also enhances proprioceptive feedback from the trunk. Most athletes use the belt only on heavy warm-up and work sets, and novice lifters may go for months before needing a belt at all. The best belts are made of leather and are of a constant diameter. That widening you see in the lumbar area of belts hanging in your local sporting goods store adds nothing functional and is a waste of cow. We are partial to single-prong belts for their ease of use. Excellent custom-made belts can be purchased online.

**Wraps and Warmers.** Most of the people you see lifting weights with wraps on their wrists don't need wraps on their wrists. *But they look badass.* If the lifter is struggling with acute or chronic wrist problems, a wrist wrap may very well be indicated.

Knee wraps are frequently worn by powerlifters and other strength athletes at heavy weights. Most beginning and even intermediate Masters don't need them, but a few do. They are not a solution to significant knee pain that interferes with exercise performance. Such discomfort indicates either improper performance of the exercise or a need for medical evaluation, imaging, and therapy. But lifters with chronic knee issues or minor acute knee injuries may benefit from the additional support offered by knee wraps. An excellent video resource on the use of wraps can be found at the Starting Strength website.[1]

Masters often benefit from the use of knee warmers, which are cotton or neoprene sleeves that trap heat and keep the knee toasty and supple. Knee warmers *may* promote favorable changes in the consistency and amount of synovial fluid in the joint. Or they *may not.* The question has not been well-studied. If you have creaky knees, you can try knee warmers and see if they help. Sullivan won't lift without them.

**Straps.** Lifting straps are used to assist the grip for heavy pulls from the floor (deadlifts, cleans, snatches). They are not appropriate for work at low weights, or even moderately heavy weights. Heavy pulls from the floor are excellent for training the grip, and the use of straps obviates this benefit. However, when the weight gets heavy enough for the grip to become limiting, the athlete is confronted by two choices. He can lift the bar with an alternate grip – one hand prone, one hand supine – which is effective but introduces a factor of rotational asymmetry at the shoulder. This is usually well-tolerated, but can lead to technical or musculoskeletal problems in some athletes, particularly those blessed by a wide carrying angle at the elbow. Straps allow one to lift the bar without grip as a limitation, and without an asymmetrical grip. Some athletes with significant arthritis in their hands or wrists may require straps for deadlifts even at low weight, but the vast majority will not require this piece of gear until they are at least several months into their training.

**Gloves.** Gloves are not used in barbell training. They do not provide a more secure grip – that's what training chalk is for. Gloves do not permit the athlete to lift more weight, they do not promote proper execution of the exercises, and they do not enhance the safety of barbell training. Indeed, by introducing an unnecessary extrinsic factor (the glove itself) which may slip, rupture or otherwise fail under loading, they make barbell training *less* safe. You don't need them. If you've already bought a pair, just leave them in a corner of the gym with a sign saying "Free to Good Home." Somebody will think they're cute and adopt them, we promise.

**The Log Book.** This is the most important thing in your gym bag, with the possible exception of your shoes. Because the Master's athlete is engaged in *training*, rather than *exercise*, and because training entails a *program* with long-term goals, complete and accurate record-keeping is essential. Many athletes keep training logs online, or use apps on their mobile devices to track workouts. That's fine, but a written record remains essential. Devices fail and databases get hacked. A simple composition book, available at most office supply shops or drugstores for a couple of bucks, will serve for several years, and allow athlete and coach to monitor progress, diagnose problems, and make intelligent decisions about programming. Record-keeping is described in detail in Chapter 17.

## Barbell Training Safety

As we saw in Chapter 2, barbell training is just about the safest form of physical exercise available. But human beings can screw up anything, and it is in fact possible to injure, maim, disfigure or kill yourself and others in the weight room if you don't pay attention to a few simple safety principles.

It goes without saying that lifting weights while intoxicated with drugs and alcohol is not a bright idea. Seriously: *You should not drop acid and lift.* We trust we need not belabor this point.

Athletes won't get injured by overloading if they stick to their program, don't get greedy, and don't try to show off by lifting more weight than they are trained to handle. Athletes must warm up with light weight, always starting with the empty bar (except for deadlifts) before progressing to heavier loads or performing the exercises at the weights prescribed for that day. Increases in weight over time must always be judicious, and are guided by the *program*, not by the athlete's exuberance or ego.

In general, lifting by yourself is not ideal, especially for novice lifters. We leave enumeration of the *many* reasons why this is so as a stimulating thought-exercise for the reader. That being said, it is true that lifting alone is sometimes unavoidable. In these circumstances, squats and bench presses should be performed in a power rack with ***safety pins*** set to the appropriate height.

When performed outside the power rack, very heavy bench presses and squats require competent ***spotters*** – individuals who are ready and able to *assist* the athlete in returning a failed rep safely to the rack. Deadlifts and overhead presses *do not* require spotters, and any attempt to recruit spotters for these exercises is likely to lead to misadventure.

Barbells are secured at the appropriate height on a power rack using ***hooks***. Athletes must never attempt to deliver the barbell directly to the hooks when returning the bar to the rack. The bar is first delivered to the metal ***uprights*** and then allowed to slide down into the hooks. Aiming for the hooks instead of the uprights will inevitably lead to a miss one day, with unfortunate results.

Of all the exercises performed in the weight room, the bench press is without a doubt the most deadly. The bench press *should* be safe, but there is just *something* about this exercise that compels people (especially young men) to go fantastically stupid when they lay on their back to lift. We shall have more to say about bench press safety in the bench chapter. But we'll take this opportunity to emphasize that the bench should *never* be performed alone outside the power rack, it should *never* incorporate a thumbless grip, it should *never* be performed with collars on the bar, and the elbows must *always* be locked while the bar is moving horizontally (i.e., anytime the bar is moving over the face, on the way to or from the hooks).

Bars, plates, and other equipment must not be allowed to clutter the working area of the gym. It is common practice to leave bars, plates, collars, belts, and wraps adrift, on the rationale they will be needed again during the workout. That may be so, but until they *are* needed again they are subject to damage. More to the point, they constitute trip hazards in an environment full of hard surfaces and heavy moving objects. When you're done with a piece of equipment, or when you pull a plate off the bar, *put it back where it belongs, now*, or someday you'll be sorry.

For more on barbell safety, we direct the reader to the very thorough and very poignant article penned by our colleagues Matt Reynolds and William McNeely, available at StartingStrength.com.[2]

## Special Topic: The Valsalva

The ***Valsalva maneuver*** is one in which the breath is held forcefully against a closed glottis. Named after the 18th century Italian physician and physiologist Antonio Maria Valsalva, this maneuver is simply the common, everyday procedure that humans use to "bear down" against a heavy resistance: pushing a car, lifting a keg, turning a stiff crank, or giving birth to a big, fat, screaming baby. It is a natural and instinctive component of our response to loading.

It is also, to hear some people tell it, universally lethal when used as an adjunct to lifting weights. The reasoning goes like this: lifting weights causes an *acute* rise in blood pressure, whether you hold your breath or not. (As we have seen, lifting weights does not cause a long-term increase in blood pressure). When we hold our breath while lifting, our blood pressure goes up even more.

*All of this is true.* Lifting weights while holding your breath ("under Valsalva") does in fact briefly drive up your blood pressure. And that's bad, we're told, because it will inevitably lead to the rupture of blood vessels in your head, causing you to have a *hemorrhagic stroke*, or bleeding in your brain.

There are three problems with the idea that lifting under Valsalva promotes a particular form of hemorrhagic stroke (*subarachnoid hemorrhage*). First of all, it ignores that the vast majority of these *fantastically rare* events occur in those uncommon and unfortunate individuals with pre-existing congenital or acquired vascular lesions – arterial aneurysms or arteriovenous malformations.

The second problem with this idea is that it presents an incomplete model of the biophysics of aneurysmal rupture (Figure 7-1). For an aneurysm to rupture, the *transmural pressure*, the pressure difference across the wall of the aneurysm, must be high enough to breach the integrity of that wall. This transmural pressure is the difference between two factors: the pressure on the inside of the aneurysm, which is increased by lifting *with or without* Valsalva, and the pressure outside of the aneurysm, *which is also increased by Valsalva.* In other words, holding your breath while lifting *increases the pressure on both sides of the artery and actually works to decrease transmural pressure and inhibit rupture.*[3]

The third problem with the idea that lifting under Valsalva is dangerous is the most damning: *It has never been shown to be true in any population, in any study, anywhere, ever.* The available data on subarachnoid hemorrhage shows that such strokes are associated with the entire range of human activity. Yes, it's true: People with aneurysms suffer strokes while exercising. They also blow their O-rings while doing many other things, or nothing at all.

To cite just one example, a case-crossover study by Vlak et al. looked at 250 survivors of intracranial hemorrhage to identify precipitating factors.[4] Eight triggers increased risk for this event: coffee, cola, anger, startling, straining to poop, sexual activity, nose blowing, and vigorous exercise. (This sounds to us like the agenda of a day well-spent.) Valsalva during lifting was associated with a lower risk than during sex, masturbation, anger, and blowing one's nose. Other studies and case series have reported similar results.[5]

The natural history of these uncommon lesions, if they are large enough, is to grow and to finally rupture. Some will rupture while their owners are working out, just by chance. But they were going to rupture anyway.

Still, one might ask, if there's even a tiny risk, why do it?

We hold our breath while lifting weights because it increases the pressure in the thorax and abdomen and thereby helps to support the thoracic and lumbar spine (Figure 7-2). This is not a serious point of contention in the sports science literature, and it is the universal practice of athletes who train for strength. Indeed, the very ubiquity of this practice is the best possible evidence of its safety. Millions of people all over the world perform billions of heavy repetitions under Valsalva *every day.* Yet the incidence of stroke in these populations is so vanishingly small, so indistinguishable from statistical noise, that opponents of the practice must resort to inappropriate and misleading manipulation of incomplete data from large electronic databases to make their case.[6]

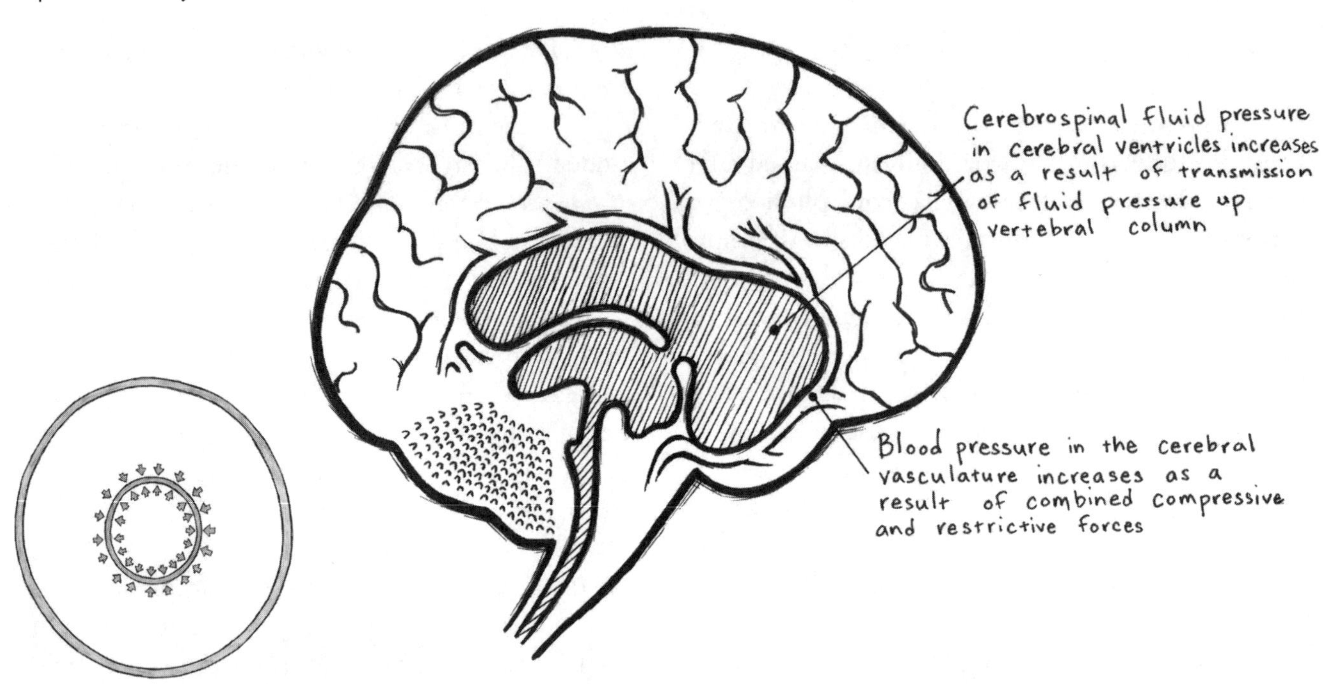


***Figure 7-1.*** The Valsalva maneuver moderates transmural vascular pressures. Cerebral vascular pressure increases with strain or effort, with or without the Valsalva maneuver. However, the likelihood of vascular rupture is mitigated by a simultaneous increase in cerebral ventricular pressure transmitted up the cerebrospinal fluid column in the spinal canal. This simultaneous increase in cerebrospinal fluid pressure is provided by the Valsalva. The volume of the skull limits these two pressures and stabilizes vessel structures, rather than predisposing them to rupture. Figure by Jason Kelly from *Starting Strength: Basic Barbell Training, 3rd edition,* by Rippetoe, 2011 by The Aasgaard Company; used with permission.

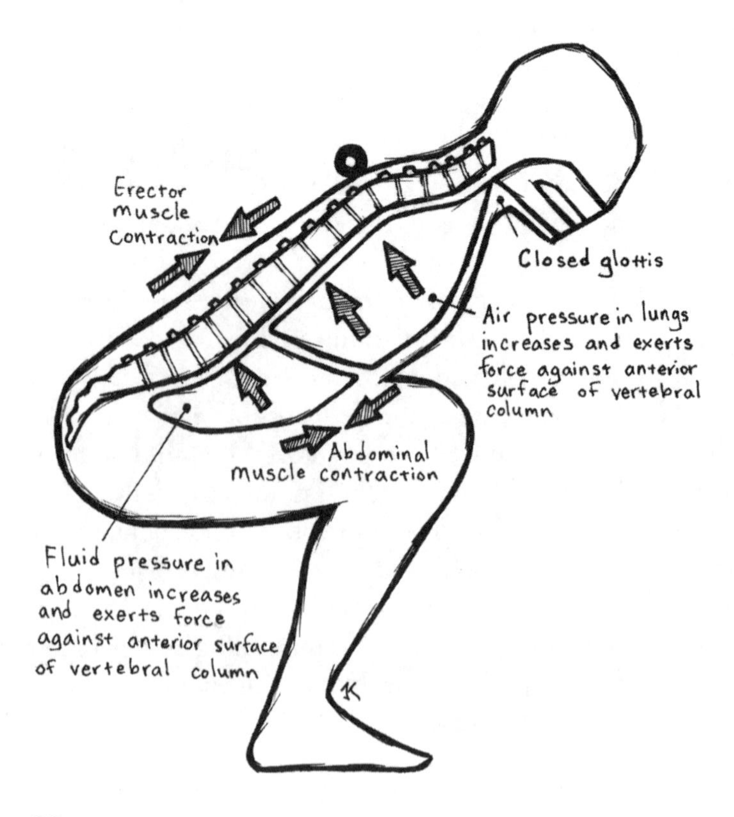


***Figure 7-2.*** The Valsalva maneuver optimizes spinal stability and support. The combined effects of increased lung (intra-thoracic) pressure, intra-abdominal pressure produced by abdominal contraction, and spinal erector contraction create spinal stability during loading. The Valsalva maneuver increases the ability to produce this pressure and stability. Exhalation during heavy efforts prevents the development of sufficient pressure to stabilize the spine. Figure by Jason Kelly from *Starting Strength: Basic Barbell Training, 3rd edition,* by Rippetoe, 2011 by The Aasgaard Company; used with permission.

*There is absolutely no good clinical evidence that lifting under Valsalva increases the risk of stroke*, and considerable evidence, both clinical and physiological, to the contrary. Sullivan has examined this issue in rather more excruciating detail in an article published by The Aasgaard Company in 2012.[7]

With all of that out of the way, we can begin our overview of the barbell exercises: the ***squat***, the ***deadlift***, the ***press***, the ***bench press***, and the ***power clean*** or ***power snatch***. All of these exercises demonstrate the attributes we've been talking about: they are all big multi-joint movements that recapitulate whole-body, functional movement patterns. All of them (with the exception of the bench press) are structural exercises, loading not just the limbs but the axial skeleton as well, conferring a training benefit to the spine and the hips. And all of them can be trained for many years with progressive overload, with weight added in measured increments so that the trainee can get stronger and stronger.

We'll begin with the exercise that forms the keystone of strength training: the squat.

# 8

# A Brief Overview of the Squat

The Squat is the cornerstone of the strength training program for the Masters Athlete. No other exercise allows as much weight to be lifted through a more complete range of motion, trains as much tissue, or drives as much improvement in overall strength as the squat. The squat is safe, comprehensive, and subject to precise dosing. It attacks the Sick Aging Phenotype, and is learned quickly by most trainees. This chapter covers the essentials of performance of the squat and discusses remedial variations.

## What is a Squat?

No exercise is as misunderstood or generates as much controversy as the venerable barbell back squat. Misinformation abounds, improper or even dangerous instruction is common, the misinformation results in any number of useless or counterproductive variants, and the most fervently held and passionately argued opinions about squats are usually the ones most devoid of any evidence whatsoever. We hope to convince you to squat as part of your training for the extreme sport of aging, to dispel some of the nonsense about squats you may have heard, and inoculate you against some of the mythology you are likely to encounter.

Let's get some terminology out of the way. A ***squat*** is an exercise in which a load is held stationary by the hands, the upper extremities, or the body itself, and the hips are then lowered and raised. For example, a ***bodyweight squat*** is one in which no external load is carried; the trainee's own bodyweight constitutes the load. A ***goblet squat*** is one in which a load, such as a dumbbell, is carried in the hands on the chest as the trainee squats. A ***barbell squat***, obviously, is a squat in which the load to be lifted is a barbell. Barbell squats will be the focus of our discussion.

Barbell squats come in a variety of flavors. A ***front squat*** is one in which the barbell is carried on the front of the shoulders, held in place by raising the elbows and locking the bar onto the anterior deltoids. An ***overhead squat*** is one in which the bar is carried overhead with the elbows locked out. The front squat and overhead squat are variations with particular applicability to Olympic weightlifting.

A ***back squat*** is one in which the barbell is carried on the back, either high on the traps at the base of the neck (a ***high-bar squat***) or lower on the shoulders, just below the scapular spines (a ***low-bar squat***).

Whether the back squat is high-bar or low-bar, it can be further characterized by the depth to which the trainee squats. For our purposes, we can consider two depths: partial squats and full squats.

*Partial squats* are squats in which the hips do not descend below a line formed by the patella (the kneecap) that is parallel to the horizontal reference – the floor. Different authors define partial squat variants (half squats and quarter squats) as occupying different joint angles, which tells you something about the poor reproducibility and consistency of these exercises. Because these exercises do not express the full range of motion, trainees can always partial squat *much* more weight than they can full squat. Many people are under the impression that this is a good thing. They are mistaken.[1]

*Full squats* are squats that are performed to below parallel. Like half- and quarter-squats, these squats can also *describe* a variety of joint angles, but they are not *defined* by joint angles. Full squats are defined by an *anatomical relationship*: The hip joint drops below the top of the kneecap. Once that has occurred, the trainee is at the bottom of a full squat. He may or may not go deeper, but he *need* not go deeper to perform the full squat, partake of its joys, and derive its many benefits. In short, a full squat is just that: a squat that expresses *the complete and natural range of this fundamental human movement pattern.*

We therefore assert that a back squat performed to full depth is the most general case, while quarter-squats and half-squats are truncated variants of this general case. Hence, full back squats will be referred to simply as *back squats.*

Of all the squat variants, the one that is most suitable for general strength development is the low-bar back squat. We maintain that the high-bar back squat is a special variant of back squat, and so from now on the term ***squat*** will refer to the low-bar back squat, performed to full depth. All other squat variants will be referred to by their respective qualifiers: high-bar squats, quarter-squats, front squats, etc.

*The squat (the low-bar back squat performed to depth) is the most general and useful of squat variants because its more-horizontal back angle recruits the largest mass of muscle tissue over the longest range of motion, and therefore provides the most intense stress for adaptation, driving the greatest increases in general strength.*[2]

Squatting is a fundamental human movement pattern. Everybody does it – or used to do it – and in some cultures it is (or was) second only to standing as the posture one most frequently assumes while awake. The bottom of the squat is the position people all over the world and throughout history assume for working, eating, voiding, talking, and having babies. The ability to squat below parallel and stand up again is fundamental to human physical existence even in cultures that have recliners and indoor plumbing, because the inability to get up from a chair or toilet can have significant negative implications for one's quality of life.

## Essentials of Performance

When you learn the squat properly, on your own or under the instruction of a qualified coach, you should undergo the ***standard teaching progression***, which starts without the bar. This teaching progression is detailed in Rippetoe's *Starting Strength: Basic Barbell Training, 3rd edition,*[3] and will not be described here. Our purpose is to give you a description of the exercise and what it is like to do it, so that we can talk about its usefulness, benefits, safety, and special challenges.

Early in the standard teaching progression, before you put the bar on your back, your coach will have you squat without any specific instructions. *You'll almost certainly do it incorrectly, because of the picture in your mind of the movement placed there by your exposure to the exercise in magazines and videos.* As a result, your back angle will be too vertical, and your knees will be in an unfriendly position, too far forward. It is a testament to the perverse inventiveness of humans in general and personal trainers in particular that such a simple and natural thing as using the hips gets so frequently and so abhorrently screwed up.

The squat is a ***hips*** exercise, not a *legs* exercise. The main reason the squat is perfectly safe is that the

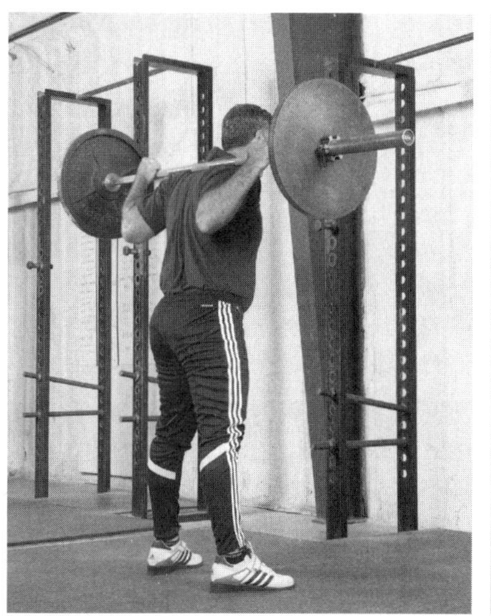

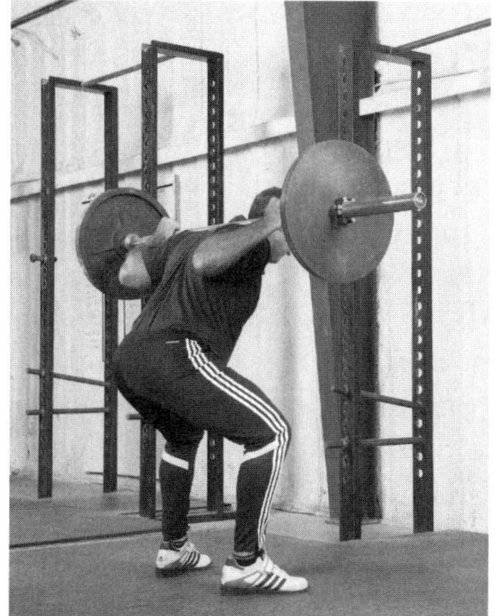

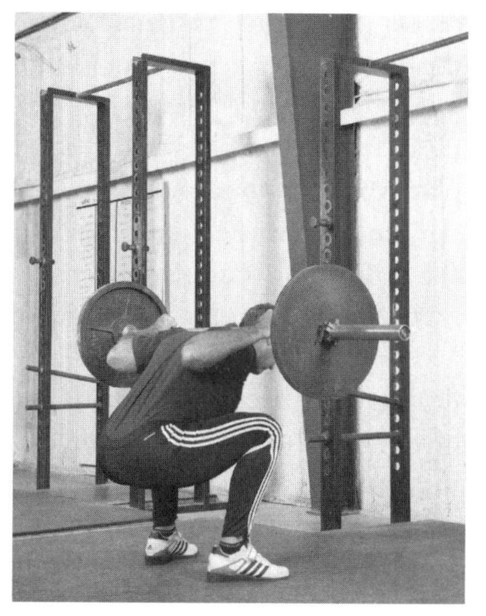

***Figure 8-1.*** The squat. *Left,* Top position. *Center,* Middle position. This position is passed through again when the lifter comes out of the bottom. *Right,* Bottom position ("the hole").

hips are capable of squatting safely, while the knees may not be. So our squat will emphasize the hips by incorporating a more horizontal back angle, which keeps the load on the hips where it belongs.

The squat is performed with a shoulder width stance *with the toes pointing out at about 30 degrees.* This is critical: your toes will *not* point straight forward. When you squat, you will drive your knees out so that your thighs are parallel with your feet (Figure 8-2). As you descend you will open your hips, you will *bend over,* you will stick your butt back and point your nipples at the floor, and you will keep your head in a neutral position. By the time you are about a third of the way down, your back angle will be set, and your knees will be as far forward as they will ever get, no more than an inch or so beyond your toes, with your shanks (your tibias or lower legs) set like rigid posts. Your hips will drop below your knees.

At this point, your back angle has pointed your chest at the floor, your hips are open, your thighs spread out, and your groin muscles and hamstrings will approach their full extensibility, triggering a ***stretch reflex*** (the "bounce") that will help drive you up out of the "hole." You will call upon this ***hip drive*** by thinking about driving your butt straight up, as if there were a winch on the ceiling attached to your sacrum, pulling you out of the bottom. By the time you are two-thirds of the way up, your back and shank angles begin to change as you assume an upright position. You stand up. You let out your wind. You take a deep breath. And then you squat again.

This method of performing the squat maximizes range of motion and recruits more muscle

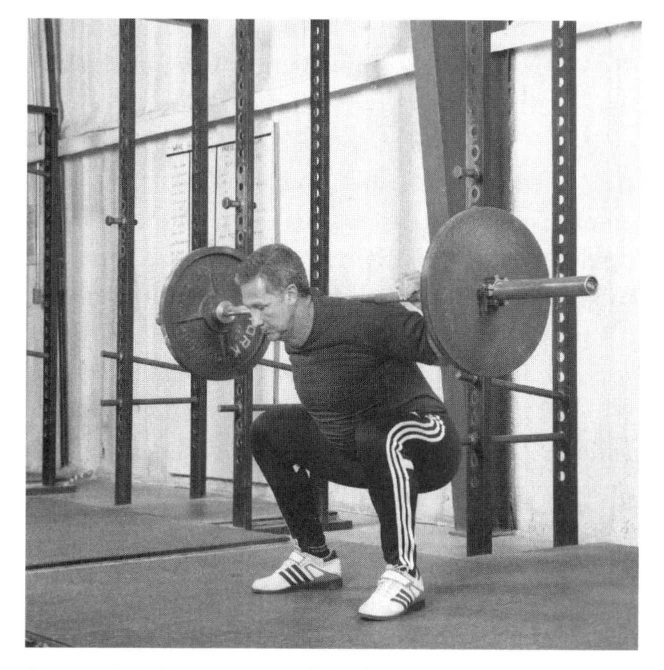

***Figure 8-2.*** Front view of the bottom position. The thighs should be parallel to the feet and the knees should point out over the toes.

tissue than other variants because it incorporates the ***active hip***,[4] which transforms the squat from a leg exercise to a movement that trains the entire posterior kinetic chain. The active hip comes into play when we point our chest at the floor and drive our knees out over our toes as we descend into the bottom of the squat. The effects of this simple maneuver are manifold and profound.

The most mechanically obvious advantage of driving the knees out is that it gets your thighs out of the way. If you don't drive your knees out, your thighs will be pointing more or less forward, and you will impinge soft tissue between your femurs and pelvis. Simply put, your belly and your thighs will run into each other well before you get below parallel. The active hip relieves this impingement and allows you to squat to full depth.

But the active hip goes much deeper (if you will) than that. Driving out the knees, bending over, and squatting to depth recruits a *vast* amount of muscle tissue into the exercise. Opening the hip angle in this manner is what an anatomist would call *femoral abduction* and *external femoral rotation.* Abduction of the femurs, which is the act of simply spreading the thighs, is an intrinsically weak movement, and the muscles dedicated to this movement are small.

External femoral rotation is another story. As you sit reading this, roll your thighs outward, as if you were opening the pages of a book. You will observe that this rotation is unavoidably accompanied by abduction (separation of the thighs). And this movement of femoral external rotation, unlike pure abduction, is driven by a large amount of muscle mass around the hips: the *gluteus maximus, gluteus medius, gluteus minimus, piriformis, gemellus superior, gemellus inferior, quadratus femoris, obturator externus, psoas major, psoas minor,* and *sartorius* muscles all contribute to this movement.[5] The contribution of so many muscles and so much contractile tissue to this one component of the movement underscores its importance and power. At the bottom of the squat, these muscles work hard to hold the femurs in external rotation and abduction.

It doesn't end with the femoral rotators and abductors. Opening the hips also brings in the femoral adductors, the "groin muscles," which include *adductor brevis, adductor longus, adductor magnus, adductor minimus, pectineus,* and *gracilis* muscles.[6] This important group of long, powerful muscles is prone to atrophy and injury in the sedentary and the aged. At the bottom of the squat, the adductors are stretched tight, and are therefore subject to a stretch-shortening stimulus, which means they contribute to the bounce out of the hole. This is important, because the thigh adductors attach to the pelvis, which means they cross the hip joint, which means they also serve as extensors of the hip.[7]

All of which is a fancy way of saying that *your groin muscles help you stand up out of the squat.*

Still deeper: because the active hip allows you to slide your middle-aged belly between your thighs and drop your hips below parallel, it permits a more horizontal back angle that pulls your hamstring muscles to their full extensibility, activating the stretch reflex that helps drive you out of the hole. The "hammies" (*biceps femoris, semitendinosis, semimembranosis*) are a group of very large, powerful muscles in the back of the thigh. They are often thought of as primarily flexors of the knee. This is actually kind of silly, because nobody ever *just flexes their knee against resistance* as an isolated movement in nature. The hamstrings cross the hip joint in addition to the knee joint, which means that when they contract against a rigid shank (knee held in flexion, as in the bottom of the squat), they perform two functions: they support the back angle in its more horizontal position, and they extend the hips.[8]

All of which is a fancy way of saying that *your hamstrings enable your hips to help you stand up out of the squat.*

And deeper yet: because the hamstrings are pulled tight and activated at the bottom of a squat properly augmented by the proper back angle and the active hip, and because they cross the hip to attach to the pelvis, they will tend to pull the pelvis forward and result in flexion (rounding) of the lower back – *if you let them.* Put another way, rounding of the lower back at the bottom of the squat will slacken the hamstrings, which will kill your hip drive. And rounding any part of the spine under a load is a bad idea in any event. So the squat performed with an active hip demands that the spine be held in rigid extension. In other words, the *active hip requires the spinal erectors to participate in the exercise.* Successful use of the active hip in the squat mandates the strong isometric contraction of these back muscles to keep the vertebrae locked together into a single rigid unit that *transmits* force, instead of bowing to it.

All of which is a fancy way of saying that your back muscles, by locking your spine into extension, help you recruit your hamstrings and your adductors, *which help you stand up out of the squat.*

So you begin to see that the squat is not a "quad" exercise. Of course, the quadriceps, the primary extensors of the knee, are vital to performance of the squat. But they are only one component of a movement that, properly performed, recruits many muscle groups through a large, natural range of motion. The active hip demands contributions from the calf, the groin muscles, the hamstrings, the femoral rotators of the hip chassis, and the spinal erectors. This is a *huge* volume of muscle – all trained with a single exercise. No other exercise comes close to training such a large amount of contractile tissue through such a large range of motion with such intensity. This is why the squat is the cornerstone of strength training.

## Exercise Rx: Squats for the Masters Athlete

The squat fits the requirements of our General Exercise Prescription. Indeed, it forms the cornerstone of that prescription.

### THE SQUAT IS SAFE

Properly performed, the squat is simply the loaded version of a normal human movement pattern. It is a movement that you were *designed* to perform. You will perform the movement the same way each time, with the bar balanced over the middle of the foot, over a normal range of motion, on a stable surface, at manageable loads, without unpredictable forces.

The squat is frequently libeled as being dangerous for the knees or back. The available evidence in the literature[9] and a vast body of coaching experience indicates otherwise. Athletes all over the world, and of all ages, use the squat to get stronger. Unlike quarter squats and half squats, the low-bar back squat performed below parallel produces balanced forces about the knee joint, and promotes strong isometric contraction of the spinal erectors. The squat *strengthens* the knees and the back.

### THE SQUAT HAS A WIDE THERAPEUTIC WINDOW

Training begins with a bodyweight squat – the squat is first taught without a barbell. In fact, the squat can be trained at *less* than bodyweight, in the form of assisted squats, chair squats, and the like. When the barbell is introduced (usually, but not always, on the first day), it can be as little as 10 pounds in weight. We've taught particularly weak people with a broomstick or a PVC pipe, although this is rarely required and the need is usually psychological more than physical. Once the athlete is training with a barbell, weight can be added in increments of as little as 1 pound at a time. However, most trainees, even the very weak and aged, can make jumps of 2.5 to 5 pounds without difficulty, and during early training jumps of 10 pounds or more are not at all unusual. From the empty barbell, the squat can be loaded progressively to any weight the trainee can safely manage. The dosing range runs from ultra-low dose to ultra-high dose.

### THE SQUAT IS A BIG MULTI-JOINT EXERCISE

This makes the squat a major contribution to our **comprehensive** exercise prescription. No other exercise recruits so much muscle tissue through such a large range of motion as the squat, or induces such comprehensive anabolic and adaptive responses at the tissue and molecular levels. For overall strength acquisition, the squat is king.

### The squat attacks the sick aging phenotype

The squat is even more important for the Masters Athlete than it is for the professional linebacker. The squat places a profound stress on the metabolism, skeleton and neuromuscular system of the trainee, forcing an equally profound adaptation to that stress. As the trainee progresses, the squat becomes a high-dose exercise medicine, with favorable implications for glucose flux, insulin sensitivity, muscle mass, strength, bone density, mobility, balance and function.

### The squat is simple

It must be learned properly, and it must be performed properly, with constant attention to correct, balanced, efficient form. And while it is *simple*, it isn't *easy*. Squats get very hard, very quickly. But it really is nothing more than a normal human movement pattern performed with a barbell on your back. Its elegant simplicity is part of its power to transform the athlete.

## Modifying the Squat to Your Circumstances

It is a wretched but undeniable fact that a few unlucky souls will be unable to perform the squat at first – or at all. Injuries, loss of mobility, certain musculoskeletal issues, or simply profound weakness may preclude the low-bar back squat. When you get on the platform with a qualified coach and find that you are physically unable to perform the squat, it isn't a reason not to train. It's a sign that you are in exactly the right place.

The governing principle in such circumstances is that it's always *better to squat than not to squat*. What this means is that if you can't low-bar squat because your arms aren't flexible enough to rack the bar on your back, then you high-bar squat until they are. If you can't high-bar back squat, then you perform front squats or goblet squats until you can. If you can't do front squats because you're too weak, then you do bodyweight squats, or bungee squats (below), or chair squats (just stand up out of a chair without using your arms). Or *assisted* chair squats.

At the time of this writing, Sullivan has been training a 67-year-old woman for three months who was unable to stand up out of a chair without using her arms or assistance. We started her with simple assisted chair stands, 5 sets of 5. Then we went to unassisted chair stands. Then bungee squats for range of motion. Then goblet squats for more strength. Finally, we put a 10-pound bar on her back. Once that happened, we were off to the races. Last week she squatted 40 pounds for 3 sets of 5. *This lady's legs weren't strong enough to get her out of a chair three months ago*. Having her do a low-bar back squat was unthinkable. It's not any more.

The foregoing is typical of our experience as coaches: The majority of Masters, particularly those under 60, will ultimately be able to perform the low-bar squat (*the* squat) and partake of its many wonders. Many will have difficulty performing the squat at first. In almost all cases this is due to limitations in *strength*, not *mobility*. These deconditioned individuals do not require training in a modified squat *exercise* over the long term. They require modified squat *programming* in the short term, with remedial exercises designed to strengthen the squat's range of motion so performance can be attained. This can mean the incorporation of leg presses, bungee squats, chair stands, and goblet squats as a prelude to training in the regular squat. These approaches are discussed in the *Remedial Squat Programming* section of Chapter 21.

Some athletes, however, will have true, uncorrectable limitations in mobility that preclude proper performance of the squat. These individuals can almost always train with one of the squat variants described in the next section.

## Variations of the Squat for Mobility Limitations

Here we will present a number of variations of the squat suitable for the training of selected athletes with mobility limitations. As with our presentation of the squat itself, this section is not intended to constitute instruction in these variants. The indication for, selection of, and instruction in these squat variants is most properly a matter for a strength and conditioning coach with experience in training Masters Athletes.

The exercises described here are indicated for athletes with significant mobility limitations due to fixed, uncorrectable structural issues, who therefore cannot and will not be able to perform the squat. This is almost never due to immobility of the lower body. (Athletes who cannot achieve the bottom position of the squat due to true immobility or pain usually require medical evaluation, imaging, and treatment, up to and including hip or knee replacement.) Rather, a truly uncorrectable inability to perform the low-bar back squat is almost always due to mobility limitations of the shoulder girdle and upper extremities.

The inability to carry the barbell in the low-bar position is the most common limitation prohibiting this version of the squat for Masters over 60 years old. Even if the position can be achieved, the discomfort may be acute enough to interfere with the athlete's ability to focus on other, more important elements of the exercise.

Limitations in the ability to carry a barbell in the low-bar position, just beneath the scapular spine, varies from trainee to trainee. In the best case scenario, the trainee is just "tight." In this case, the culprit is simple muscular tension, which can be stretched out and improved. It may take several training sessions to get the shoulders completely stretched out, but improvement can be made, even within the first workout. It is not uncommon for the first set or two with the bar to be carried in a high-bar position, and a low-bar position to have been achieved by the final work set of the day. Muscular tension may make the low-bar position uncomfortable, but not painful. Over time, the position will become easier and more natural. Such individuals should train the low-bar squat. They do not require a squat variant.

In some cases, however, improvement in shoulder mobility is not possible, and attempts to achieve greater flexibility can be dangerous. Mild shoulder arthritis is common in most adults over 50, and severe shoulder arthritis becomes increasingly common with every passing decade. Shoulders locked into a shortened range of motion due to degenerative changes in the glenohumeral joint, the joint capsule, or the ligamentous structures of the shoulder cannot be "stretched out." Athletes who have had rotator cuff surgeries (very common among the Masters population) tend to demonstrate decreased range of motion, and it is unwise to attempt to "stretch out" a structure that may have been artificially shortened during a surgical repair.

Athletes who cannot maintain the low-bar position have a number of alternatives available. In order of decreasing preference, these are the high-bar squat, the front squat, the goblet or dumbbell squat, and the leg press. Athletes who cannot train any of these exercises in the absence of correctable pathology are rare, and they will require special programming and coaching, probably as deadlift specialists.

## The high-bar squat

Training the high-bar squat is indicated for the Master who truly cannot carry the barbell stably in the low-bar position. Coaches who routinely work with Masters will find that a significant percentage of their athletes need to use the high-bar squat.

While squats are preferred to high-bar squats, high-bar squats still rank far ahead of other squat alternatives. The primary disadvantage of the high-bar squat is that, because of the more vertical back angle and the resultant effects on the recruitment of the muscles of the hips and back, it trains less muscle mass than the low-bar position, does not train the back and hamstrings as intensely, and does not allow the trainee to use as much weight. Nevertheless, high-bar squats are the preferred alternative if the squat is unattainable. They still train a large volume of muscle, and many lifters, young and old, have put up impressive weights using high-bar mechanics.

The difference in carrying position between high-bar and low-bar may seem relatively minor and inconsequential. It isn't. Even a few inches of change in bar position on the torso (from just beneath the scapular spine to the top of traps) significantly shifts how the bar will align with the athlete's center of gravity during the exercise. This affects the back angle – and the effectiveness of the movement – quite profoundly.

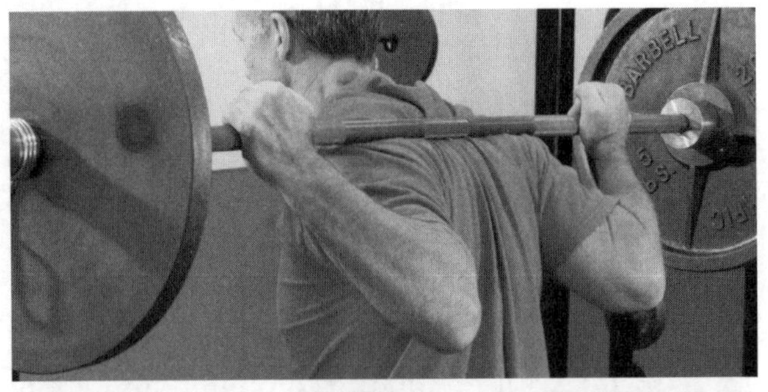

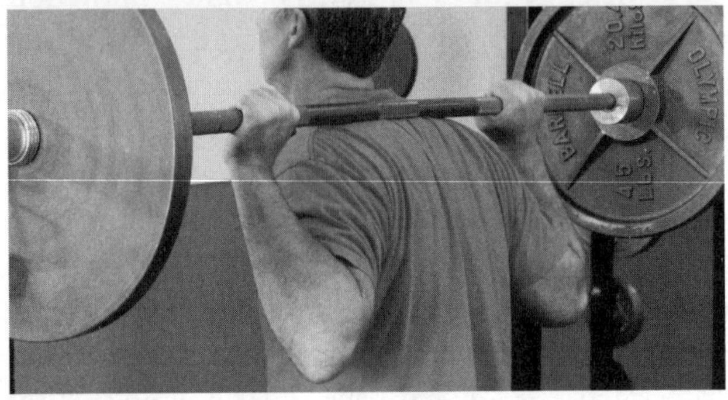

***Figure 8-3.*** Bar position in the squat *(top)* and the high-bar squat *(bottom)*. In the squat, the bar is carried on a "shelf" of muscle formed by the posterior deltoids and the trapezius, just beneath the spines of the scapulas. In the high-bar variant, the bar is held well above the scapulas, high on the trapezius. Both positions are stable, but produce markedly different back angles and therefore different muscle recruitment patterns.

Safe and efficient execution of *any* squat requires that the barbell stay in alignment with the mid-foot. Even a small shift backwards or forwards of the mid-foot position can throw the entire system off balance. The change in bar position on the torso may be as little as an inch or two of actual distance. However, considering that the actual mid-foot position is quite small, a 1 to 2-inch shift relative to that position is significant. In practice, this means that if the athlete is forced to carry a barbell in the high-bar position, he must alter the mechanics of the movement pattern. The position of the bar on the back therefore determines the back angle during the movement, which therefore determines the pattern of muscle mass activation during the exercise.

If the trainee attempts to squat a barbell carried on top of the traps with low-bar mechanics he will throw the barbell well forward of the mid-foot. Low-bar requires the lifter to push the hips *back* while allowing the torso to lean *forward,* thus balancing the barbell over the middle of the foot.

In the high-bar squat, the athlete will think more about squatting *down* instead of *back* (Figure 8-4). The less the hips travel backward, the less the torso needs to lean forward as a counterbalance. High-bar will produce a much more upright torso than low-bar. Most of the other cues remain the same. The lifter will still try to maintain tight shoulder blades under the bar, keep an arch in the lower back, and shove the knees out to the side. The stance may be slightly narrower for the high-bar squat.

Another significant difference between high-bar and low-bar is how the lifter ascends out of the hole back to the upright position. As described previously, hip drive occurs when the athlete leads out of the bottom of the squat position by driving their hips straight up while maintaining a relatively horizontal back angle. However, exaggerated hip drive during a high-bar squat is not particularly useful and can even be dangerous. Trying to powerfully drive the hips *up* during a high-bar squat can throw the lifter's torso abruptly forward, placing the bar well forward of the mid-foot. Instead, trainees should come out of the high-bar squat bottom position by leading up with their chest. The coaching cues for the high-bar squat and the low-bar squat are exactly opposite: "*Chest up!*" and "*Hips up!*" produce dramatically different effects.

Use of the high-bar squat has implications for programming. The high-bar squat is often said to be more "quad-dominant" than the squat. It would be more correct to say that high-bar squats are less hamstring-dominant, leaving the quads with more work than in the squat. Because high-bar squats utilize less muscle mass than low-bar squats,

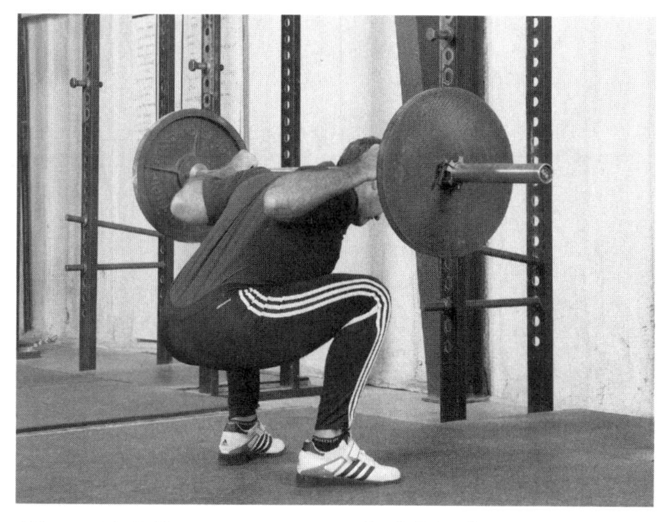

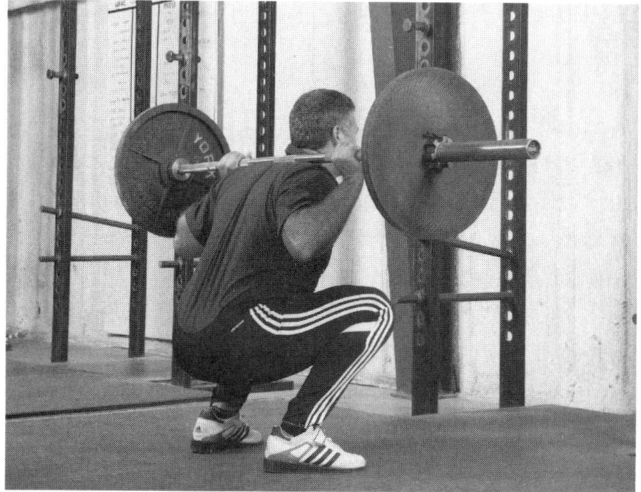

***Figure 8-4.*** Bottom position. *Left,* The bottom position of a properly executed (low-bar) squat. *Right,* The bottom position of a properly executed high-bar squat. Note the pronounced difference in knee, hip and back angles.

they will progress more slowly. As a rule, the less muscle mass an exercise uses, the slower and more conservative the rate of progression must be. A trainee that might be capable of 10-pound jumps per session with the squat might be constrained to 5-pound jumps or less with a high-bar squat.

High-bar squats put more stress on the knees and less stress on the hips compared to the squat. The hip chassis is bigger, more muscular, more mobile and far more powerful than the knee apparatus, can absorb far more training stress, and is more important to general athletic development. Athletes using the high-bar squat, especially those with sensitive knees, must take care to avoid excessive volume and frequency. For example, the standard 3-day novice program incorporates 3 heavy squat sessions per week, each consisting of 3 work sets of 5 repetitions each, for a total of 45 heavy repetitions (Chapters 19-21). A Master using high-bar squats might consider reducing that schedule to just twice per week or perhaps only performing 2 work sets at each session. Further programming adjustments at the late stage novice, intermediate, and advanced levels will be dependent on the individual trainee. The important point for those using high-bar squats is to remember to watch for knee strain and inflammation, and make programming adjustments accordingly. For the Master who is using the high-bar squat, we strongly recommend a thick, tight pair of knee sleeves and/or knee wraps.

The high-bar squat also introduces the risk of hip flexor tendonitis. This condition can develop *easily and rapidly* as a result of the excessive depth invited by the high-bar variant. With older trainees, excessive depth is usually not a problem, but a small proportion of Masters are very flexible – most of them female. Because the trainee is not *sitting back* and *leaning forward* during a high-bar squat, less tension builds in the hamstrings during the eccentric (descending) phase. So there is less hamstring rebound to "catch" the athlete in the hole, resulting in a squat that is too deep, or "ass-to-grass." Excessively deep squats are usually exacerbated by a forward knee slide that will promote soreness and inflammation of the hip flexors within just a few workouts. Inflamed hip flexors are *no fun at all.* They're miserable, they take a long time to heal, and training around them is difficult to impossible. It's best to avoid getting them in the first place. Hyper-mobile trainees should take extra care to not squat any further than just below parallel. The *"Knees Out!"* cue becomes incredibly important to these trainees. Forcing the knees out to the side prevents the knees from going forward and builds tension in the adductors which can help to "catch" the lifter in the hole.

## The front squat

Rarely, an athlete will be too immobile in the shoulder girdle to perform either a low-bar or high-bar back squat. In such cases, the barbell cannot be carried stably on the back, and will consistently gravitate to a position on the posterior neck, over the cervical vertebrae.

*This is categorically unacceptable and must not be permitted under any circumstances.* Carrying the barbell on the cervical spine is intrinsically dangerous at *any* load. This situation demands *immediate* termination of the set, very careful reassessment, and strong consideration of abandoning the back squat in favor of a front squat variant.

Front squats are carried on the anterior deltoids, just below the lateral clavicle (Figure 8-5). Front squats share some of the characteristics of a high-bar squat, and have very little in common with the squat. Front squats require the athlete to keep his torso almost perfectly erect with a very vertical back angle during the eccentric and concentric phase of the lift, in order to keep the barbell centered over the mid-foot. As with the high-bar squat, the lifter will lead up out of the hole with the chest, and hip drive is not a central component of this movement. The athlete must fight to not tip forward during the exercise. Even a slight tilt forward of the mid-foot or a relaxation of the upright chest position or the upper extremities will cause the barbell to fall in front of the athlete.

The primary challenge of the front squat for most Masters is exactly analogous to the challenge they faced in the back squat: finding a grip that is comfortable enough and strong enough for them to actually train in the exercise. Athletes who cannot even high-bar squat due to mobility issues will often struggle with the front squat as well. The ideal front squat position will utilize a grip that requires flexible shoulders, elbows, and wrists. Pictured below are 3 different potential grip positions with which trainees can experiment, in order of decreasing difficulty.

**Standard front squat.** The ideal front squat grip racks the barbell on the front of the shoulder with the elbows high and the hands simply securing the weight as it is carried on the anterior deltoids. This is a very stable position, provided the back remains erect, and is in fact the position in which Olympic weightlifters receive and recover a clean in competition and practice. Unfortunately, it requires considerable mobility of the upper extremity, particularly the wrists and shoulders, and wrist and shoulder mobility were the problems with the back squat. Some individuals cannot achieve a good standard rack under any circumstances due to their anthropometry. A very long forearm relative to a short humerus essentially precludes a satisfactory standard rack.

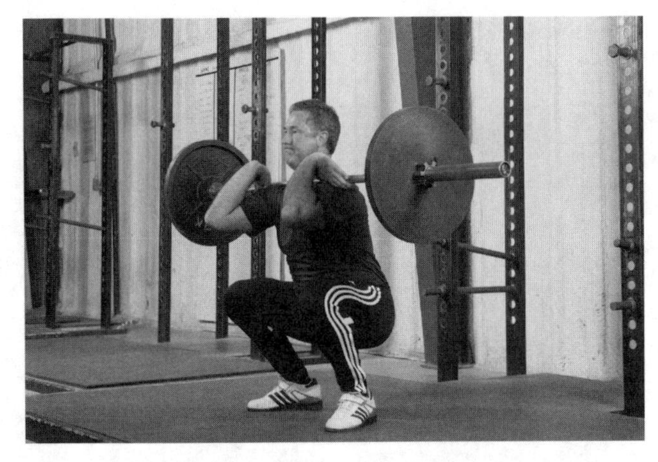

***Figure 8-5.*** The bottom position of a properly executed front squat. Notice that the bar is carried on the front of the shoulders (anterior deltoids), the elbows are up, and the wrists are extended. The hands do not hold the bar – they trap the bar on the shoulders. Note the very acute knee angle and open hip angle of this squat variant and compare with Figure 8-1.

Less flexible trainees will wind up carrying the weight of the barbell in the hands with the elbows down, under the barbell. This position becomes untrainable as weight increases and the increased load will pull the barbell and lifter forward.

**California front squat.** This position requires far less flexibility than the standard rack. In the California, the bar is again carried on the anterior deltoids, with the elbows held high and the arms crossed and parallel to the floor (Figure 8-6). This option may be useful for athletes who cannot back squat due to

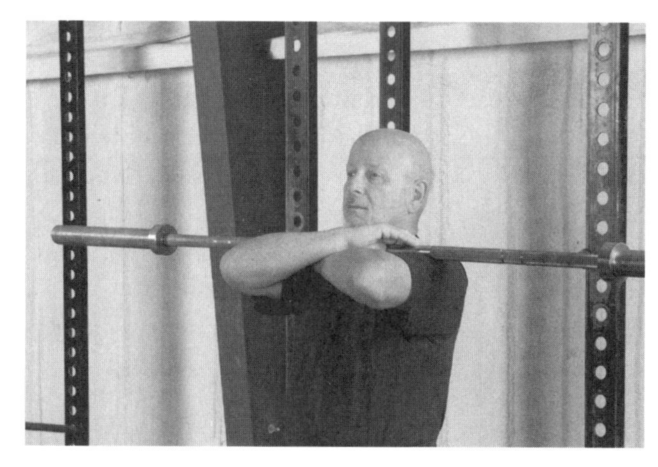

***Figure 8-6.*** The California variant of the front squat allows the athlete to hold the bar for the front squat without strain on the wrists, but with less security for the bar.

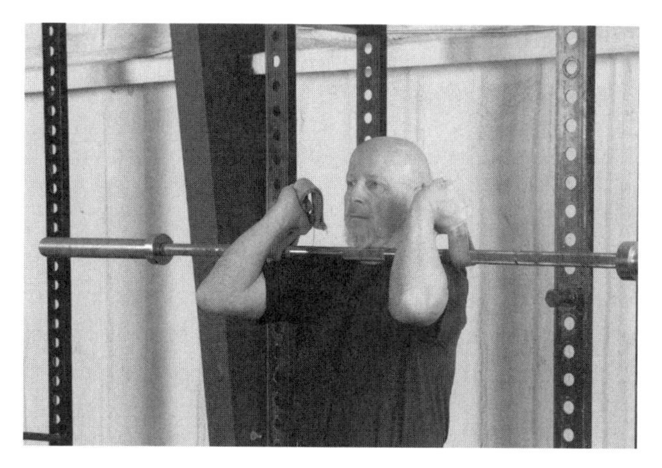

***Figure 8-7.*** The strap-assisted rack for the front squat is less stressful for the wrist, elbow and shoulder joints, but closely mimics the mechanics of the standard front squat.

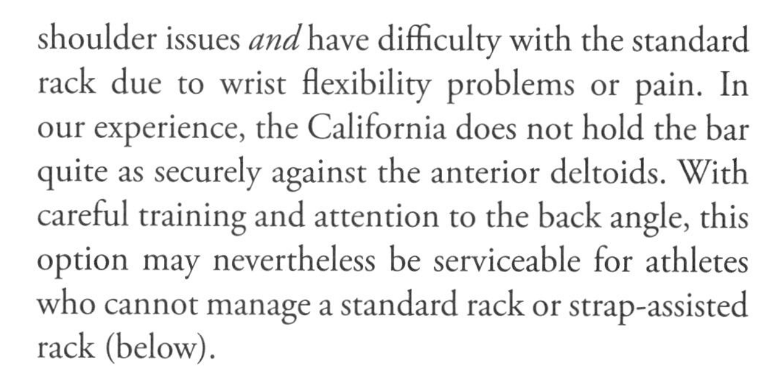

shoulder issues *and* have difficulty with the standard rack due to wrist flexibility problems or pain. In our experience, the California does not hold the bar quite as securely against the anterior deltoids. With careful training and attention to the back angle, this option may nevertheless be serviceable for athletes who cannot manage a standard rack or strap-assisted rack (below).

**Strap-assisted front squat.** This variant of the front squat is stable and recapitulates the mechanics of the standard rack far more closely than the California. Lifting straps, usually used for deadlifts and other pulls, are secured to the bar just lateral to the contact points with the shoulder, and the strap ends are gripped firmly by the trainee (Figure 8-7). The elbows are held high, as in the standard rack, but the length of the straps takes considerable tension off the shoulders in anterior flexion and the wrists in extension, making this position more tolerable and accessible to most Masters with upper extremity mobility limitations. The use of this option requires some practice and should ideally be implemented under the supervision of a coach experienced in its use. Programming should be especially judicious, with weights kept light until the athlete is skilled in the use of this variant and confident of the security of the bar.

The front squat will bring in the same programming considerations as the high-bar squat. Front squats place even more stress on the quads, and therefore the knees. Volume and frequency must be adjusted if front squats are to supplant back squats in any of the programs in this text. Moreover, many Masters cannot maintain proper bar position for sets of five. The bar has a way of working its way down the delts and into the chest and arms. This usually results in a dropped rep or a rep performed with very poor technique. The proper bar position of a front squat can also make it difficult for a trainee to breathe for a long set, as the bar sits very close to the throat. For these reasons, front squats are generally kept to 2–3 reps per set.

For any of the programs in this text where front squats will supplant back squats, the Master need not and must not try to maintain equivalent volume. Using the basic novice linear progression as an example, the squat is prescribed for 15 total reps per session (3 sets x 5 reps). Using 3-rep sets, front squatters might be tempted to do 5 sets of 3 reps. This will likely be excessive if squats are to be performed multiple days per week. As a rule of thumb, 3 to 4 work sets of 2 to 3 reps will be sufficient for a front squat. A proven and practical method is to start a program with 3 sets of 3 reps as the target goal for each session and then switch to 4 sets of 2 reps as weights become heavier and harder to hold.

## Eliminating the Squat

An exceedingly small number of trainees who can perform the other movements will, for one reason or another, be incapable of performing barbell squats. These people will, if possible, become deadlift specialists. This is not at all ideal, but it will still make them very strong indeed. Programming options for these individuals are examined in Chapter 21.

We must emphasize that such individuals are *incredibly rare*. With a good coach (especially critical for such trainees) and the principles of adaptation and progressive overload always in mind, almost anybody with legs can make progress in the squat or one of its variants. That, indeed, is part of its unrivaled power as the King of Exercises.

# 9

# A Brief Overview of the Deadlift

The deadlift is the simplest exercise in the training program, and consists merely of lifting a very heavy barbell from the floor and standing straight up with the load held in the hands. It permits the athlete to lift more weight than any other exercise, albeit through a shorter range of motion than the squat. The deadlift trains the legs, hips, and trunk muscles, and it is the back-strengthening exercise *par excellence*. The deadlift is safe, comprehensive, and has a wide therapeutic window. It fights the Sick Aging Phenotype, and is learned quickly by most athletes. This chapter covers the essentials of performance of the deadlift and discusses remedial variations.

## What is a Deadlift?

Few movement patterns are more natural than bending over and picking something up off the floor. Everybody does this. Most adults, in our century, in our part of the world, don't squat down on their haunches very often. But even in the West, we still have to bend over and pick stuff up. This is unlikely to change, although we have seen people waddling around with special pick-up sticks that allow them to avoid such an ordeal, in the tragic event that they drop their cigarettes, their mega-burrito, or their Vicodin.

The deadlift is nothing more than this natural movement performed correctly, with a loaded barbell held in the hands. It describes a shorter range of motion than the squat, and it probably does not produce the same degree of anabolic response as the squat (good data on this point is lacking, even while long experience demonstrates it). But it allows human beings to develop more force than any other exercise – in other words, to lift more weight than anything else you can do. And it allows you to do it safely as part of a rational program that will get you stronger and stronger. A huge amount of muscle is involved, including the muscles of the legs, hips, buttocks, lower back, abdomen, upper back, and chest.

The squat may be the King of Exercises, but the deadlift is the Queen, and like many great Queens she is stronger than the King. And tougher. And, well, *a Mother*.

As with the squat, there are numerous variations of the deadlift. For example, the ***hex***

***bar deadlift*** uses a special bar with a central open hexagon with handles. One essentially stands inside the bar and pulls it up with the handles, as if putting on a particularly heavy pair of pants. In the ***sumo deadlift***, the lifter stands with feet very wide apart and grasps a standard bar with a narrow grip in the center. Both the hex bar and the sumo permit the deadlift to be performed with a more vertical back, which misses the point. In the case of the hex-bar apparatus, there is no bar in contact with your legs as the weight is lifted from the floor – thus its mechanics differ fundamntally from a barbell deadlift, where the movement is constrained by the presence of the bar on the legs, and whose stability in the lockout position is enhanced therewith.

We will here reserve the term ***deadlift*** for a movement in which a standard barbell is positioned directly over the middle of the feet, and the bar is lifted straight up, in contact with the legs, with a grip that is just slightly wider than the stance. At the top of the movement, the lifter is standing perfectly erect, head neutral, with straight knees and no bend at the waist. (Another completely natural position – they keep showing up, don't they?) At the beginning of the movement, the back is not vertical, but it is held in rigid extension throughout the exercise. The bar is lowered quickly to the floor by reversing the movement, the trainee breathes and resets his position, and the exercise (the "pull") begins again – from a dead stop each time.

That's right. Each repetition of the deadlift occurs from a *completely dead stop* (hence the name), with the bar just sitting there on the floor. You may have seen people at ***the Circus*** (your local commercial franchise gym) or on the Interwebz "bouncing" deadlifts off the floor. These people are not role models. They are job security for orthopedic surgeons. But we're getting ahead of ourselves.

## Essentials of Performance

We again emphasize that this material does not constitute instruction in the deadlift, but rather an introduction, an overview, and an indication of what to expect when you receive competent instruction in the exercise. Rippetoe's *Starting Strength: Basic Barbell Training, 3rd edition,* is the definitive analysis of this lift, at both the instructional and biomechanical levels.

With a good coach in a well-equipped gym, one can learn to deadlift correctly in about 10 minutes, and with very low weight indeed. With a lightweight aluminum bar and plastic technique plates, instruction can begin with as little as 20 pounds. Most trainees, even the aged and weak, can begin with more than this.

A competent coach will instruct you in the proper setup for the exercise. You will begin with a stance much narrower than the squat and toes and knees pointed slightly out. The bar will be over the middle of your foot, about an inch or so away from your shins. Keeping your knees as straight as possible and keeping your hips high, you will bend at the waist and take the bar low in your hands (toward the fingers, not the wrists) with straight arms. Without moving the bar, you will then bring your shins forward just until they come into contact with the bar. Then, without moving the bar or lowering your hips, you will raise your chest and tighten your entire body, locking your entire spine into rigid extension.

This will be uncomfortable, because the deadlift starts at the point of maximum tension – tension in the back, hamstrings, butt, arms, everything. But this procedure, when performed every single time you approach the bar for a set of deadlifts, will produce a combination of hip, knee and back angles that are exactly correct *for you.*

This is critical to understand. There is no ideal set of such diagnostic angles for the deadlift (or any other exercise), because everybody is built differently. A lifter with short legs, long arms and a long torso will simply have a more vertical back angle and a more closed knee angle at the bottom of a deadlift than a lifter with a short torso and long legs. For one lifter to try to emulate the diagnostic angles that are correct for another is a serious mistake. Following the procedure above is dependent at every step upon *your* anthropometry, and so the result will be correct for *you.*

This correct result, much to the alarm of misinformed people who may be watching, will

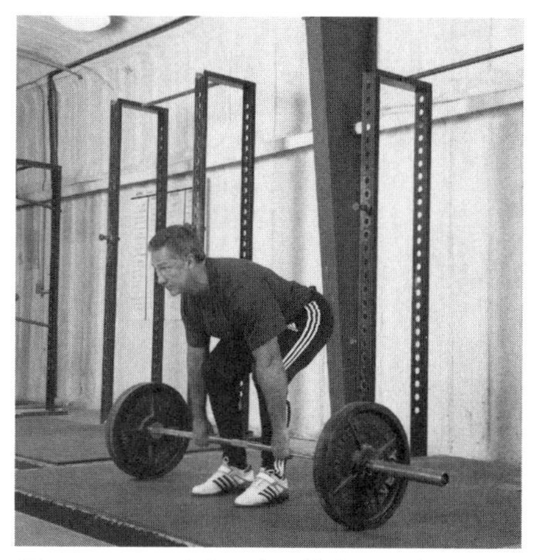
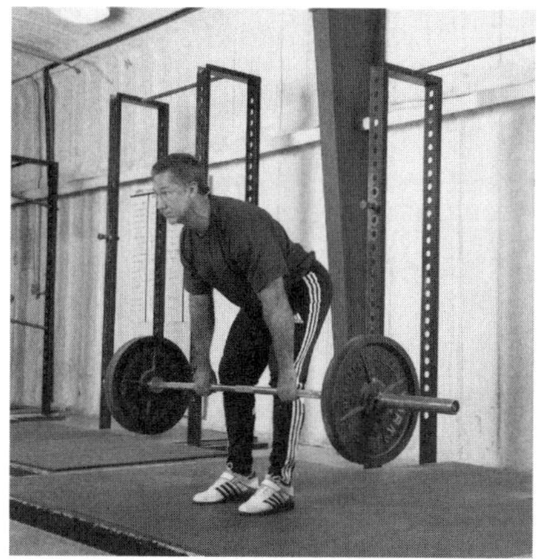
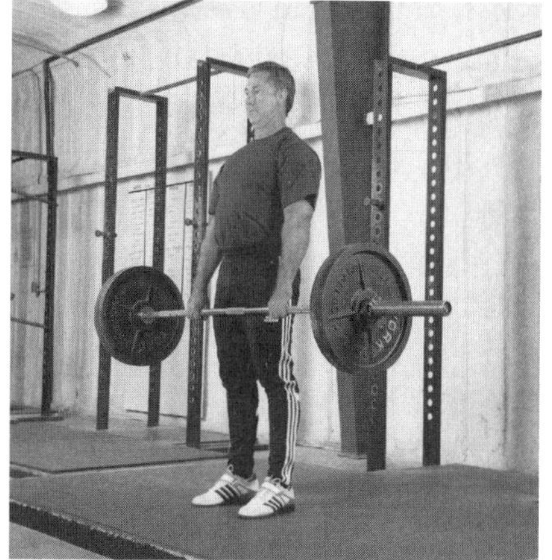

***Figure 9-1.*** The deadlift. *Left,* Starting position, with the back in full extension, the bar over the middle of the feet and against the shins, the hips held high, the elbows and wrists straight, the arms describing a slight posterior angle from the shoulder to the bar, and no slack anywhere in the system. *Center,* On the way up, the back is held in extension and the bar is kept in contact with the legs. *Right,* The top position, in which the athlete merely stands straight up, with knees and hips locked in extension and the bar still balanced over the middle of the foot.

not include a vertical back. Your back angle will be somewhere not vertical to just about perfectly horizontal, depending on how you're constructed. **The purpose of good deadlift technique and setup isn't to make your *back* vertical. It's to make the *bar path* vertical – to lift the bar straight up over the middle of the foot.**

In the process of doing so, you will have to stabilize your back and your trunk with strong isometric contractions of your spinal erectors and other so-called "core" muscles. The properly performed deadlift doesn't try to *reduce* the shear forces acting on the non-vertical spine. The properly performed deadlift just *deals with and adapts to* the shear forces acting on the spine. What this means is that, as your deadlift gets stronger, your back gets stronger. This would seem to be a desirable feature of the exercise.

With the bar in your hands, your back locked in extension at some non-vertical angle, and everything tight, you take a deep breath (the Valsalva) and "squeeze" the weight off the floor, dragging the bar straight up your legs as you stand up. At the top, you simply stand up straight, locking your knees and hips into extension, not shrugging, not leaning forward or back. After a brief pause, the weight is lowered quickly but in a controlled fashion by reversing the movement, again maintaining contact with the legs. It is here, and only here, that you breathe – not at the top.

If you have performed the movement correctly, the bar will end up where it started, over the middle of your feet. Keep your grip on the bar, keep your hips up, get tight, raise your chest, *lock your back into extension*, take a deep breath, and pull again (Figure 9-1).

## Exercise Rx: Deadlifts for the Masters Athlete

The squat and the deadlift are the alpha and omega of strength training. Increasing your deadlift strength drives up the strength in your squat, and vice-versa. These two exercises make *everything* stronger, because they both allow so much weight to be lifted, because they demand the recruitment of so much muscle tissue, and because together they describe such an extensive range of motion. For the Athlete of Aging, the deadlift is critical not only as a strength-builder, but also a confidence-builder. Most trainees think it feels "safer" than the squat. Of course, both lifts are incredibly safe. But one isn't "under" a deadlift. It is held in the hands, which most people find less disconcerting at first, and it allows the Master to very quickly reach the point where he can lift more weight than he ever dreamed possible.

But what about our exercise prescription?

### The deadlift is safe

Again: the deadlift is simply a natural human movement pattern loaded with a barbell. You will perform the movement the same way each time, with the bar balanced over the middle of the foot, over a normal range of motion, on a stable surface, at manageable loads, without unpredictable forces. If you don't put more weight on the bar than you're ready for, if you don't jerk the bar off the floor on the way up or bounce it on the way down, if your setup is the same each time, and if you keep it on your legs throughout the pull, your risk of even minor injury is several orders of magnitude removed from the unspeakable perils you will face in traffic on the way home from the gym.

### The deadlift has a wide therapeutic window

There is no "bodyweight deadlift," but as we have noted training can begin with very light weights indeed. Particularly weak individuals quickly attain minimal deadlifting strength with lightweight kettlebells or dumbbells (Figure 9-2). At the high end of the dosing spectrum, the sky is the limit with consistent training, rational programming, and a bit of determination. People in their fifties and beyond can work their way up to deadlifts of 300, 400, 500 pounds and more. Adaptation to progressive overload is second only to compound interest as a real-life miracle.

### The deadlift is a big multi-joint exercise

This makes the deadlift a major contribution to our **comprehensive** exercise prescription. Although the range of motion is shorter than the squat, it recruits a vast volume of tissue from the floor to the shoulders, including muscles of the legs, hips, abdomen, chest, shoulders and the entire back. By training the ability to rigidly stabilize the spine and the trunk, the deadlift promotes stability in all other movement patterns as well. Because it allows so much weight to be lifted and generates so much ***work*** (force x distance), it also increases ***power*** (work/time, or force x velocity). No serious athletic training program can be considered complete without this exercise.

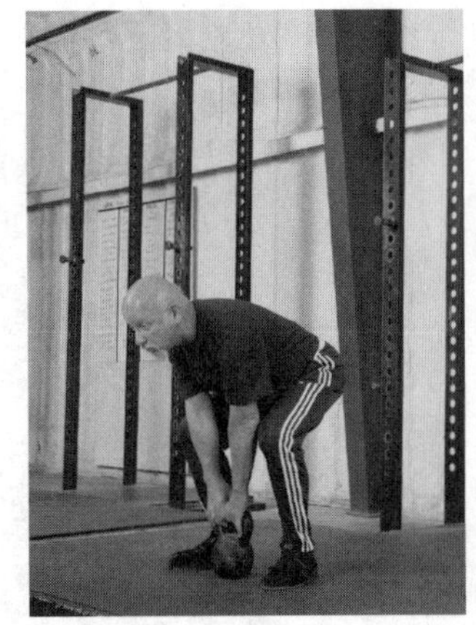
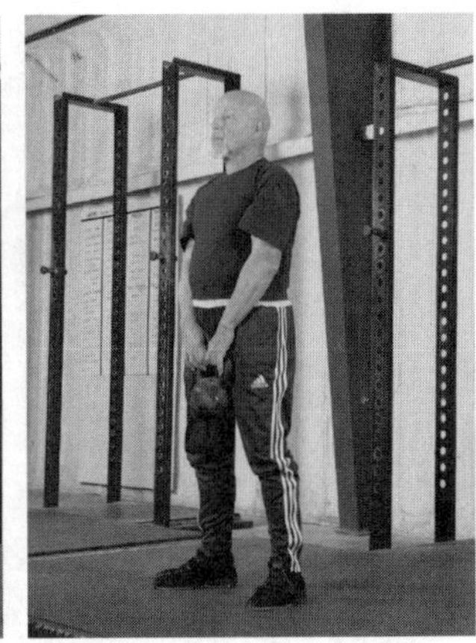

***Figure 9-2.*** An athlete performs a 12 pound kettlebell deadlift. Extremely low doses can be used with this exercise.

### The deadlift attacks the sick aging phenotype

Rippetoe is fond of saying that the weightlifter with the bigger deadlift will also have a bigger clean. Sullivan likes to say that the grandma with the bigger deadlift can snatch the bigger grandchild. She'll also have thicker bones, more muscle, better mobility and balance, and a twinkle in her eye. Like the squat, the deadlift is a structural exercise, exerting deep compressive and distracting stresses on the entire skeleton, thereby forcing bone adaptation. Stronger bones in the spine come with stronger spinal erector muscles attached to the spine. *Nobody* has a stronger back than a deadlifter, except a stronger deadlifter. As an intense resistance exercise, the deadlift will increase insulin sensitivity, stress the entire bioenergetic spectrum, and promote healthy cardiovascular and metabolic adaptations. It forces muscular and neuromuscular adaptations to handle the increasingly heavy weights, and reaches such a high dosing intensity that it must be relegated to once-weekly performance fairly early in training.

### The deadlift is simple

In fact, we're unable to think of a more simple training movement. Some people seem to think the deadlift is terribly complicated, but about a quarter-hour with a good coach will convince you that it's the most straightforward exercise you will ever do. Complicating the deadlift is the key to screwing it up. Yes, deadlifts are hard – *very* hard. That's why we do them. Yes, after a few months of training you'll look at that loaded bar on the floor with a mixture of dread, wonder, and exhilaration. And yes, you have to set it up right and pay attention to your form. But really, lifting a heavy bar off the floor for a few warm-up sets and a single work set of five repetitions, once a week, has to be the *ne plus ultra* of training simplicity.

## Modifying the Deadlift to Your Circumstances

As rare as it is to encounter an individual who can't do a barbell squat, it is even more uncommon to encounter a trainee who cannot deadlift at all. And of course, the overlap between these two small populations is considerable, but here we're getting into a very rare demographic, composed primarily of people who will never walk into a gym anyway. We know people with spinal fusions and spinal rods who deadlift, people with artificial knees who deadlift, and people with heart failure and diabetes who deadlift. And a cursory search of the internet will reveal no shortage of incredibly beautiful septuagenarians and octogenarians squeezing heavy bars off the floor, not to mention a "disabled" young lady performing a one-legged deadlift in competition.

So there really aren't a lot of good excuses available for avoiding deadlifts. Sorry.

If an individual cannot bend over to lift a 5-pound weight off the floor, he will not be able to perform a good, safe deadlift. A person with such a profound limitation in strength and/or mobility is not suitable for barbell training, and will require specialized rehabilitation, probably under physician guidance, before any sort of General Exercise Prescription can be contemplated. Individuals who experience pain in the deadlift, despite good instruction and proper form, need to see a physician for further evaluation, very likely including diagnostic imaging, to rule out a structural lesion.

Just about everybody else can deadlift, with occasional minor adjustments. In our experience, a trainee who can lift a 5-pound kettlebell or dumbbell from the floor without pain can almost always lift a 10-pound bar loaded with 5-pound technique plates during the same session or the next. From there, progressive overload takes over, and a small amount of weight can be added each time until one day the trainee realizes that he has become very, very strong.

The deadlift relies heavily on a strong grip, and trainees with grip problems due to aggressive diseases such as rheumatoid or psoriatic arthritis may need lifting straps or lifting hooks to deadlift without pain. This is not ideal, because the deadlift is a wonderful exercise for strengthening the forearm and the grip, and should be used as such by those with osteoarthritis or other more common, more indolent hand and wrist problems. But if the grip is painful, this equipment should be used so the athlete can focus on the movement. It's better to deadlift than not.

It is not uncommon for trainees of any age to experience light-headedness after a heavy set of deadlifts. This is almost always very brief, and tends to be more uncommon as training progresses. It is important not to hold your breath for more than a single rep, and to breathe normally after the set is over. Standing up slowly after your last rep is a good practice. If you're like us, standing up quickly after a set of heavy deadlifts wasn't high on your agenda anyway.

The uncommon trainee who cannot squat and is a "deadlift specialist" should generally train the deadlift more frequently than an individual who does both exercises. Because the deadlift is heavy and places a high demand on recovery, this is a situation

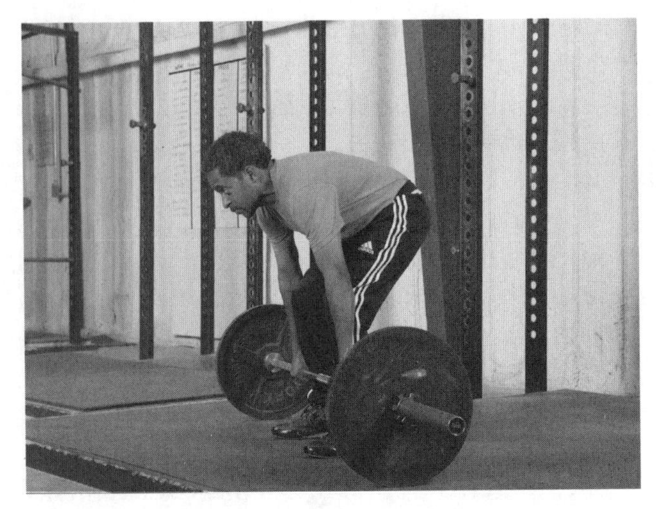

***Figure 9-3.*** An unacceptably rounded back during the deadlift. This athlete has no structural issues underlying his spinal flexion; he is merely demonstrating poor form due either to weak paraspinal muscles or inattention to correct setup and execution (compare with Figure 9-1 above). This situation demands correction for the deadlift to be trained productively and safely.

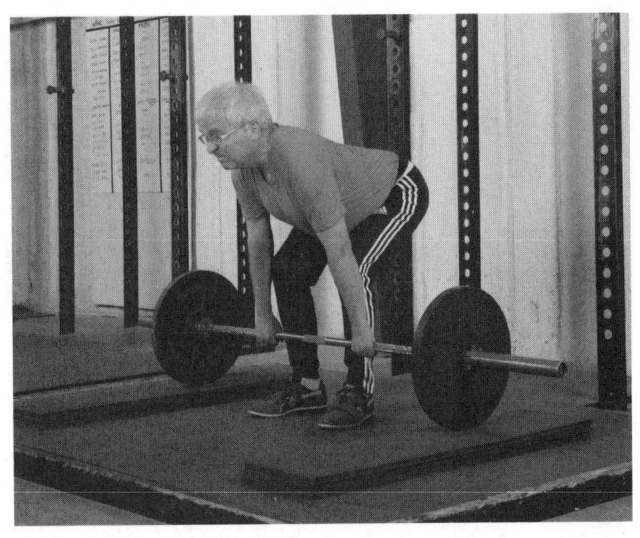

***Figure 9-4.*** Elevated deadlifts. The loaded bar sits on a stack of ¾" gym floor mats (or horse stall mats). Elevation of the bar allows the athlete to attain full spinal extension for the pull, so the deadlift may be trained safely.

that requires considerable care and attention to programming, especially in the Masters Athlete. The input of a coach experienced with older trainees is important in such circumstances.

## Deadlift modifications

Many Masters, especially men, and especially tall men, may have difficulty setting their back into proper extension in preparation for a deadlift. If a lifter cannot set the back, he cannot deadlift. Injury is the inevitable consequence for an older lifter deadlifting with a loose, rounded back (Figure 9-3).

Sometimes the athlete is simply struggling with neurological control of his paraspinal muscles. He may *know* what he is supposed to do, and may have the flexibility to achieve the task, but neuromuscular control makes consistent extension difficult. Other trainees may have underlying structural issues that inhibit or prevent proper spinal extension in the setup position.

**Elevated Deadlifts.** Elevation of the barbell is an easy fix for the Master with recalcitrant spinal extension issues. If the athlete displays a minor degree of flexion despite proper setup technique and coaching, even after several sets or several training sessions, an elevation of just a few inches can help him cross the threshold into a quality start position with good spinal extension. The easiest way to do this is with stacks of cut out sections of ¾ inch rubber mats. 2–4 rubber mats placed under each side of the bar usually gives enough elevation to get the lifter in position (Figure 9-4).

The athlete struggling with hamstring flexibility may not need the risers after a few weeks of training the squat and deadlift, as this work will improve hamstring flexibility quickly. Deadlifts elevated by just a few inches can be programmed in the same way that regular deadlifts are.

**Rack Pulls.** For athletes with very poor mobility or very poor neuromuscular control, the ***rack pull*** is indicated. The rack pull is a deadlift performed inside the power rack with the bar set somewhere between the middle of the tibia and the bottom of the patella. This elevated starting position often makes spinal extension during the setup and performance of the movement more attainable. (Figure 9-5). It should be noted however that rounded-back rack pulls

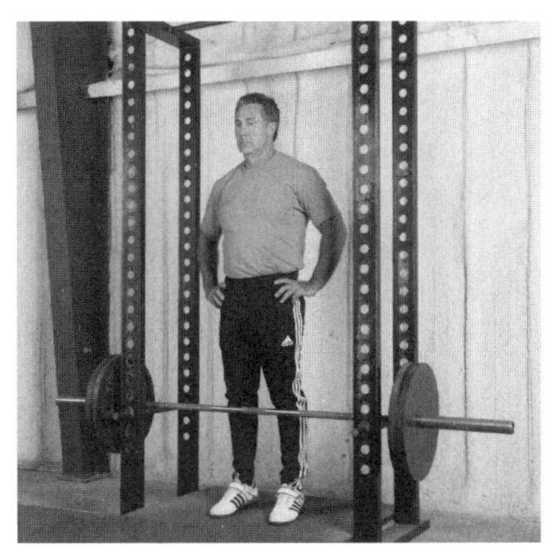
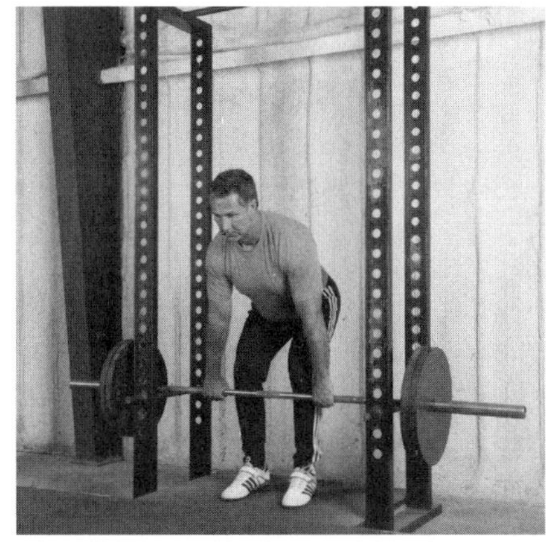
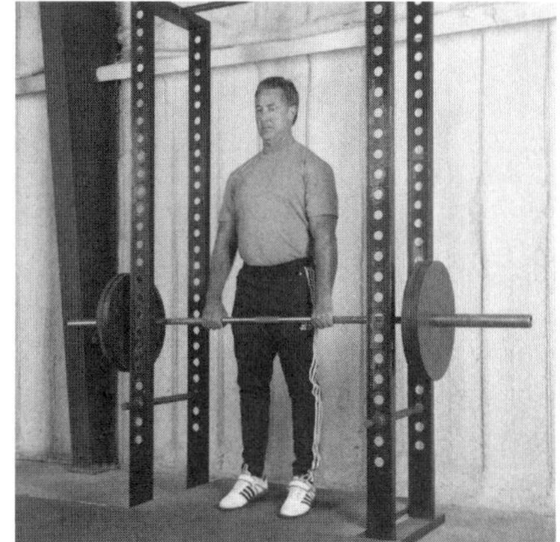

***Figure 9-5.*** Rack pulls. This exercise is simply a higher version of the elevated deadlift, and permits athletes who have particular difficulty with spinal extension to perform the exercise safely. Rack pulls are also an excellent assistance exercise for more advanced athletes.

can result in injury just as easily as rounded-back deadlifts. Although the range of motion is shorter in a rack pull, there is arguably just as much if not more stress on the lower back than in a deadlift. In a deadlift the bar is squeezed off the floor and moved through the first few inches predominantly by the legs. In a rack pull, the back is more heavily involved in "breaking" the bar off the pins, as the use of the legs is de-emphasized. Rack pulls can be invaluable for Masters with mobility issues, but they must be used carefully, preferably with the oversight of an experienced coach. Rack pulls are also useful as assistance exercises in conjunction with halting deadlifts, for advanced athletes who cannot tolerate heavy pulls on a weekly basis. Additional discussion on rack pulls and their programming are to be found in Chapter 13 and in relevant sections on programming.

**Sumo Deadlifts**. A *very few* individuals with particularly weird *Tyrannosaurs Rex* anthropometry (very long legs with very short arms) may find it quite difficult to perform standard deadlifts and might be better served by using the sumo variant. The sumo stance produces a more vertical back angle by artificially "shortening" the legs by widening the stance and narrowing the grip, and as such it is frequently and inappropriately prescribed on the rationale that it therefore avoids the deadly levels of spinal shear produced by the standard deadlift setup. What it really avoids is the opportunity to train the spinal erectors and make the back as strong as it can possibly be.

Sumo deadlifts are so rarely indicated for general strength training that we will not address them in any detail here. The decision to use the sumo for general training should be made only with the input of an experienced coach, because the vast majority of people who *think* they have to use a sumo stance actually *don't.* They just need to work on their setup, and/or get over the idea that lifting must always be done with the most vertical back angle possible. The World does not accommodate this misinformed biomechanical ideal. Training the deadlift as we have described it *loads* the back, and therefore *strengthens* the back, and makes the athlete stronger and *harder to break*. And that is the whole point.

# 10
# A Brief Overview of the Press

The standing overhead press (or simply *the press*) is an exercise in which the bar is held in the hands at the shoulders and lifted overhead, to a position directly above the shoulder joints and over the middle of the foot. For general strength training, the press can and should be performed so as to recruit muscle tissue from the entire body. Because the press describes such a long range of motion and such a long potential moment arm, it demands balance and stabilizing contributions from the muscles of the lower extremities, hips, back, abdomen, chest, shoulders, and arms. It is an excellent exercise for the development of upper body strength, balance, mobility, and proprioception. The press is safe, and when properly performed does not produce shoulder impingement in those without underlying structural abnormalities. The press meets all other requirements of the General Exercise Prescription. Some Masters will have difficulty with the press due to shoulder mobility issues, and for a few the exercise will not be accessible. Press alternatives for these athletes are described.

## What is a Press?

As with the other exercises in our prescription, the taxonomy of the press is extensive. There are seated presses, standing presses, military presses, push presses, Olympic presses, dumbbell presses, and machine presses. And of course there is the ubiquitous bench press and all of *its* variants. We will consider the bench press in the next chapter, and confine our discussion here to what some call the "shoulder presses." In the Starting Strength system of exercises, we train the *standing overhead press,* and we simply call it ***the press.***

The press is of course an upper body exercise, but it isn't *just* an upper body exercise. Like the squat and deadlift, it is a whole-body, multi-joint exercise that beautifully recapitulates a fundamental human movement pattern: lifting a heavy object overhead, as high as possible. The press, performed so as to exploit the center of human power – the hip chassis – recruits an enormous mass of muscle tissue from the feet to the forearms. Legs, glutes, abdominals, back muscles, shoulder and arm muscles, spinal erectors, pectorals, and traps all get a workout from loading this movement pattern, all contributing their correct share of the work to get the bar locked out overhead. The press doesn't just train upper body strength. The press demands and therefore builds precision, grace, timing, power, mobility, and terrific truncal stability (so-called "core strength"). If you can stand up and lift a broomstick straight up over your shoulders, you can train this indispensable movement pattern.

## Essentials of Performance

As we have emphasized, most individuals are better off learning the deadlift and squat under the supervision of a qualified coach. This goes doubly for the press. We have coached many talented lifters who have done a not-half-bad job of teaching themselves to squat and deadlift, but who have made a total botch of the press. We believe this is because people assume there just isn't that much to it. Pick up the barbell and lift it overhead. How difficult can it be?

You will quickly learn that, while the press may be *simple*, and can be taught quite quickly, it demands good technique. And once the movement is mastered and weight is added, the press rapidly becomes very difficult indeed. The long range of motion and the heavy reliance on the muscles of the upper extremity (which are smaller and weaker than the legs) means the press gets heavy in a hurry. It is the exercise in which you will lift the least weight with the most effort. You will be able to lift more if you learn to do it right, and you have the best chance of learning to do it correctly in the presence of a coach who has learned to *teach* it correctly.

With that in mind, this description will be quite basic. The press begins with the bar set in the rack as for a squat, at about the height of the middle of the sternum. The trainee takes a grip that is just a little more than shoulder width, closer than most people would think necessary, with the bar on the heel of the palm.[1] The bar is taken out of the rack and held close to the lifter's body, as close to the shoulders as possible, and balanced directly over the middle of the foot. Depending on the lifter's anthropometry, it will either rest on the anterior deltoids or it will "float" above the deltoids, under the chin. The trainee steps back into a stance that is identical to, or slightly wider than, the squat stance.

The lifter tightens his entire body, systematically and forcefully eliminating any slack anywhere in the system. Calves, quads, hams, butt, and abs are tightened. *The knees are locked tightly in extension.* Chest is held high. The upper back is tight. This position is very important, and may be one of the most difficult aspects of the press to learn – there are no relaxed muscles in the body at the start of the press.

The lifter then pushes the hips forward, creating some clearance between the bar and the chin, and then he drives the bar *straight up*, keeping it close to his face. As the bar just begins to pass the lifter's head, he drives his torso forward to get his shoulders beneath the bar. The bar moves upward in a straight vertical line. The press is finished with a forceful shrug that completes the rotation of the scapula to support the humerus, which supports the forearm, which supports the bar. The top position, with its vigorous shrug and the bar locked out as high as possible directly over the shoulder joint, recruits intense contributions from the upper body musculature, and especially the trapezius, a great mass of tissue that rotates the scapulas and stabilizes and strengthens the upper back (Figure 10-1).

Later, as the lifter becomes more skilled under the bar, the movement may become more dynamic, using the hips in creative ways that generate a little momentum at the start of the movement. But for now, just concentrate on keeping the bar close to the face, and therefore the shoulders, which keeps the mechanics of the movement efficient and the bar moving in a straight line directly over the middle of the foot.

## Exercise Rx: The Press for the Masters Athlete

When people think of upper-body exercises, they think about bench presses, flyes and curls. But the standing overhead press is the paragon of upper body strength exercises, because no other upper body exercise describes such a long range of motion, recruits so much muscle mass, demands so much balance and coordination, or recapitulates such a

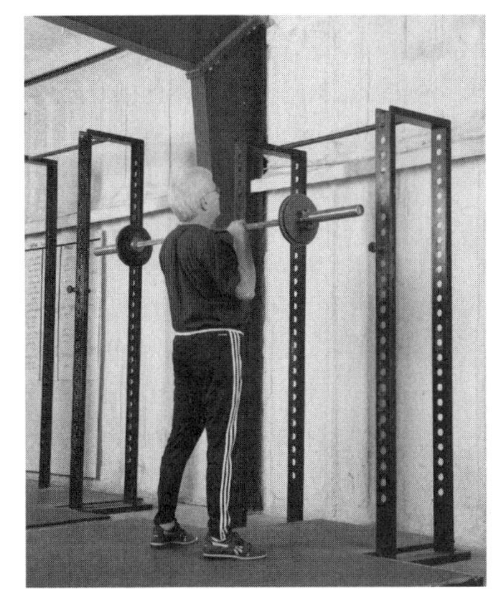
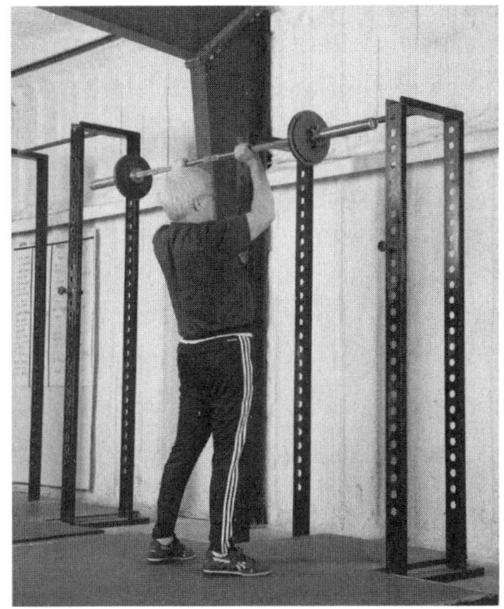
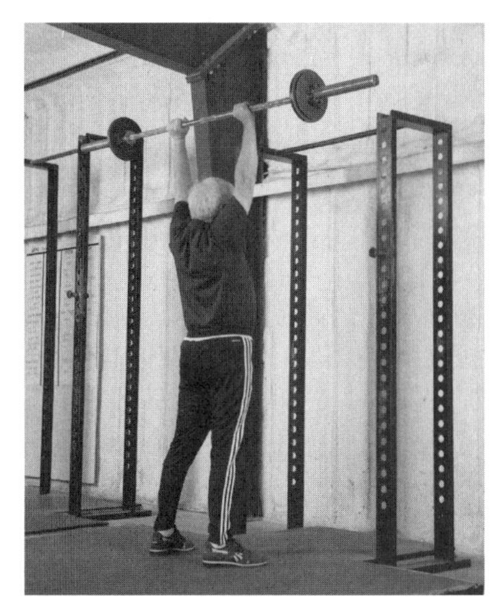

***Figure 10-1.*** The press. *Left,* Bottom position, with the bar low in the grip, elbows slightly in front of the bar, and forearms vertical. *Center,* The bar path is vertical and stays close the athlete's face. At this point the athlete is preparing to move his torso forward to bring his shoulders under the bar. *Right,* The press finishes with the bar balanced over the shoulder joint and the mid-foot, with a vigorous shrug.

universal human movement pattern. If you think about it, curls and flyes are a bit silly when viewed through the prism of everyday function. Nobody does anything even remotely resembling deltoid flyes in their daily life. But useful human beings have to lift stuff overhead all the time.

Which brings us, of course, to our exercise prescription.

## The press is safe

Not to sound like a broken record, but the press is simply a natural human movement pattern loaded with a barbell. You will perform the movement the same way each time, with the bar balanced over the middle of the foot, over a normal range of motion, on a stable surface, at manageable loads, without unpredictable forces.

The press is frequently maligned as having the potential to cause damage to the shoulder's *rotator cuff* and other structures by producing a *shoulder impingement syndrome*, colloquially known as "swimmer's shoulder" or "thrower's shoulder." Setting aside the medical literature casting doubt on whether this condition actually exists at all,[2] it is supposed to arise when soft tissue passing through the narrow *subacromial space*, between the lateral superior tip of the shoulder blade and the top of the humerus, is compromised by any phenomenon that causes narrowing of that space. On this model, elevation of the arms, as in the press, will cause the humerus to bang up against the tip of the acromion, a bony hook that curves over the subacromial space, thereby crushing the tissue passing through that space.

Whether or not there is a shoulder impingement *syndrome* resulting in chronic rotator cuff pathology, it is certainly the case that *the shoulder can impinge.* It is easy to demonstrate this to yourself by bending your elbows to 90 degrees, placing your arms parallel to the floor and at right angles to your torso, and then raising your elbows slightly. Unpleasant, isn't it? But if you drop your elbows slightly, so that your arms describe a slight downward angle, this impingement is relieved. This has implications for the performance of the bench press, as we shall see in the next chapter.

In the absence of shoulder pathology, however, a similar demonstration of impingement with an overhead pressing movement is difficult. This is because when we raise our arms overhead, as in the press, we also rotate our scapulas upward, *as an unforced, natural, intrinsic component of the movement pattern.* This rotation of the scapula causes the shoulder joint to "point" upward, at the ceiling. The entire shoulder apparatus, including the scapula, swings up, and impingement of the humerus on the acromion does not – *and cannot* – occur.

In other words, Mother Nature doesn't *want* your shoulder to impinge, because She loves you, and She designed the movement pattern so it *wouldn't* impinge. We can help Her help us, by shrugging hard at the top of the press, emphasizing the contraction of the trapezius, which drives this rotation of the scapulas.

In the absence of significant shoulder pathology, if you perform it as described in *Starting Strength: Basic Barbell Training, 3rd edition,* and as taught by a competent coach, if you don't put more weight on the bar than you're ready for, and if you set it up the same way each time with proper grip, breathing and stance, the press won't hurt your shoulders. The press won't hurt your elbows. The press won't hurt *you.* It will, in fact, *prevent* you from getting hurt, by strengthening the shoulder girdle and improving your ability to express useful force over your full range of motion.

### The press has a wide therapeutic window

Training in the press can begin with a stick of bamboo, if necessary, and proceed from there. In practice, even very deconditioned, very frail, very elderly women can usually press a 10-pound bar for repetitions and make excellent progress in the exercise. With regular long-term training, men in their 50s or 60s can aspire to the lifetime goal of a bodyweight press. They may never get there, but traveling the road will make them strong indeed. Women should shoot for a ½ or ¾ bodyweight press. Early increases will be dramatic. Later gains will demand consistent, dedicated training.

### The press is a big multi-joint exercise

The press makes a major contribution to our **comprehensive** exercise prescription. The press recruits a vast volume of tissue from the floor to the forearms, including muscles of the legs, hips, abdomen, chest, shoulders, and the entire back. As with the deadlift and the squat, the press trains the ability to rigidly stabilize the spine and the trunk. This means that a strong deadlift makes for a stronger press. Because the press lifts a load so high over the middle of the foot (the fulcrum of the barbell-lifter-floor system), it creates the longest moment arm ("lever arm") of any of the barbell exercises. This creates the kind of "core stress" and "instability" that personal trainers are always trying to produce with their goofy bosu balls, their ridiculous balance boards, and their silly one-legged exercises. Pressing a heavy weight high above your head means that considerable effort is devoted to stabilizing the load with the muscles of the trunk and shoulder girdle – without having to stand on a big stupid rubber ball.

### The press attacks the sick aging phenotype

Like the squat and the deadlift, the press is a structural exercise. Because the exercise is performed standing, compressive loads are delivered to the entire skeleton – arms, spine, hips, legs – and training loads are imposed on the muscles that attach to the bones. A heavy press is intense, using a large muscle mass, with all the usual implications for insulin sensitivity, bioenergetics, and cardiovascular, neuromuscular, and metabolic adaptation. Most importantly, the press is profoundly functional, for reasons we have belabored quite enough.

### The press is simple

It's not as simple as most people think, but it's pretty simple. It's not as simple as a deadlift, but it's arguably less complicated than a squat, and is quickly and easily learned with proper instruction. Sullivan has taught fairly uncoordinated people to do an excellent press in one session, and Baker can get it done in ten minutes. The biggest problem with very weak or deconditioned people is bar path. Weaker trainees require instruction with loads they can move around their head, rather than straight up, which makes instruction a bit of a challenge for these athletes. As they get stronger, and the weight gets heavier, it becomes rather more easy to convince an athlete's spinal cord that the weight really does need to go straight up.

## Modifying the Press to Your Circumstances

Most athletes, even very aged Masters, can press. Nevertheless, a significant proportion of individuals with advanced arthritis in the shoulders or elbows are unable to perform the movement. Some are unable to grip the bar. Trainees who are unable to perform the complete movement pattern with a very light bar require special interventions, beyond the scope of this book, to correct these issues. In the meantime, they should not press except under the supervision of a very alert and knowledgeable coach. Such a coach will not permit you to train the press at significant intensity unless and until you demonstrate an ability to properly grip the bar, describe a vertical bar path, and lock the load at full extension over the middle of the foot.

### The seated dumbbell press

In circumstances where shoulder mobility or lower back health will not allow for effective training of standing barbell presses, seated dumbbell presses may be a serviceable alternative (Figure 10-2). As a general rule, trainees who do not have the mobility to press overhead with the barbell will not be able to press overhead with dumbbells either, since the lockout position will usually be forward of the desirable balance point directly over the shoulders. However, when barbell presses are unattainable, coaches and trainees should at least experiment with dumbbells to see if some overhead work is still possible. In some cases the change in angle of the upper arm relative to the torso will allow a trainee to press dumbbells overhead with a full range of motion. A proper overhead barbell press is performed with the elbows tucked in (*adducted*) and positioned slightly forward of the barbell – just in front of the upper body. In contrast, a dumbbell press flares the upper arms out (*abducted*) to the side of the body – in line with the torso. For some this makes mobility of the shoulder worse, while for others there is dramatic improvement. A single experimental set is all that is needed to determine the usefulness, or lack thereof, of the exercise.

Doing the exercise seated (with a back support) helps the trainee keep the dumbbells aligned over the shoulder joints instead of drifting out in front of their body, as usually happens with trainees struggling with tight shoulders. A seated position also allows the coach to *carefully* pull *back* on the lifter's arms at the elbow joint. Even the lightest pull backwards by the coach allows the trainee to keep the barbells traveling vertically. We hasten to emphasize that this technique is only to be used *gently and only on those with mild to moderate shoulder immobility.* The coach must never attempt to *force* the shoulder to move through a range of motion that it mechanically cannot achieve or is painful for the trainee to perform.

The seated dumbbell press is also good for those trainees dealing with pain in the lower back. Squats and deadlifts already put training stress on the low back and under some circumstances the coach may decide to give the back a break by allowing the trainee to remove the standing overhead press from the program for a time. Switching to a seated pressing version for a few weeks can provide valuable recovery for a tired lower back. In our experience the trainee will often return to the barbell press and set

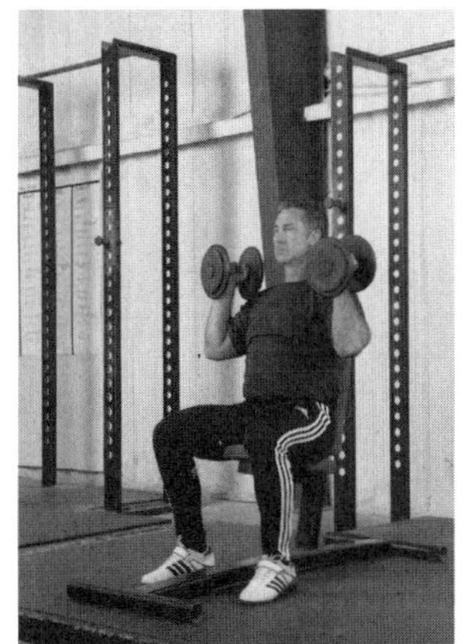
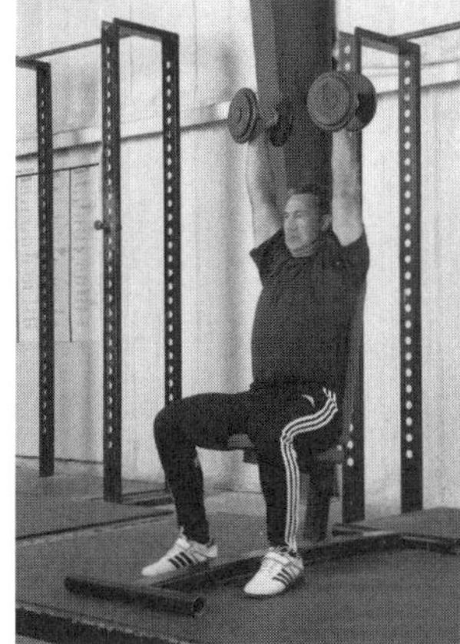

***Figure 10-2.*** The seated dumbbell press.

an immediate personal record, reaping the rewards of enhanced recovery and the training effects of the dumbbell work.

Seated dumbbell presses are best programmed within a range of 3 to 4 sets of 6–8 reps.

### One-arm overhead press

Another option for those with poor shoulder mobility is to perform all overhead pressing one arm at a time. This technique can be performed standing utilizing the end of a standing T-Bar Row machine. If a T-Bar is not available, a barbell set on the floor with the opposing end secured against a heavy dumbbell or other heavy object can also be used (Figure 10-3).

When using the T-Bar machine or the barbell, the trainee will stagger the stance a little (the foot on the side of the working arm is back) and lean at about a 10 degree angle. By doing so, an athlete with shoulder mobility restrictions can often extend the arm directly above the deltoid, even though he cannot do so with a dumbbell or barbell. An added benefit is that the trainee is standing and able to deeply engage the abs and obliques. A unique feature of this exercise is that trainees have to resist the forces of rotation during the concentric and eccentric phase of the lift. This results in a strong isometric contraction of the obliques and transverse abdominals. Coaches will often find that weak and deconditioned trainees requiring substitution of this movement for the press also have limitations on their squats and perhaps their deadlifts. Such trainees are not doing as much heavy standing work as we would like. The more heavy work that can be performed on two feet the better. This exercise allows the trainee to stand and lift even when overhead barbell pressing is restricted. For an older trainee, 2 to 3 sets of 6–8 reps is appropriate.

## Eliminating the Press

*A correct press will not hurt you.* But a press performed in the setting of significant structural or functional shoulder pathology may prevent the bar from traveling vertically to a balance point above the shoulders, without the scapulas rotated upward, without the elbows locked into extension, and without the wrists in a neutral position. In this situation, the athlete runs the risk of developing chronic or acute injuries. Surgery or aggressive therapy may help some of these people get under the bar and press correctly. Others may have to become bench press specialists, although this presents its own problems. Still others may have to perform some other upper body exercise to increase strength in the shoulder girdle, either as a substitute or preparation for the press. Again, oversight by a qualified coach is critical.

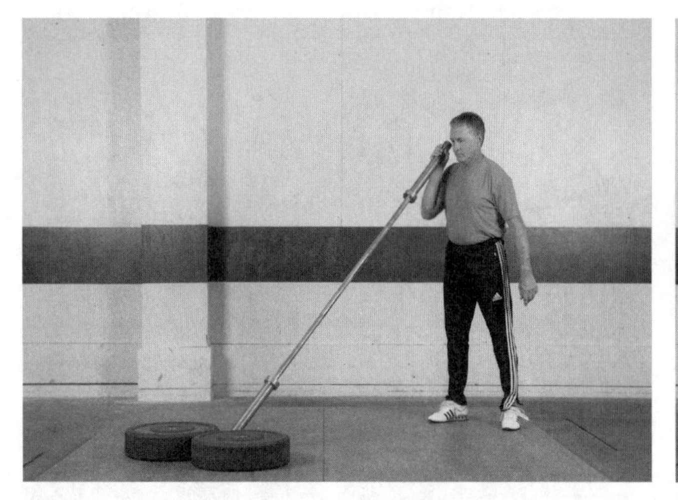

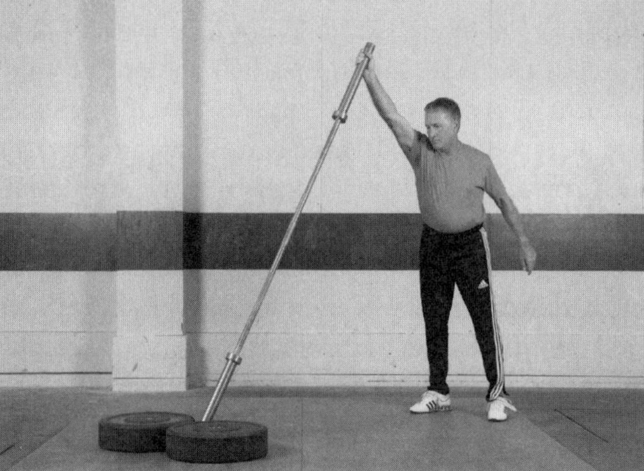

***Figure 10-3.*** The standing one-armed press, using an anchored barbell. *Left,* Bottom position. *Right,* Completed position. A T-bar machine may also be used.

# 11

# A Brief Overview of the Bench Press

In the bench press, the athlete lays on his back on a bench and lowers and raises a barbell over the chest, describing a *nearly* vertical path from the mid-sternum at the bottom to a position directly over the shoulder joints at the top. Of the four primary barbell exercises, the bench is the only one that is not a structural exercise, and it describes the shortest range of motion. However, it allows considerable weight to be handled, and produces marked improvements in upper body strength. The bench trains the anterior muscles of the chest and shoulders, and also trains the muscles of the upper extremity, particularly the triceps. When performed with proper equipment, correct technique, and attention to simple, common sense precautions, the bench press is a completely safe and powerful addition to the General Exercise Prescription. Some Masters will have difficulty with the bench press due to mobility or back health issues, and for a few the exercise will not be accessible. Remedial exercises and bench press alternatives for these athletes are described.

## What is a Bench Press?

A bench press is quite simply a pressing exercise performed while lying supine on a bench. As with all the other exercises we have discussed, the bench press has multitudinous variants. Some of them are quite useful when indicated. Some are fantastically silly. Our attention will be focused on the most prototypical form of the bench press, in which the athlete's torso is parallel to the ground, his feet are flat on the floor, and his grip is of such width as to permit the forearms to be oriented perpendicular to the floor at the bottom of the movement. This model of the bench press is most suitable for general strength acquisition.

The bench press is the most kinetically truncated and limited of the primary barbell exercises presented in this text. It describes the shortest range of motion, has the shortest ***kinetic chain***, uses the least amount of muscle mass, and does not apply a significant load to the axial skeleton, meaning it is not a structural exercise. This makes the bench press the most *theoretically* dispensable of the barbell exercises we have described.

However, the bench press allows very heavy weights to be handled, and therefore produces massive increases in upper body strength. Moreover, for those Masters who cannot perform the press due to mobility issues, the bench is indispensable. And while the squat, press, and deadlift certainly train more muscle, the bench is not to be dismissed in this regard, either. The *pectoralis* muscles, *deltoideus anterior*, *corachobrachialis*, *triceps brachii*, *anconeous*, *trapezius*, the lats, and scapulohumeral muscles all get a workout. In addition, so-called "core" muscles are recruited to stabilize the trunk: *erector spinae*, *serratus anterior*, *transversus abdominus*, *multifidus*, *quadratus lumborum*, and the obliques are involved. This is not an insignificant volume of muscle tissue.

The bench press is therefore a *pretty* big multi-joint exercise that loads a fundamental human movement pattern: pushing hard against a heavy resistance.

## Essentials of Performance

The bench press is a simple exercise, but not without its technical subtleties, as described in detail in *Starting Strength*. We will very briefly review the essentials of performance and touch upon a few points of technique to optimize the mechanics of the lift. But because this exercise is favored by silly people hell-bent on disabling, disfiguring, or dispatching themselves and others, any discussion of the bench press must begin with the primary consideration of safety.

### How not to get killed or maimed

The bench press is the single most dangerous barbell movement, in terms of actual havoc wrought and total body count.[1] This is not the exercise's fault, but is entirely due to human carelessness and stupidity. If we observe a few very simple precautions, the bench is an entirely safe, productive, and enjoyable exercise.

**Bench With a Spotter, or in the Rack.** Ignoring this rule is how most people get themselves hurt on the bench. If the bench press is performed alone, it *must* be performed inside a power rack with the pins set so as to prevent the athlete from being trapped under the bar. If the bench press is performed on a dedicated pressing bench, without safety pins, then a competent spotter is mandatory, to assist the athlete in the event he fails a rep. In such an event, *the athlete must not abandon the bar*. The spotter *helps* the athlete return the bar to the rack.

**Do Not Use a Thumbless Grip.** The bench press must *never* be performed with a thumbless grip. Take a walk through The Circus and you will see people – mostly young males – using such a "suicide grip" on the bench. This is either straightforward testosterone encephalopathy or a misguided approach to positioning the bar over the forearm for better mechanics. This laudable technical goal can be achieved without a thumbless grip, as briefly described below and in definitive detail in *Starting Strength*. Athletes who use a thumbless grip are literally *begging* for disaster. One day, their dreams will come true, much to the delight of a maxillofacial surgeon, neurosurgeon, or undertaker.

**Lock Your Elbows**. The performance of the bench press will require the athlete to unrack the bar from the hooks and then move it into a position over the shoulder joints, where the exercise can begin. This positioning of the bar necessarily entails movement of the load over the face and neck. Regardless of whether this is done in the power rack or with a handoff from a spotter, it must be done *with straight elbows*, locked in extension. Locked elbows are much stronger than "soft" elbows. If the elbows are not locked and the weight is heavy, the arms can fail to support the weight and the bar could come crashing down onto the face, mouth, or throat. This is not ideal.

**Don't Aim for the Hooks**. This is a corollary of the previous rule. The last rep of a bench work set is *heavy*, and there is a natural inclination to aim this rep at the hooks. This cannot be permitted. It is extremely dangerous, for two reasons. First, aiming for the hooks introduces a curved bar path that invites unlocked elbows – and we've seen where *that* can go. Second, if you aim for the hooks, especially as an intrinsic part of a maximal effort (last bench rep), *you could miss.* And you don't want to miss. The results of missing are suboptimal. Always lock out each rep and then aim the bar at the upright part of the rack, *above the hooks.* If you touch the uprights, you're above the hooks, and you won't miss them when you set the bar down.

**Do Not Bounce the Bar Off Your Chest.** In the *Starting Strength* model of the bench, we do not pause at the bottom, as in most powerlifting competitions. But we don't bounce the bar, either. Go to The Circus and you will observe this foolishness: smacking a damn heavy bar against the sternum to harvest a bounce that helps the lifter get the weight out of the hole. This not only dissipates the training effectiveness of the exercise, but it is also dangerous, for reasons we should not have to elaborate. *Touch* the bar lightly to the chest, then drive up.

**Do Not Collar the Bar.** The bench press must never be performed with collars on the bar. If the rep is failed and the lifter is caught under the bar with collars, he cannot unload the bar by tilting off the plates, thereby escaping this deadly predicament. In our opinion, this safety rule holds *even if the athlete is being spotted*, because spotters have an unfortunate tendency to be distracted by the very beautiful young ladies working their Downward Dog stretches on the yoga mats across the room.

## Now that you're safe, you can bench

The bench press begins with the bar set in the hooks of a rack or pressing bench at appropriate height. If in a rack (benching alone), safety pins are set at a height such that, if a rep cannot be completed the bar can be lowered onto the pins safely, just *below* where the top of the chest is positioned during the exercise, by relaxing the arch in the chest. This is because the chest will be more elevated during benching than in a relaxed supine position. Setting the pins at this height will allow full range of motion during the exercise, but still permit the lifter to escape if a failed rep ends up on the pins.

Position yourself on the bench such that the bar in the rack is just above the eyebrows in the horizontal plane. In other words, if a spotter standing behind you at the head of the bench were to look straight down at the bar, your eyes would be just on the other side of the bar. Your feet are flat on the floor with lower back arched and chest elevated. Your upper back at the shoulder blades and the buttocks must remain in contact with the bench, but the lumbar spine should be arched such that a coach could pass a hand between the bench and your lower back.

The shoulders are pulled *down* and *back,* as if you are attempting to hold an object pinched between your shoulder blades. Not only does this enhance the raising of the chest, which improves the angle of chest muscle engagement with the humerus, it also decreases the distance the bar has to travel.

Assume a grip of such a width that, at the bottom of the movement with the bar touching your chest, your forearms will be perpendicular to the ground. This will almost always be about one hand width wider than the press grip. The distance between the hands and the sleeves of the barbell must be equal on both sides, so that each hand carries the same amount of weight. As in the press, carry the bar in the hand over the heel of the palm with your thumb wrapped around the bar, right over the bones of the forearm. *Optimizing the position of the bar over the forearm does not require a thumbless grip.*

With the feet flat, the back arched, the chest high, the shoulder blades retracted, and the proper grip established, take a deep breath and unrack the bar, pushing it straight up out of the hooks, against the uprights. Do *not* attempt to unrack the bar and bring it into position in a single curved movement. Lift the bar straight out of the hooks with the elbows extended and move the bar over the face and throat and into position over the shoulder joints *with locked elbows.* This is the case whether or not there is a spotter to hand off the bar.

With the bar locked out over the shoulder joints, take note of the position of the bar against the ceiling. *Keep your eyes on this point during the*

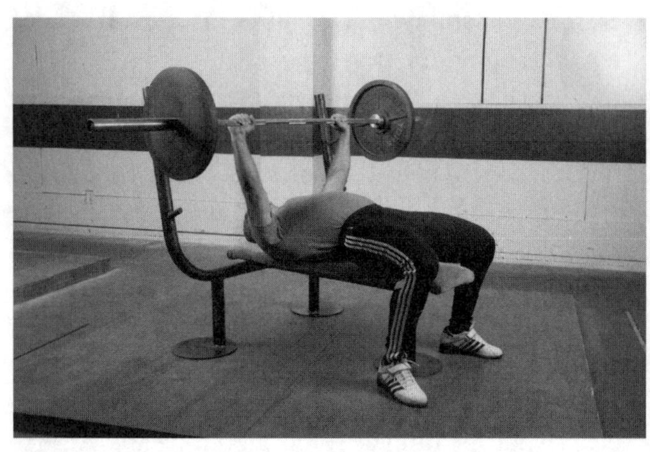
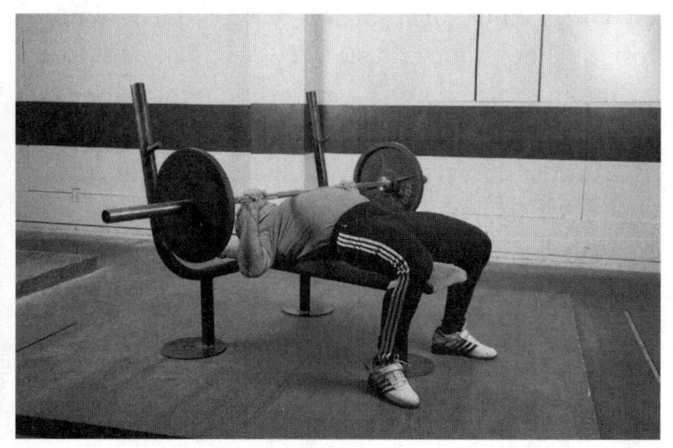

***Figure 11-1.*** The bench press. *Left,* Top position. The bar has been unracked and brought to a position over the shoulder joints on locked elbows. *Right,* Bottom position. The bar has been lowered to the chest at mid-sternum, such that the forearms are vertical and the upper arms describe an angle of about 75 degrees to the torso.

*entire set, bringing the bar to this same point at the end of every repetition.* Lower the bar slowly to touch the middle of your sternum *lightly*, then drive up hard. The mid-sternum position drops the elbows to about 75 degrees of humeral abduction and prevents shoulder impingement. There is no relaxation during the lowering (eccentric) phase. The athlete is always pushing hard against the bar. Do *not* watch the bar, but rather keep your eyes fixed on the stationary reference (that point on the ceiling) and "stare" the bar into place at the top. Breathing occurs *only* at the top of every rep, after the bar is locked out with straight elbows, shoulders still shrugged together against the bench.

The last rep does not aim for the hooks, but rather locks out at the same position as every other rep. Move the bar back to the uprights on straight, locked elbows. Once the bar strikes the uprights, you know it is over the hooks and it can be safely lowered into them.

## Exercise Rx: The Bench Press for the Masters Athlete

We believe the bench press is not as important as the press, which has a longer range of motion, a longer kinetic chain, a longer moment arm, and demands more coordination, timing, balance and mobility. But the bench is nevertheless an extremely useful exercise, and for those who cannot perform the press due to mobility issues it is essential for the development of upper body strength. It is a powerful addition to our General Exercise Prescription.

### The bench press is safe

With the simple precautions previously discussed, the bench press is entirely safe. *You can't even fall down.* You will perform the movement the same way each time, in the rack or with a spotter, over a normal range of motion, on a stable surface, at manageable loads, without unpredictable forces.

### The bench press has a wide therapeutic window

Training in the bench press can begin with a half-pound piece of PVC pipe, if necessary, and proceed from there. In practice, even very deconditioned, very frail, very elderly women can usually bench press a 10-pound bar for repetitions and make regular, steady progress in the exercise. Over the long term, the Masters Athlete can train to put up very impressive weights with this exercise.

### The bench press is a *pretty* big multi-joint exercise

Which makes it a major contribution to our **comprehensive** exercise prescription. Although it has a shorter kinetic chain than the other primary lifts, it nevertheless trains a large volume of tissue in the chest, shoulders, arms, neck, and back. Properly performed, it even recruits a major contribution from the lower extremities. The bench recapitulates a completely natural and useful human movement pattern, that of pushing against a heavy resistance. It allows very heavy weights to be lifted, and develops both strength and power. It digs deep into the high-intensity end of the bioenergetic spectrum.

### The bench press attacks the sick aging phenotype

The bench press is intense, recruits a large volume of muscle, and builds tremendous upper body strength and power. As such, training in this exercise will have beneficial impacts on glucose disposal, insulin sensitivity, neuromuscular and bioenergetic adaptation, cardiovascular health, frailty, and function.

### The bench press is simple

But as should now be apparent, it's not as simple as you probably thought it was. Biomechanical and safety considerations dictate certain technical requirements for the bench, and it must be taught and performed properly. That all being said, the bench can be learned as quickly as any of the other exercises in our prescription, and for athletes with significant limitations in lower body mobility or balance it can produce tremendous increases in strength and confidence early in training, while the standing lifts are still being mastered. This has huge implications for Masters who are particularly physically challenged. Progress in the bench press gives them the confidence and sense of accomplishment they need to stick with the program and continue their training long enough to overcome difficulties they may have with the other exercises.

## Modifying the Bench Press to Your Circumstances

It is uncommon, even among the Masters population, to encounter individuals who cannot perform the barbell bench press. Nevertheless, shoulder mobility issues or chronic low back problems can interfere with performance. For these athletes, the careful substitution of commonly used assistance exercises can confer some of the benefits of the bench press.

### The close-grip bench press

For intermediate and advanced athletes, the close-grip bench press can be a valuable assistance exercise for the upper body. The simple adjustment of narrowing the standard bench press grip (usually to about 12–16 inches apart) imposes significant

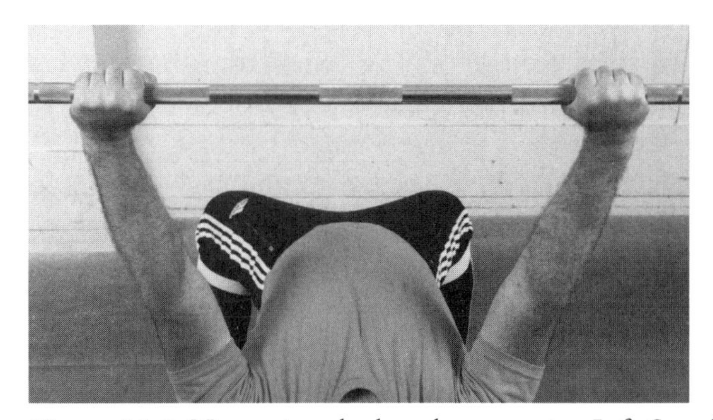

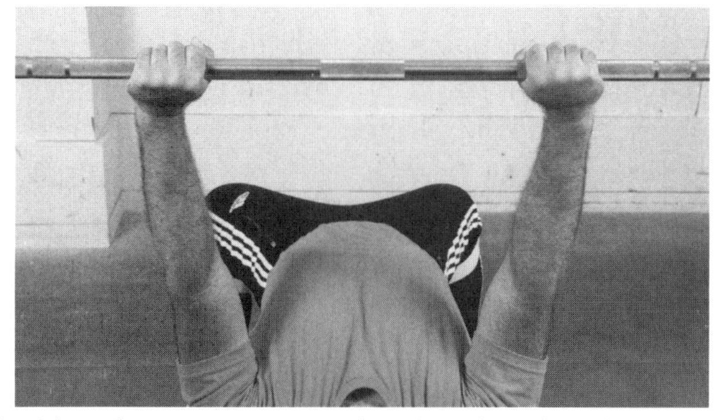

***Figure 11-2.*** Narrowing the bench press grip. *Left,* Standard bench press grip. Note that the edge of the little finger is next to the score in the lateral knurling for this athlete. *Right,* Close grip. Note that the inner edge of the index finger is positioned at about the edge of the lateral knurling. Depending on the needs of the athlete, the grip could be narrowed further.

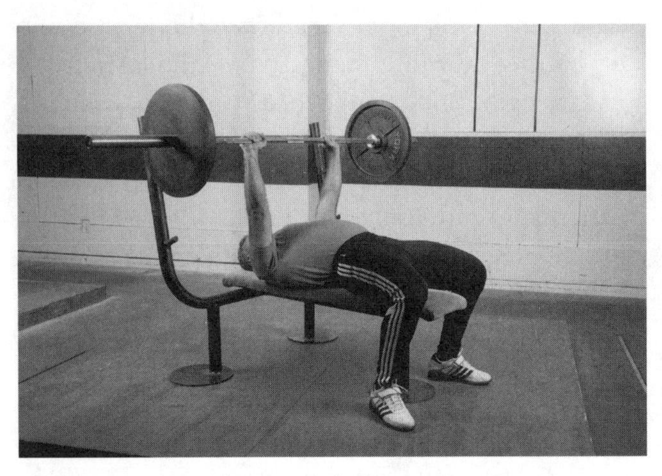

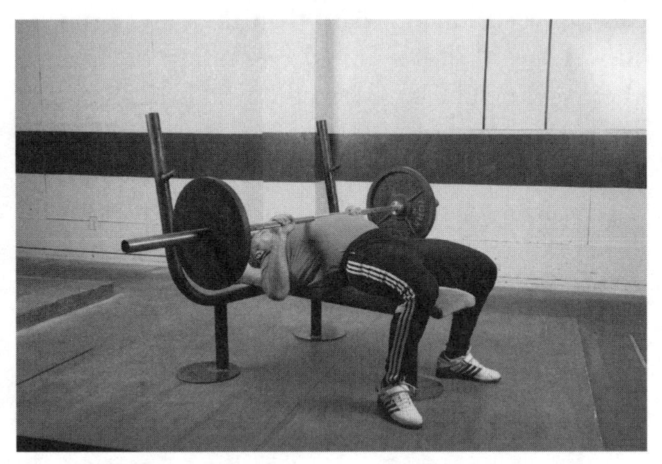

***Figure 11-3.*** Tucking the elbows. In this variation, the athlete combines a close grip with tucked elbows at the bottom of the movement to accommodate decreased mobility or pain in the shoulder. It is instructive to compare this figure with Figure 11-1.

training stress on the triceps. This can have huge returns for a more advanced athlete who is struggling to increase his bench or press (Figure 11-2).

The exercise can also serve as a replacement for the bench in selected trainees. A few novice Masters will have shoulder issues that make bench pressing with a shoulder-width or wider grip painful. In these situations, the easiest fix is usually to narrow the grip.

If the athlete is using the close grip bench press as an *assistance exercise* to regular bench presses, then he will want to move the hands in quite a bit to force the triceps to take on more of the load. He will usually begin by experimenting with a grip that puts his index fingers at the inner border of the lateral knurling – on a bar with industry-standard markings, this dimension is about 16.5 inches. For a larger athlete this is probably the closest he can comfortably set his hands without undue strain on the wrists and elbows. A smaller athlete may experiment with an even narrower grip, adjusting one finger-width at a time. Even the smallest of trainees will never have a grip more narrow than about 10 inches.

In contrast, the athlete who is *replacing* the bench press with a close-grip bench press because of shoulder pain will want to narrow his grip *as little as possible.* Remember, we always want to use the exercise or exercise variant that recruits the largest volume of muscle and allows the heaviest weights to be lifted. The closer the grip on the bench press, the less pectoral muscle mass that can be recruited and the lower the weight that can be handled. Starting with pinkies on the scores, the athlete should experiment at first with a grip that is thumbs-distance from the smooth part of the bar. If this grip is still too wide and pain in the shoulder still occurs, then slowly move the grip in 1 or 2 finger widths at a time until a comfortable position is found.

In addition to using a closer grip, athletes dealing with shoulder pain should also avoid touching the bar too high on the chest. In our experience, this is a more common culprit for shoulder discomfort. With as much of an arch in the back as possible, bringing the bar down below the sternum – just to the very top of the abdominals – often resolves shoulder discomfort on the bench. Further reduction of stress on the shoulder can be achieved by "tucking" the elbows instead of allowing them to flare out to the sides (Figure 11-3). A combination of these 3 techniques – close grip, touching the bar to the upper abs, and tucking the elbows will allow almost any trainee to safely and effectively bench press a barbell.

## The Dumbbell Bench Press

In the uncommon instance that a barbell cannot be effectively utilized, trainees might experiment with flat dumbbell bench presses, using a semi-pronated

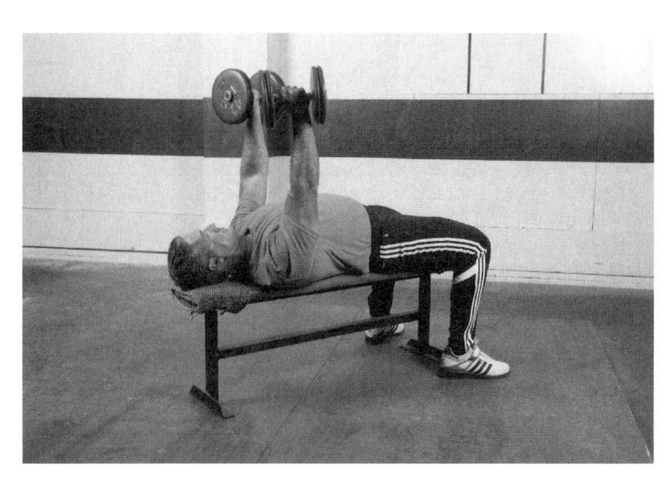

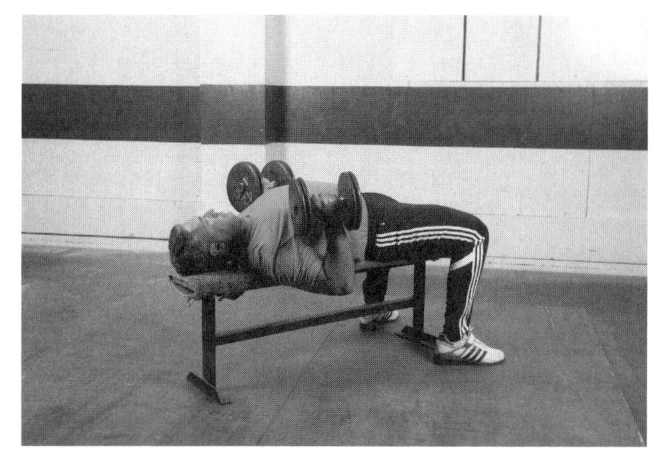

***Figure 11-4.*** The dumbbell bench press. In this case, the trainee is performing the exercise using a neutral grip, as described in the text.

or neutral grip (palms facing each other). Keeping the palms facing each other and the elbows tucked may allow the trainee to bench without shoulder pain (Figure 11-4).

Dumbbell bench presses require programming modifications. They demonstrate erratic progress and are extremely sensitive to small weight increases. Fixed-repetition-number sets across (Chapter 17) are not a good idea for dumbbell work. Instead, trainees should operate within a range. Three to four sets of 6 to 8 reps are effective for dumbbells. Progression can occur when at least one set within the workout achieves 8 reps, and no set drops below 6. Microloading should be used to the extent possible. For most Masters, 5-pound increases on a barbell bench are significant; for dumbbell bench presses 5-pound jumps will frequently be unworkable. In some well-equipped gyms sets of dumbbells in 2.5-pound increments are available. If not, then trainees should invest in a set of magnetized 1.25-pound PlateMates (available on Amazon) that can be stuck to the sides of each dumbbell and allow for 2.5-pound increases.

### Back pain: shimming and the incline bench press

Some trainees cannot tolerate a flat barbell bench press. In some rare cases issues other than shoulders make the flat bench a problem. Very overweight trainees (young or old) may struggle to get on and off the bench without assistance, and may have difficulty maintaining balance while on the flat bench. Some trainees with chronic pain or stiffness in the lumbar or thoracic spine may find that a completely flat position is too painful to maintain on a rigid surface. Shimming of the feet with wood blocks or rubber mats can often alleviate back pain (Figure 11-5).

Shimming tends to work well if the pain is in the hips or lumbar spine, but pain in the mid or upper back usually persists. In these instances, the incline bench press is probably indicated (Figure 11-6). Incline bench presses usually take the same standard grip as a flat bench press and operate with the same basic mechanics, but the barbell will be lowered to just below the clavicle, to the upper chest. Inclines can be programmed in the same manner as a flat barbell bench press.

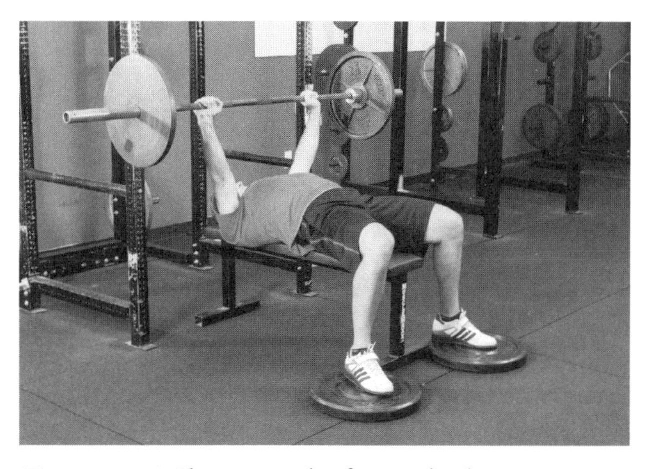

***Figure 11-5.*** Shimming the feet with plates.

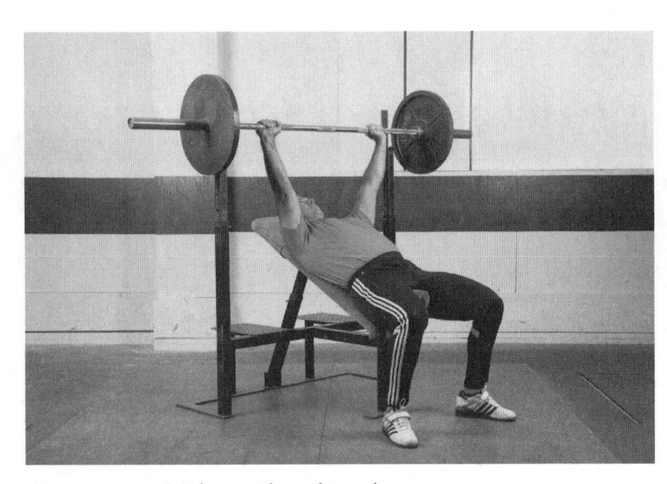

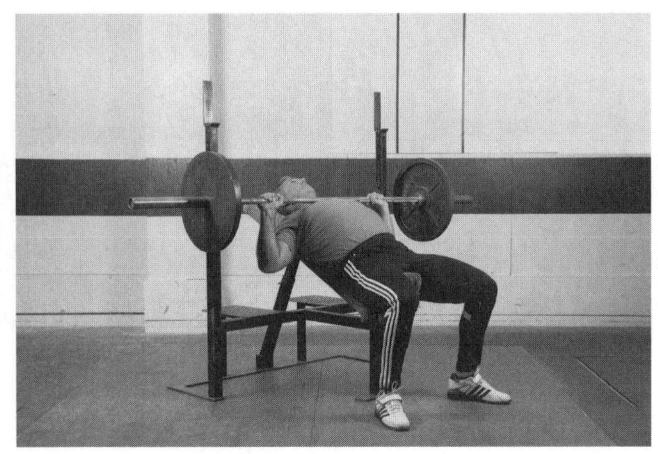

***Figure 11-6.*** The incline bench press.

# 12

# A Brief Overview of the Power Clean and Power Snatch

The power clean and power snatch are training variants of the corresponding Olympic weightlifting movements, the clean and the snatch. These exercises begin by pulling the barbell from the floor in a fashion very similar to the deadlift, but after the bar leaves the floor the lifter accelerates the load which culminates in an explosive jump that creates full extension at the ankles, knees and hips, driving the barbell upward without the use of the arms. The barbell is then caught on the shoulders (clean) or overhead (snatch). In the power clean and power snatch, the movement does not finish in a full squat or split position, as in the customary competition versions. Olympic movements train the display of power, the first derivative of strength, or "strength displayed quickly." They are more technical than the other primary barbell lifts in the exercise prescription, and rely to a greater extent on speed, agility, mobility, and timing. These Olympic variants are to be used with great caution in the Masters Athlete, and only when the trainee demonstrates the requisite desire, aptitude, and ability to tolerate and recover from such training. The power snatch and power clean are described briefly and their utility and limitations for Masters training are discussed in detail.

## What are Power Cleans and Power Snatches?

In Olympic weightlifting, the two contested lifts are the snatch and the clean and jerk. In the ***snatch***, a barbell is pulled from the floor to a position overhead in a single, uninterrupted movement. The bar is caught with straight elbows – it may not be pressed out to full extension – and it is usually (but not always) racked with the lifter in a deep overhead squat position, to reduce the distance the lifter has to pull the heavy weight. The lifter stands erect to finish the lift. In the ***clean and jerk***, the barbell is pulled from the floor and caught on the shoulders, usually (but not always) in a deep front squat position, again to shorten the distance the bar has to be pulled. This is the *clean* portion of the lift. The lifter then stands erect and slams the bar overhead in a single sharp, explosive movement (the *jerk*), once again racking the load on fully extended arms.

The ***power snatch*** is a training variant of the "full" snatch, in which the bar is pulled from the floor and racked as in the snatch, but the athlete does

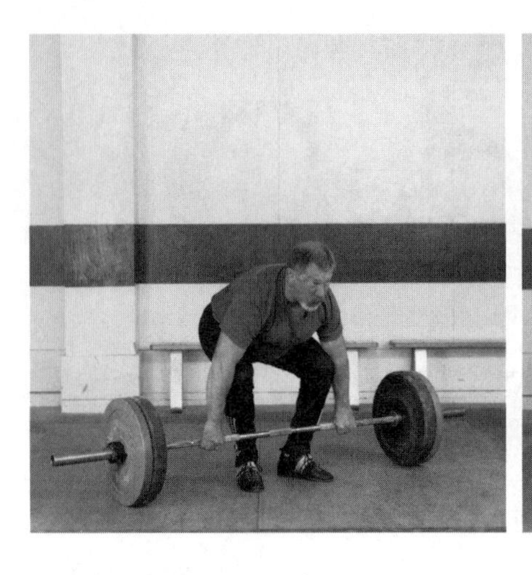

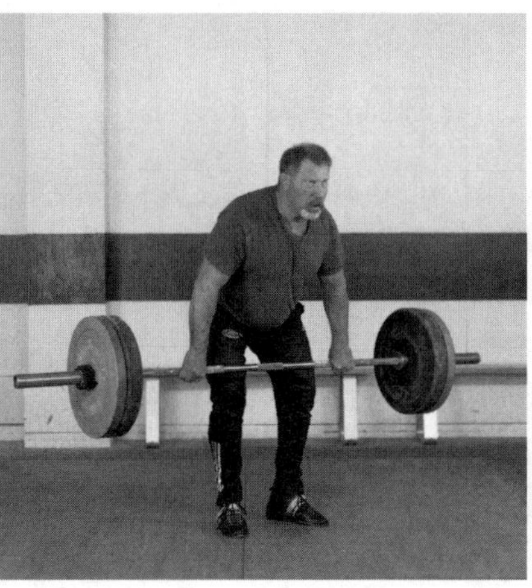

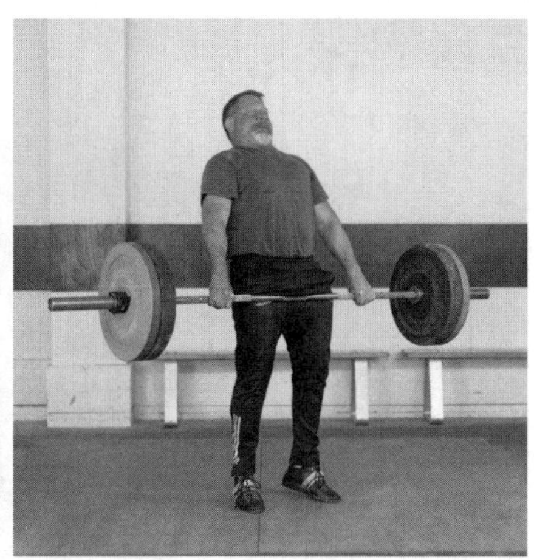

not receive the bar in a full squat position. Similarly, the ***power clean*** is a training variant of the clean portion of the clean and jerk. The athlete pulls the bar from the floor and catches it on the shoulders, but does not receive it in a full front squat. In both of these power variants, the athlete receives the bar in a high partial squat position, well above parallel. This requires the bar to be pulled higher than in the "full" versions of the lifts. Training in the power versions does not allow as much weight to be lifted, and requires a bit less flexibility, speed, skill, and mobility. And they are *probably* somewhat easier on the knees and easier on recovery capacity. The power variants therefore allow all types of athletes, not just Olympic weightlifters, to train these movements.

That's important, because cleans and snatches have a lot to offer the athlete who can train with them. Both of these movements are intrinsically explosive. They require the production of force *quickly*, which means they display and practice *power* production. For example, if we move a 100-pound bar from the floor to a position 4 feet above the floor, we do the same amount of *work* on the bar whether we lift it slowly or quickly: 400 foot-pounds (ft-lb). *Work* is not dependent on *time*. But *power* is: when we lift the 100-pound bar 4 feet in 1 second, we are expressing 10 times more power than if we do it in 10 seconds (400 ft-lb/s vs. 40 ft-lb/s, or 540 watts vs. 54 watts). The ability to express power – the ability to *explode* – is fundamental to all athletic endeavors, except for the boring ones.

In both the clean and the snatch, the bar is pulled from the floor like a deadlift, and then it begins to *accelerate* – its velocity increases the higher it moves – until it reaches a position on the thigh where the athlete must *jump,* explosively slamming hips, knees, and ankles into full and powerful extension. In a fraction of a second, the athlete transforms from a bent-over mid-pull posture into a straight-up skyrocket. This violent jump marks the end of the acceleration of the bar in the vertical direction, and if it is moving fast enough it can be racked on extended arms overhead (snatch) or on the shoulders (clean). The quest for the *jump* allows these movements to demonstrate the athlete's capacity for explosion.

It is very important to note that power is quite dependent on the inherent genetic capacity for explosion. For people who are not endowed with explosive talent – you know who you are – the ability to develop more explosive capacity, and therefore more power, is quite limited for a variety of reasons having to do with the nature of the nervous system and the intrinsic quality of muscle tissue. If a slow athlete could become a quick athlete, there would be a lot of quick athletes – there aren't.

**The power movements are important because they allow us to improve our ability to display what power we *can* produce as the strength upon which it is based increases.**

But the explosive nature of these two movements is a double-edged sword. On the one hand, their dynamic quality makes them valuable tools for matching power display to increasing strength. As strength increases, power increases, because power is strength displayed quickly, and

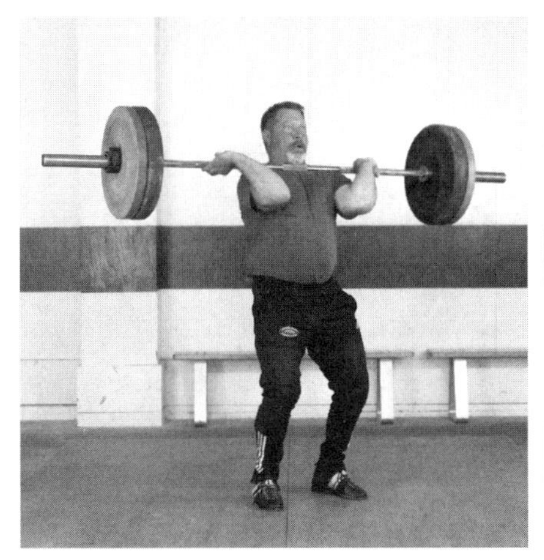
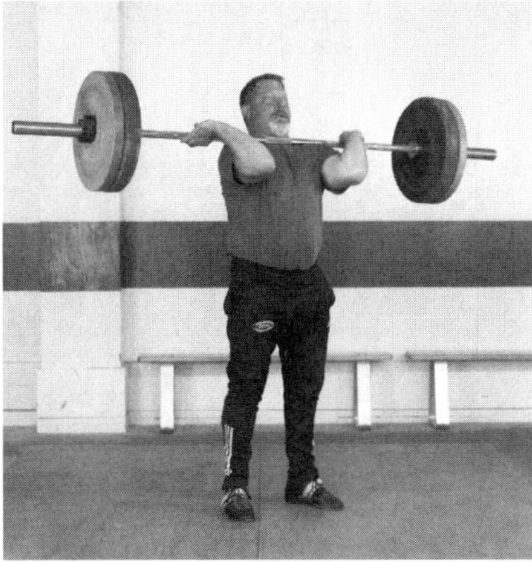

***Figure 12-1.*** The power clean.

*without strength there is no power to display.* On the other hand, these very same explosive and dynamic qualities limit their applicability and safety for Masters Athletes. The clean and snatch can be hard on aging tendons, ligaments, and joints. They challenge the older athlete's capacity to recover, and can interfere with performance and progress on the more fundamental and important exercises. And there are other alternatives, less technically and physiologically demanding, for the improvement of power display for the Masters Athlete.

Accordingly, *we consider the power clean and power snatch to be entirely optional movements for the Masters population.* They are powerful, beautiful, exciting movements, and some Masters are understandably infatuated with them. But they aren't for everybody. For those select athletes who enjoy them, who have aptitude for them, *and* who are able to tolerate and recover from them, they are wonderful additions to the program. But they must be used *with great caution* in the Masters population, and only under the direction of an experienced, judicious, and careful coach.

## Essentials of Performance

More so even than with the previously discussed exercises, we must again emphasize that it is not our purpose here to instruct the reader in how to perform the power clean and power snatch. For more comprehensive analytic and technical treatment of these movements, the reader is directed to *Starting Strength: Basic Barbell Training, 3rd edition.* For *instruction* in these movements, the reader is directed to a qualified strength coach.

Both the power clean and the power snatch are pulls from the floor, which means that, at a very fundamental level, they both recapitulate the mechanics of the deadlift.

### The power clean

In the *Starting Strength* system, the power clean is taught from the top down, and only after the deadlift has been mastered. Our purpose here is simply to describe the movement as it is performed, not as it is taught (Figure 12-1).

The power clean setup is identical to that of the deadlift, except that the grip will usually be somewhat wider. This has to do with contribution of upper extremity anthropometry to the rack position. From this deadlift setup, the athlete pulls the bar from the floor, exactly as in the deadlift, keeping the bar in contact with the legs.

As the bar rises from the floor, it accelerates, building velocity as it gets higher, all the while remaining in contact with the legs. At a discrete position in the middle of the thigh, the bar breaks contact with the thighs as peak velocity is achieved. This looks like an explosive "jump" *with straight elbows* – and indeed, this is the way the movement is taught, although the bar velocity that permits this jump was accumulated during the pull from the instant the bar left the floor.

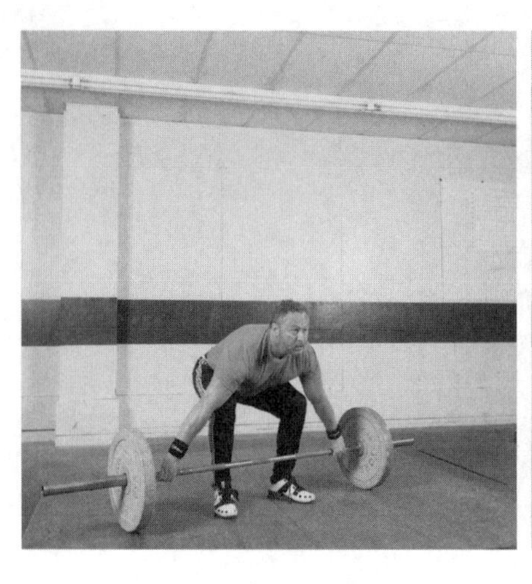
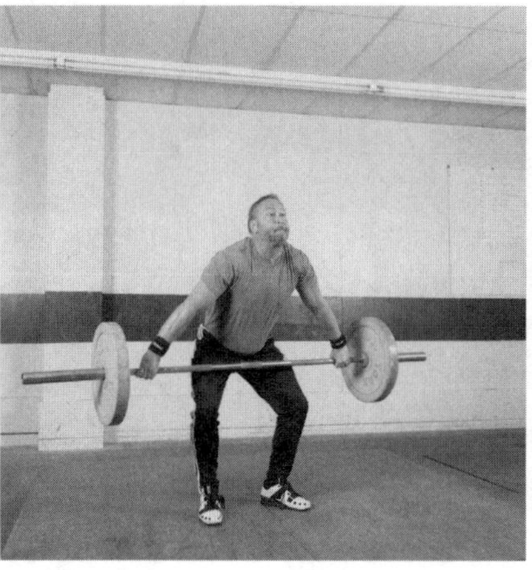
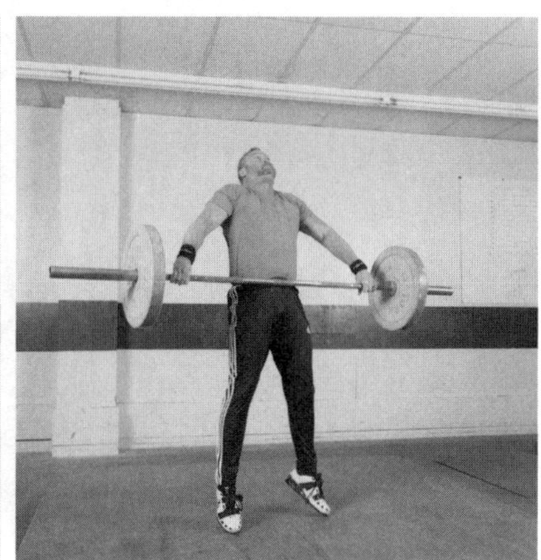

After the bar leaves contact with the thighs, it continues upward under the momentum imparted to it during the pull. *The bar is not pulled up with the arms.* The upper extremities do *nothing* during the pull except connect the bar to the lifter – the bar goes up because of the acceleration produced by the extending hips and knees during the pull. After the jump, the arms merely guide the bar onto the shoulders.

In the next few milliseconds, a lot of stuff happens, none of which need be of any concern to the athlete. The less he thinks about them, the better. From his perspective, he jumps, his feet break contact with the ground as a result of the upward momentum, and then he immediately catches the bar on the shoulders as his feet land. The elbows slam up, pointing straight forward, to trap the bar on the deltoids.

The bar is *not* received in the hands, and it should not strike the sternum or the collar bone – it lands on the bellies of the contracted deltoid muscles. The lifter receives the bar in a high quarter-squat position, with the knees and hips slightly flexed, in an erect position. His feet move from the narrower pulling stance into a wider, more stable stance (which may in fact be the same stance as the squat) as he receives the bar on his shoulders, and the receiving position should be completely stable and balanced. At the completion of the movement, the athlete stands erect with the bar still racked on the shoulders. He then either allows the bar to fall down the front of his torso to be caught in the hands (like the top of a deadlift), or drops the bar to the platform (if equipped with bumper plates).

### The power snatch

As with the power clean, the power snatch is taught from the top down, and only after the deadlift has been mastered. The snatch setup is identical to that of the deadlift, except the grip will always be much wider. When the bar is held in the hang position – the position of the lifter standing fully erect with the bar hanging from straight elbows – for the snatch, it sits just above the pubic bone and just below the "hip pointers" (the anterior superior iliac spine). From this snatch-grip deadlift setup, the athlete pulls the bar from the floor, exactly as in the deadlift, keeping the bar in contact with the legs (Figure 12-2).

As with the clean, the pull accelerates the bar off the floor, and at the top of the pull the bar velocity will bring the bar into contact with the hang position on the lower belly. From here the bar breaks contact with the body, and continues on upward under the momentum of the pull. Again, this is thought of as a "jump" even though it is the culmination of the acceleration. Elbows kept straight during the pull then break as the elbows and wrists lead the bar upward into the rack position overhead.

As the arms are changing from pulling tools to catching tools, the feet are breaking contact with the floor with the upward momentum of the pull, as the stance shifts from that of narrower pull to the wider catching stance, for stability. The elbows bend and the wrists "turn over," and *the torso drops*

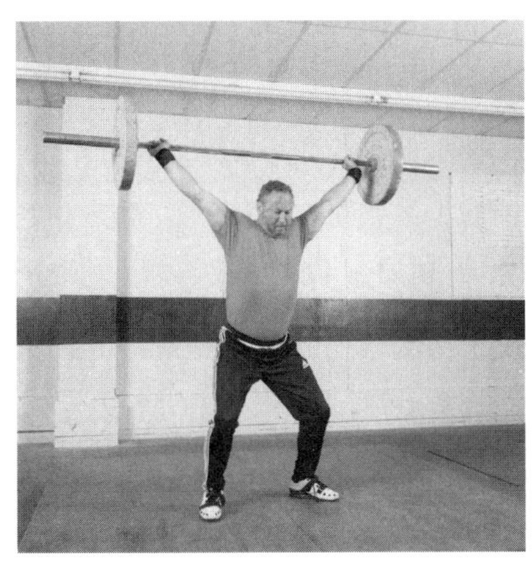
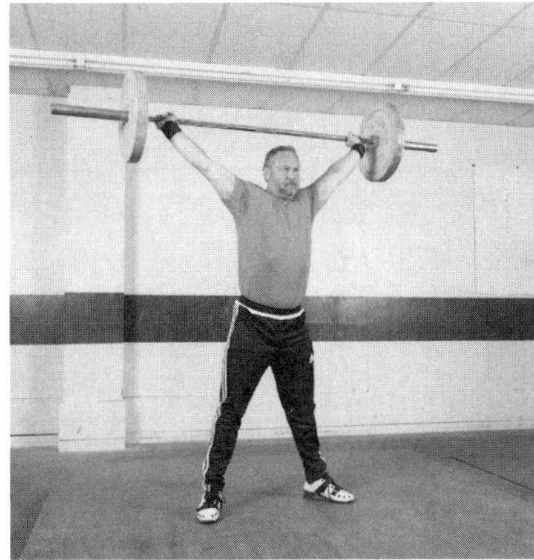

***Figure 12-2.*** The power snatch.

*down to straighten out the elbows and wrists* as the bar is finally racked overhead. This is perhaps the most important aspect of the snatch: the bar is not pressed into lockout – the *drop* straightens out the elbows and wrists, not the triceps and deltoids. Any "press-out" in this position is intrinsically dangerous, it disqualifies a snatch in competition, and it should not be tolerated in training.

As with the press, the top of the snatch balances the bar over both the shoulder joints and the middle of the foot. The lifter receives the bar in a high quarter-squat position, with the knees and hips slightly flexed. The receiving position must be stable and balanced. At the completion of the exercise, the athlete stands erect with the bar still racked overhead on straight elbows. He then either catches the bar in the hang or, if equipped with bumpers, drops it and tends it to the platform.

## Exercise Rx: Olympic Movements for the Masters Athlete

The Olympic movements are not essential components of training for the Masters Athlete. They do satisfy some criteria of our exercise prescription, but none that are not already met in full by the primary exercises already discussed. Most Masters, especially those over 50, can dispense with them entirely. But some enjoy, tolerate, and benefit from the clean and snatch. Particularly fit and active Masters who engage in sports or professions that demand expression of power (track and field, combat sports, rugby, soccer, military and police work, etc.) may productively train these movements, but these individuals tend to be the exception rather than the rule.

### THE OLYMPIC MOVEMENTS *MAY* BE SAFE, DEPENDING ON THE ATHLETE

Aging joints, ligaments, tendons, and muscles can take a real beating with the clean and the snatch. The power clean demands excellent mobility of the shoulders, wrists and elbows. The power snatch requires great flexibility and strength at the shoulder. Both movements require the lifter to receive a heavy bar in a partial squat position, which places a significant impulsive stress on the feet, ankles, knees, hips, and spine. Because these movements are intrinsically dynamic, explosive, and technically demanding, the potential for missing a rep is significantly greater than for missing a deadlift, squat, or pressing movement, even at light loads. Missed reps present the possibility, however remote, of injury. Olympic weightlifting is an *extremely* safe activity,[1] both in training and competition, and injuries tend to be minor. But Masters heal more slowly, and a sprained wrist or shoulder can wreak havoc on a training program. Masters who demonstrate the desire, technical aptitude, and capacity to recover from training in the clean and snatch can and should do so, but both athlete and coach must be cognizant of the risks, and ever vigilant.

### The olympic movements have a *fairly* wide therapeutic window

As with the other movements, training in the clean and snatch can begin at very light weight. Most Masters begin training with a 10- or 15-pound bar. The therapeutic window is rather more limited at the high end, however. Our experience shows that most Masters, even those who demonstrate the capacity to train in these movements, reach a plateau in the weights they can handle relatively early, at a time when they are still making great progress in the slow lifts. They are more constrained by mobility, recovery capacity, motor recruitment, and their innate explosiveness than their younger counterparts. But with careful, patient, regular training, select Masters Athletes can put up fairly heavy weights in the clean and snatch.

### The olympic movements are big multi-joint exercises

Which allows them to contribute to **comprehensive** exercise prescription. Both are total body movements that recruit a huge volume of muscle. They drill deep into the high-power end of the energy spectrum, relying entirely on the phosphagen system for the development of power. They emphasize grace, balance, mobility, and timing.

### The olympic movements attack the sick aging phenotype

If they can be trained productively, the Olympic movements will confer beneficial impacts on glucose disposal, insulin sensitivity, neuromuscular and bioenergetic adaptation, cardiovascular health, frailty, and function.

They can also be tremendously rewarding at a deeper level. Those Masters who *can* train the power clean or power snatch invariably derive a tremendous sense of accomplishment from mastering a technically demanding exercise, one which allows them to express strength rapidly and with grace and beauty. The potential impact of a such an achievement on a Masters' confidence and self-image is not to be dismissed.

### The olympic movements are *relatively* simple

We have stated repeatedly that these movements are technically demanding, and this alone presents a barrier to training in the clean and snatch. Nevertheless, and notwithstanding the over-emphasis on the difficulty of these movements in much of the literature, we should point out that, provided he has learned the deadlift and can demonstrate good pulling mechanics, an athlete with adequate mobility can be taught to do a reasonably adequate clean or snatch in less than an hour. The dynamic nature of these movements means that minor form errors have a disproportionate effect on performance, relative to the slow lifts, and constant refinement of technique is mandatory. But it is a mistake to assume, as some would have us believe, that these exercises require months or years of practice to achieve the requisite training proficiency to make progress. It just isn't so. In the final analysis, they're just deadlifts that become jumps to launch the bar upward to the rack position.[2]

## Use with Great Caution

We know we're repeating ourselves here, but it's important: Most Masters *need* not and *should* not train in the Olympic lifts. Their fundamental utility lies in their ability to practice power production. And power is certainly important. But there are other options available to the Master for the development of power.

For a deconditioned Master, power is best developed by increasing strength. Again, this is easy to demonstrate. Strength is the ability to develop a force against a resistance, like a heavy barbell. When we express force against a barbell, and make it move, we do ***work***:

**Work = Force x Distance**

Power is, loosely speaking, the ability to work rapidly. Technically, it is the rate at which work is done:

**Power = Work/Time = (Force x Distance)/Time**

The reader who examines the foregoing equations will readily see that the ability to produce *force* is fundamental to both strength and power. Power is the first derivative of strength. This means, very simply, that if you increase the strength of a movement pattern, you immediately increase the power of that movement pattern, even if you don't do it any more quickly, because you're doing more work in about the same amount of time.

More advanced trainees can develop the power of a strong movement by increasing the speed at which the movement is performed. *Dynamic effort training* uses this simple physical fact, and is discussed in detail in Part III: Programming.

In summary, the power clean and power snatch have limited utility for Masters Athletes. They present technical, physiological, and practical challenges, they make heavy demands on the recovery capacity of the athlete, and they address performance attributes that are more easily and safely trained with other modalities. They are not *necessary* for the realization of our General Exercise Prescription. For those Masters who are willing and able to train them productively, they can be *immensely* rewarding. But they must be learned and trained properly, with tremendous care and vigilance on the part of both athlete and coach.

# 13
# Assistance Exercises

Assistance exercises are used to supplement or replace the primary barbell exercises used in strength training. As supplements, they are usually prescribed no sooner than a few weeks after the onset of novice training. As replacement exercises, they are used as indicated to take the place of a primary barbell movement until that movement can be performed.

## The Role of Assistance Exercises

Assistance exercises are frequently misunderstood and misused. Their proper role is to supplement and support progress in the primary barbell movements, but all too often they end up becoming the core of a strength training "program." This is unfortunate, because they are completely unsuited for such a role. These movements typically recruit less muscle, use a shorter range of motion, impose less comprehensive training stresses, promote less general adaptation, and have far less potential for progressive development than the squat, deadlift, and pressing movements. When you see somebody in a gym whose workout consists of barbell curls, leg presses, lat pull-downs, dips, and maybe bench presses, you're looking at somebody who is, in the words of Jim Wendler, "majoring in the minors."

Assistance exercises are *properly* indicated in any number of training circumstances:

1. Helping particularly weak or deconditioned trainees develop the requisite strength, mobility or exercise capacity to perform the primary barbell movements. An example would be the leg press for those not yet strong enough to squat.

2. Substituting, temporarily or permanently, for a primary barbell movement that the trainee cannot perform, or to give a tired athlete a break from a particularly heavy exercise without completely detraining the movement. Close-grip bench work for athletes with

shoulder problems that prohibit standard-grip benches is a good example, as is the substitution of straight-leg deadlifts to promote recovery for an athlete who has been pulling heavy and is starting to stagnate.

3. Promoting strength gains in more advanced athletes who are on the flat part of the strength curve. Again, close-grip bench work is a good example, as are rack pulls, halting deadlifts, and dips.

4. Assistance exercises can address a particular attribute that the trainee or coach wishes to emphasize in training. Athletes interested in upper body hypertrophy, for example, will want to know how to do barbell curls.

It is not the purpose of this chapter to present the full range of assistance exercises available or all the situations in which they may be used. Our goal here is to illustrate the assistance exercises most commonly referenced in Part III of this text. The implementation, programming, and proper performance of assistance exercises demands experience and judgment, and the input and guidance of a good coach is important.

## Chin-ups and Pull-ups

The trainee should perform chin-ups and/or pull-ups if capable of doing so. They are perhaps the most valuable non-barbell movements in the entire arsenal of strength-training exercises. Most strength coaches consider them to be fundamental. The primary drawback to chin-ups and pull-ups is that many novice trainees, especially Masters, cannot do them. For these athletes there are other options, as discussed below.

Chin-ups ("chins") and pull-ups performed through the full range of motion quite thoroughly work the musculature of the lats, upper back, forearms, and biceps. Which variation you choose is not terribly important and many trainees alternate between the two. Chins are performed with the arms supinated, such that the bar is gripped with the palms facing the lifter (Figure 13-1, left panels). Pull-ups are performed with the forearms pronated, with the palms facing away (Figure 13-1, right panels). Chins use more muscle mass and are usually stronger than pull-ups. Chins recruit much greater involvement of the biceps while pull-ups place more stress on the forearms and the lats.

As with most assistance exercises, chins and pull-ups cannot be programmed at the same level of precision as big multi-joint barbell movements. Performance capabilities vary from day to day on both exercises and experience shows that a predictable linear progression is never realized. Baker is fond of telling his Masters that chins and pull-ups are a "completion grade" at the end of the workout. We do them, but are not overly concerned with the numbers improving at every session. Instead, we judge performance on a monthly basis.

An excellent way to program both exercises is through the use of ***repetition totals.*** In this approach, the trainee and coach simply select a set number of pull-ups or chins to achieve – 20, for example. The trainee tries to reach that number, performing as many sets as it takes to attain the total. Progression is monitored along two metrics: the total number of reps achieved on the first set, and the number of sets needed to achieve the target number of reps. One reason for the difficulty in assessing progress is that improvement on the first set of the day often comes at the expense of all sets that follow. For this reason, the first set is a good indicator of how chin/pull-up strength is coming along. Instead of tracking the exact number of reps on every following set, it is more useful to track the total number of sets it takes to reach a certain target. So when 20 total pull-ups can be achieved in 3 sets instead of 4, progress has occurred. Every few weeks or months (depending on the athlete and his progress) the rep totals can increase by 5 or 10.

Once the trainee has a rep total of around 50 per workout, then it is more useful to add weight to the first couple of sets than it is to add more reps. A good strategy is to perform the first 20 or so reps with added weight, and finish the rest of them off at bodyweight for higher rep sets.

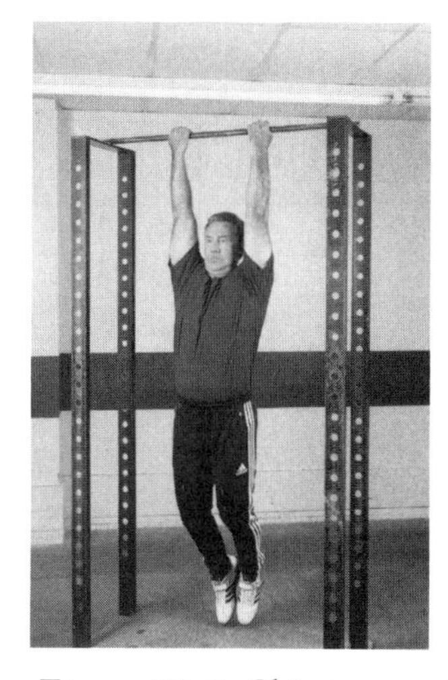
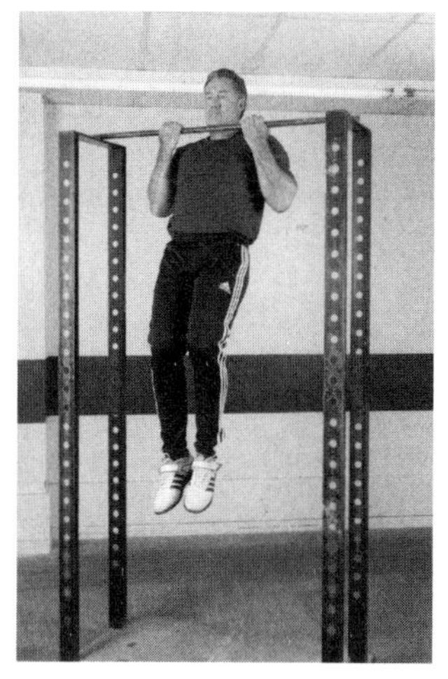
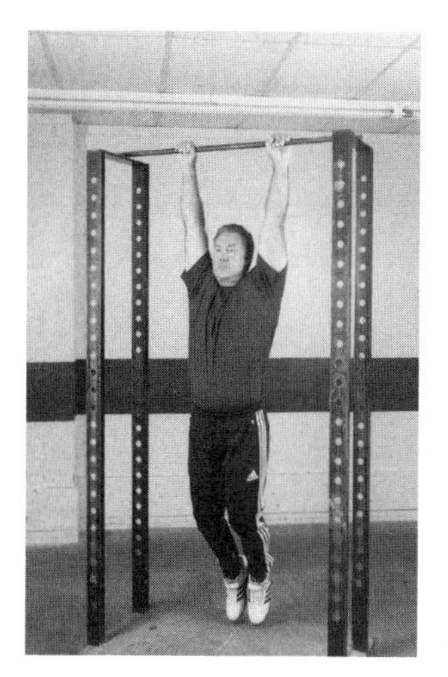
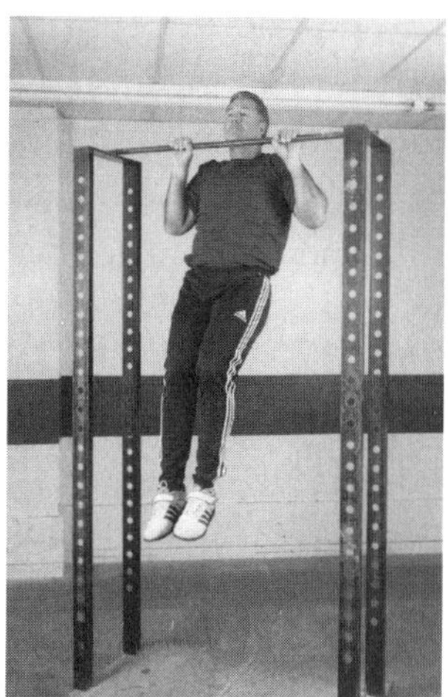

***Figure 13-1.*** Chin-ups and pull-ups. *Left panels,* Chin-ups are performed with the hands supinated, such that the palms face toward the trainee. *Right panels,* Pull-ups are performed with the hands pronated.

Even for Masters, who tend to be sensitive to volume, higher volume on chins and pull-ups is usually feasible without the soreness and inflammation seen with similar volumes on heavy barbell exercises.

## Bodyweight Rows and Lat Pull-downs

For those Masters who cannot perform pull-ups or chins due to excessive bodyweight or a lack of strength, lat pull-downs ("lat pulls") or bodyweight rows are excellent alternatives.

Bodyweight rows are best performed on a pair of straps or rings, although a barbell set in a power rack at the proper height is a suitable alternative, provided the bar is being pulled into the uprights during the performance of the set (so that the bar does not pull out of the hooks during a rep). With the rest of the body held completely rigid, the trainee pulls himself to a position where the hands are against the torso, squeezing the shoulder blades together at the top (Figure 13-2). The exercise is made more difficult by walking the feet out to the front (making the body more horizontal) and made easier by walking the feet backward (more vertical). Bodyweight rows are done for high-rep sets (around 10). Programming can use rep totals as a progress metric, as with chins and pull-ups. Alternatively, they can be programmed for 3–4 sets of a fixed number of repetitions. The feet may be adjusted between and during sets so that prescribed volume can be completed.

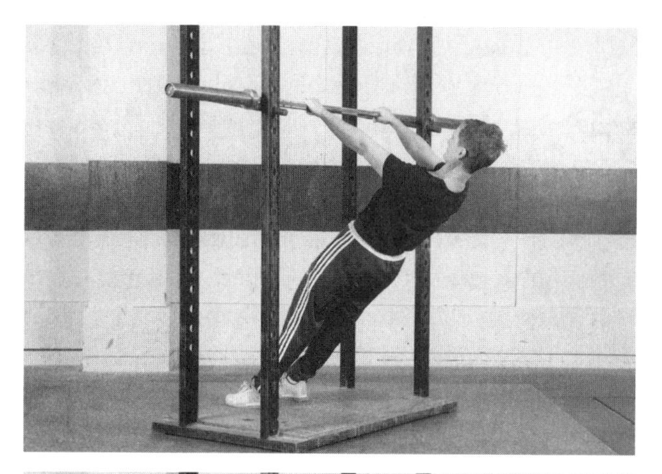
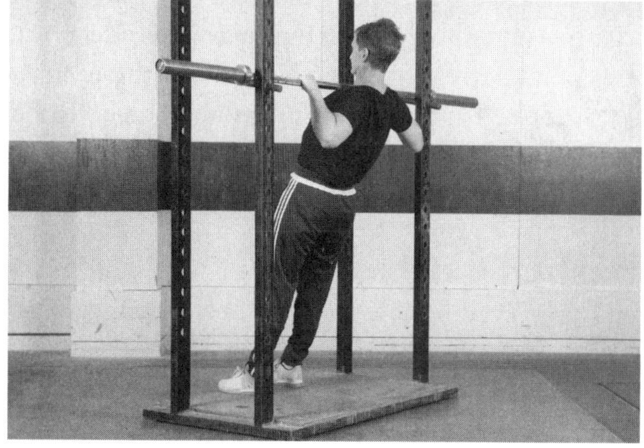

***Figure 13-2.*** Bodyweight rows.

Lat pull-downs (Figure 13-3) allow for a more precise, almost linear approach. They are indicated for Masters who are too weak to perform chins or pull-ups. These Masters will often experience tremendous improvement in their shoulder mobility with lat pull-down work over the long term.

Grips on a lat pull-down machine can vary. We prefer the reverse grip, which mimics a chin-up grip (Figure 13-3, top). This will allow for the fullest range of motion, the most amount of weight to be used, and the most muscle to be trained. It also is the easiest grip for the trainee to learn and for the coach to teach.

The slightly wider overhand grip (Figure 13-3, bottom left), which mimics a pull-up, is also useful but uses less weight and works less muscle mass. This grip is also more difficult for the trainee to "feel" working the upper back. Early novice trainees will often lack upper back muscle control and won't have much command over what their upper back muscles are doing. Most will report only feeling this exercise in their arms.

Close, parallel-grip pull-downs (Figure 13-3, bottom right) can be useful for those who experience wrist pain with the reverse grip pull-down and cannot control the wide-grip pull-down. The neutral grip puts no strain on the wrist and the close-grip allows for the exercise to be performed with a great deal of control. Older, weaker trainees may perform the other two variations with a great degree of "wobble" in the longer handle. This causes an uneven descent and can cause the exercise to become quite sloppy at heavier weights.

Whatever grip is used, good form, rather than weight, should be the primary consideration. The weight will come, but only when the exercise is performed properly. Masters will make good progress on 3 to 4 sets of 8–12 reps.

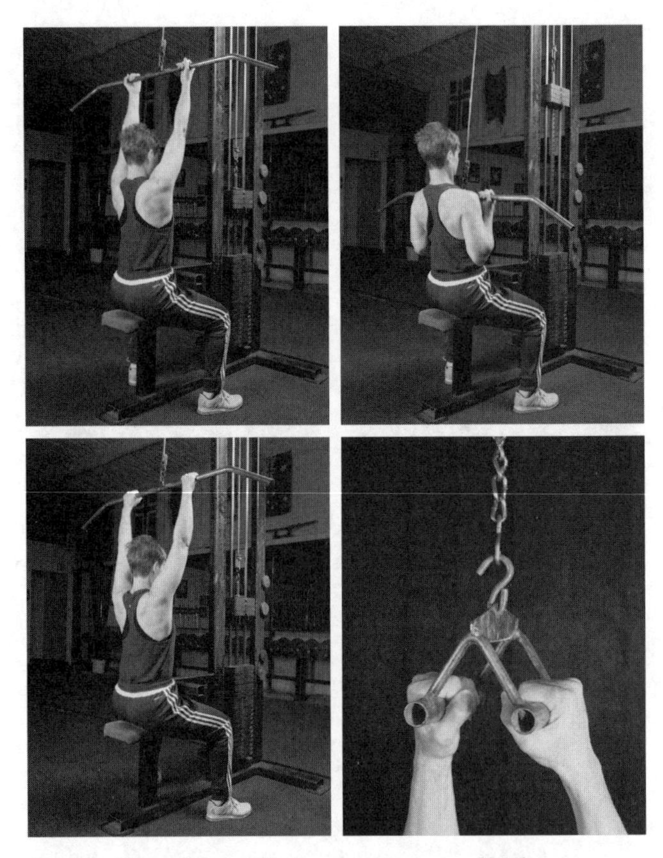

***Figure 13-3.*** Lat pull-downs. *Top panels,* The reverse grip mimics the chin-up grip, and is preferred by the authors for most Masters. *Bottom left,* The overhand grip. *Bottom right,* A parallel-grip is useful for some Masters with wrist pain.

## Barbell Curls

Curls are the very archetype of an overused exercise with limited utility, especially for those who are most prone to use them (young men). They train a very limited amount of muscle mass through a relatively short range of motion, do not promote the same tremendous gains in functional strength as the primary movements, usually confer very minimal health and performance benefits, and can easily result in overuse injuries. These latter often turn out to be quite unpleasant, stubborn, and persistent.

That all being said, curls are not *completely* useless. They promote accumulation of muscle mass, however limited, and that's always a good thing. Some trainees, even Masters, appreciate the cosmetic effects of strength training, and if it helps a Master stick with the program, that's a good thing, too. And as it happens, the barbell curl, if properly performed and programmed, can be a useful assistance exercise for selected Masters with limitations in the primary barbell movements (Figure 13-4).

Although mostly unrelated in terms of muscle groups trained, barbell curls are a useful exercise for those trainees who cannot perform the overhead press. Curls offer an opportunity to train an upper body barbell movement while standing on two feet, rather than sitting on a bench or machine. Heavy barbell curls, performed standing, not only work the biceps, shoulders, and forearms, but also the abdominals and a little of the upper back. Many will report unexpected soreness in the abs and traps after their first exposure to the exercise. And like all other barbell movements trained while standing, curls train the fitness attribute of balance. Since you have to *not fall over* to complete the exercise, increasing ability on the curl (or deadlift or squat) also represents an increased ability to *not fall over.* This is an important consideration for athletes over 60. Barbell curls make an excellent addition to the program for those older trainees who can't do a lot of other meaningful work on two feet. Barbell curls are usually accessible, even for the most afflicted of Masters.

Curls can be incrementally loaded over time, and steady progress on the exercise has excellent carryover to those whose strength on the chin-up bar or the lat pull-down machine may have stagnated.

Barbell curls should be done with a full range of motion, with a supinated forearm, and with involvement of the shoulder. The bar should be curled up to the bottom of the chin and lowered to the point where the elbows are straight, but not completely relaxed. Two or three sets of 8–10 are sufficient.

## The Leg Press

The leg press is not a useful training modality for Masters who are able to perform the squat in regular training. It is however valuable for preparing those Masters who cannot squat due to a lack of strength throughout the entire range of motion. Most Masters who are unable to squat below parallel are diagnosed by trainers and physical therapists as lacking in mobility, when in fact the problem is almost always a lack of strength, particularly at the bottom. Institution of a progressive leg press program in this situation will permit the vast majority of Masters to

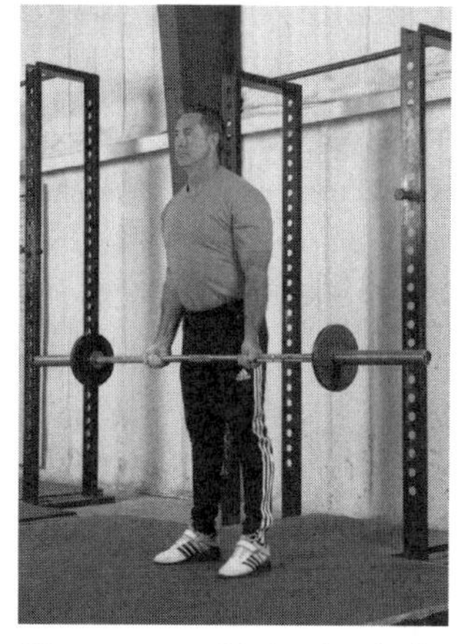
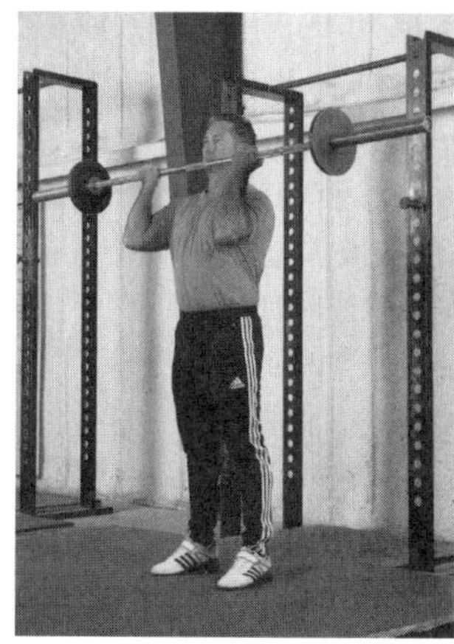

***Figure 13-4.*** The barbell curl.

proceed to the barbell squat. The apparatus is safe when used for this purpose, and easy to operate and coach. This intervention is described in detail in the section on remedial squat programming (Chapter 21).

## Deadlift Variations

Because the deadlift poses such a demand on the recovery capacity of the trainee, intermediate or advanced trainees will occasionally benefit from avoiding regular deadlift training for a period of several weeks or even months. During a deadlift hiatus, however, trainees will still need to pull heavy. Abandoning all heavy pulling exercises will leave the movement detrained and regression will occur. But there are ways to pull heavy without actually deadlifting.

One popular method, covered in detail in *Starting Strength: Basic Barbell Training, 3rd edition,* is a weekly rotation between halting deadlifts and rack pulls. These exercises split the range of motion of the deadlift into two overlapping components which can be trained heavily but separately, reducing the demand on recovery capacity. Both exercises use partial ranges of motion – but when combined they cover the complete range of motion from floor to lockout. Halting deadlifts begin on the floor and are pulled to just above knee height and then returned to the floor. Rack pulls begin just below the knees (set on the pins of a power rack) and are pulled to

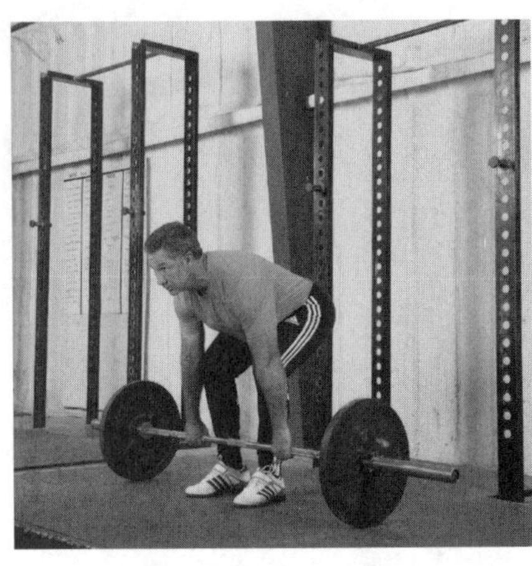
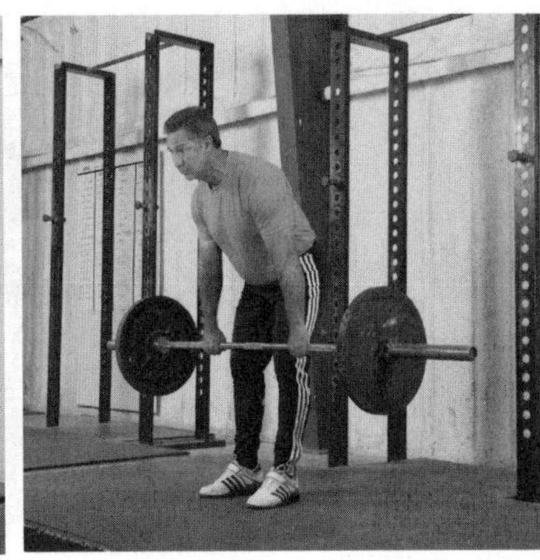

***Figure 13-5.*** The halting deadlift. The exercise begins exactly as for the standard deadlift *(left)*, but terminates just above the kneecap *(right)*.

lockout. Alternating these two exercises allows the trainee to pull heavy on a weekly basis without overtraining on the full movement.

## Halting deadlifts

Halting deadlifts begin exactly as a regular deadlift, and the pulling mechanics will be identical to the first part of a deadlift. This variant brings the bar to a point just above the kneecap (Figure 13-5). On a regular deadlift, as the barbell begins to clear the knees, the back angle will become more vertical as the lifter attempts to lock the weight out. In a halting deadlift, the lifter will attempt to keep the shoulders out over the bar for an extended period of time, even as it approaches knee height. Maintenance of a more horizontal back angle for the duration of the exercises will impose a heavy and beneficial training stress on the erectors and lats. The lats will work to keep the barbell actively over the mid-foot, just lightly in contact with the legs at all times during the lift. It is best to perform halting deadlifts with a double overhand grip, and because the weights will likely be in excess of what the trainee can deadlift, straps are usually required to perform sets of 5–8 reps. Halting deadlifts should be treated as a *concentric-only* lift. This means that the trainee will not be actively lowering the barbell slowly through the eccentric phase of the lift, which will quickly overtrain the lower back. Think of the eccentric phase as a "controlled drop" that maintains control of the barbell but lets the bar fall quickly to the ground after the repetition has reached a point just above knee height. This will require the athlete to reset each rep at the bottom, as in a regular deadlift.

## Rack pulls

Rack pulls reconstitute the top half of the deadlift and begin with the bar elevated either inside of a power rack or on pulling blocks (Figure 13-6). In either case, the barbell should be set just a couple of inches below the kneecap. Trainees commonly make the mistake of setting the barbell up too high in the rack, either right at the knee or even above the knee. Doing so does not actively engage enough hamstring and glute into the movement to be an effective replacement for the upper half of the deadlift. Begin with only a moderate amount of knee bend, keep the shoulders out over the barbell to begin the lift, and they should stay out over the barbell as it travels up the thigh. Avoid allowing the knees to travel forward as the barbell ascends. This will allow the back angle to go vertical and bring the quads back into the movement, and most often results in a "hitching" of the weight into lockout – a series of pulls that rest the bar on the thighs on the way up. The point of the rack pull is to force the hamstrings to extend the hips under very heavy load. Prematurely straightening out the torso by shoving the knees forward and under the barbell disengages the hamstrings from the pull, thus defeating the purpose of the exercise.

Rack pulls will be done with very heavy weights for sets of 5 reps, and a double overhand grip with lifting straps is preferred.

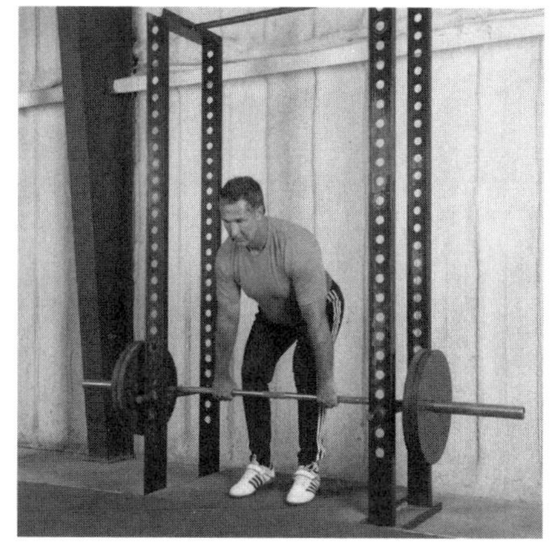

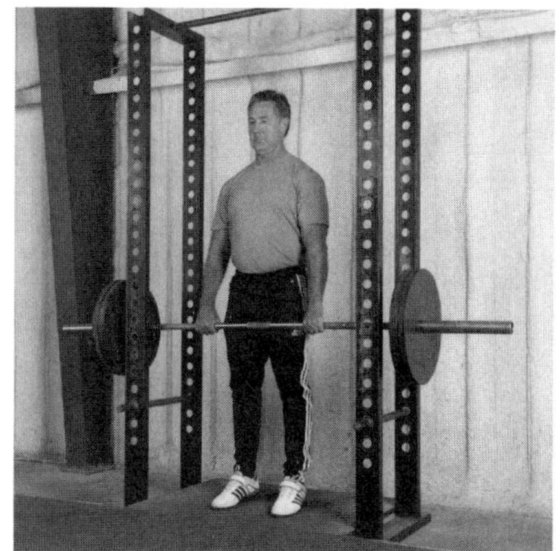

***Figure 13-6.*** The rack pull. The bar is set in the rack to a position just below the patella, such that the range of motion will overlap with that of the halting deadlift *(left)*. The exercise is finished exactly as a standard deadlift *(right)*.

Rack pulls and halting deadlifts can be alternated for many weeks without actually doing any direct deadlift training, and the deadlift will not regress in this situation. Every 4–12 weeks, the trainee and coach may decide to instead pull a heavy set of regular deadlifts just to ensure the programming is working as it should, and then return to the halting/rack pull rotation.

Both lifts should be programmed for just one work set after warm-ups. Both lifts can be trained for sets of 5 reps, but many have found that using slightly higher reps for the haltings is preferred due to their short range of motion. Up to 8 reps is appropriate for haltings.

Example 13-1 illustrates a an 8-week progression for an intermediate Master who has stalled on regular deadlifts at 365x5.

### Stiff-leg deadlifts and Romanian deadlifts

Stiff-leg deadlifts (SLDLs) can be used in place of or in conjunction with regular deadlifts. Although SLDLs are lighter and less stressful, they can produce memorable soreness in the hamstrings, especially when they are first introduced into the program.

SLDLs begin on the ground, from a dead stop, just like a regular deadlift. The SLDL will begin with knees that are *slightly bent,* not totally straight. For those who don't know better, stiff-leg deadlifts are often referred to as *straight*-leg deadlifts – but this is incorrect. Performing a deadlift with knees completely straight is both dangerous and ineffective.

**Example 13-1: Making Progress with Halting Deadlifts and Rack Pulls**

|  |  |  |
|---|---|---|
| Week 1: | 135x5, 225x3, 275x2, 315x1, 355x1, **385x8** | Halting deadlift |
| Week 2: | 135x5, 225x3, 315x1, 365x1, **405x5** | Rack pull |
| Week 3: | 135x5, 225x3, 275x2, 315x1, 365x1, **390x8** | Halting deadlift |
| Week 4: | 135x5, 225x3, 315x1, 365x1, **415x5** | Rack pull |
| Week 5: | 135x5, 225x3, 275x2, 315x1, 365x1, **395x8** | Halting deadlift |
| Week 6: | 135x5, 225x3, 315x1, 385x1, **425x5** | Rack pull |
| Week 7: | 135x5, 225x3, 275x2, 315x1, 365x1, **400x8** | Halting deadlift |
| Week 8: | 135x5, 225x3, 315x1, 365x1, 395x1, **435x5** | Rack pull |

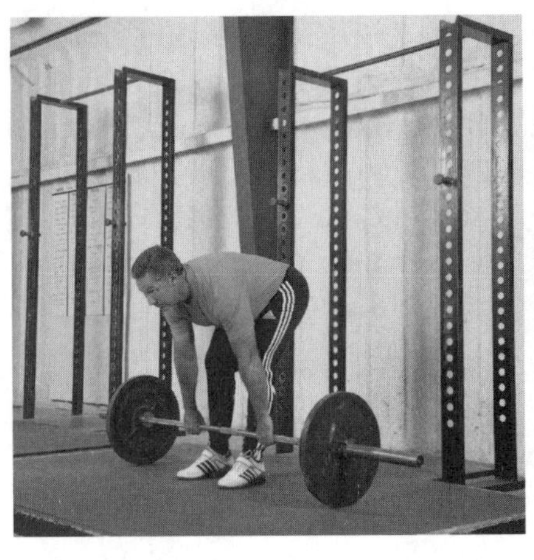
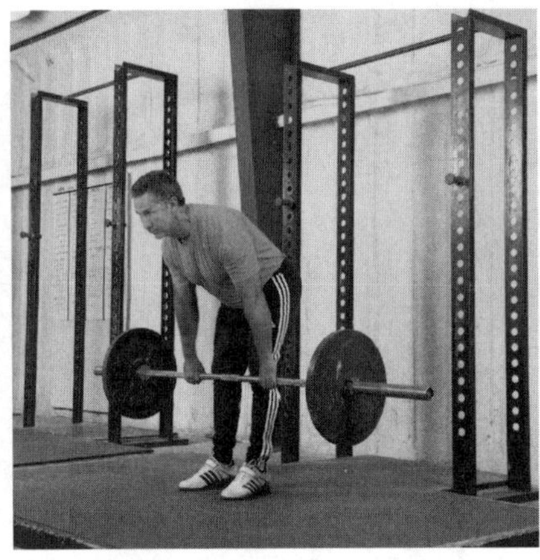
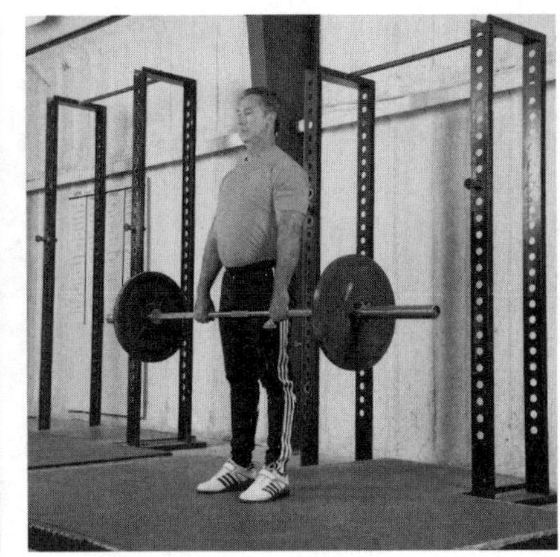

***Figure 13-7.*** The stiff-leg deadlift.

The degree of knee bend in an SLDL will be dependent on the mobility and anthropometry of the individual trainee. SLDLs are performed with the hips high and a back angle that is as horizontal as possible. The trainee *must* perform this exercise with rigid extension of the low back. The knee angle will bend enough to allow the trainee to set the back into rigid extension, but no more. This will usually leave the shins almost vertical, and if the bar is in balance over the mid-foot it will therefore not be in contact with the shins as it moves up through the bottom of the range of motion, but will meet the thigh just above the knee. The trainee thus breaks the bar off the ground with very little involvement from the quads (Figure 13-7).

SLDLs can be used in place of a regular deadlift as part of a bi-weekly rotation. This allows the trainee to pull relatively heavy and still work the hamstrings and erectors thoroughly without the stress of heavier conventional deadlifts. Unlike rack pulls and haltings, SLDLs will likely be much lighter than regular deadlifts. A good starting point is 60–70% of an athlete's regular 5-rep sets. SLDLs are effective in a range of 5–8 strict reps for 1–3 total work sets.

Romanian deadlifts (RDLs) are another deadlift variation, and the two exercises are often referred to interchangeably. But RDLs actually begin in the hang position rather than on the floor. RDLs are different in that they are actively lowered down the legs with a very controlled eccentric and then utilize a stretch reflex in the hamstrings to return the barbell back to the top of the movement. Because of the eccentric lowering and the stretch reflex, they produce exquisite hamstring soreness, so use them carefully. RDLs are typically done with a shorter range of motion as the barbell is lowered to just below knee height or perhaps mid-shin (Figure 13-8).

Either SLDLs or RDLs are effective for adding work to the hamstrings. For older, more inflexible Masters RDLs might be safer than an SLDL. Unless the trainee can set up in absolutely perfect position in the bottom of the movement, SLDLs should be avoided. RDLs have the benefit of being able to be lowered to a point just before a trainee loses his ability to hold the low back into rigid extension. Therefore an RDL can be used even by less-flexible older trainees, the range of motion titrated to their individual levels of flexibility or lack thereof.

Using a pair of dumbbells for RDLs (Figure 13-8, bottom panel) is an excellent way for the busy traveler to get in some hamstring and erector work while at an ill-equipped hotel where regular barbell training cannot be performed due to equipment limitations. They can also be used for much older Masters trainees who may have a variety of limitations that make any sort of barbell-based deadlifting difficult to perform.

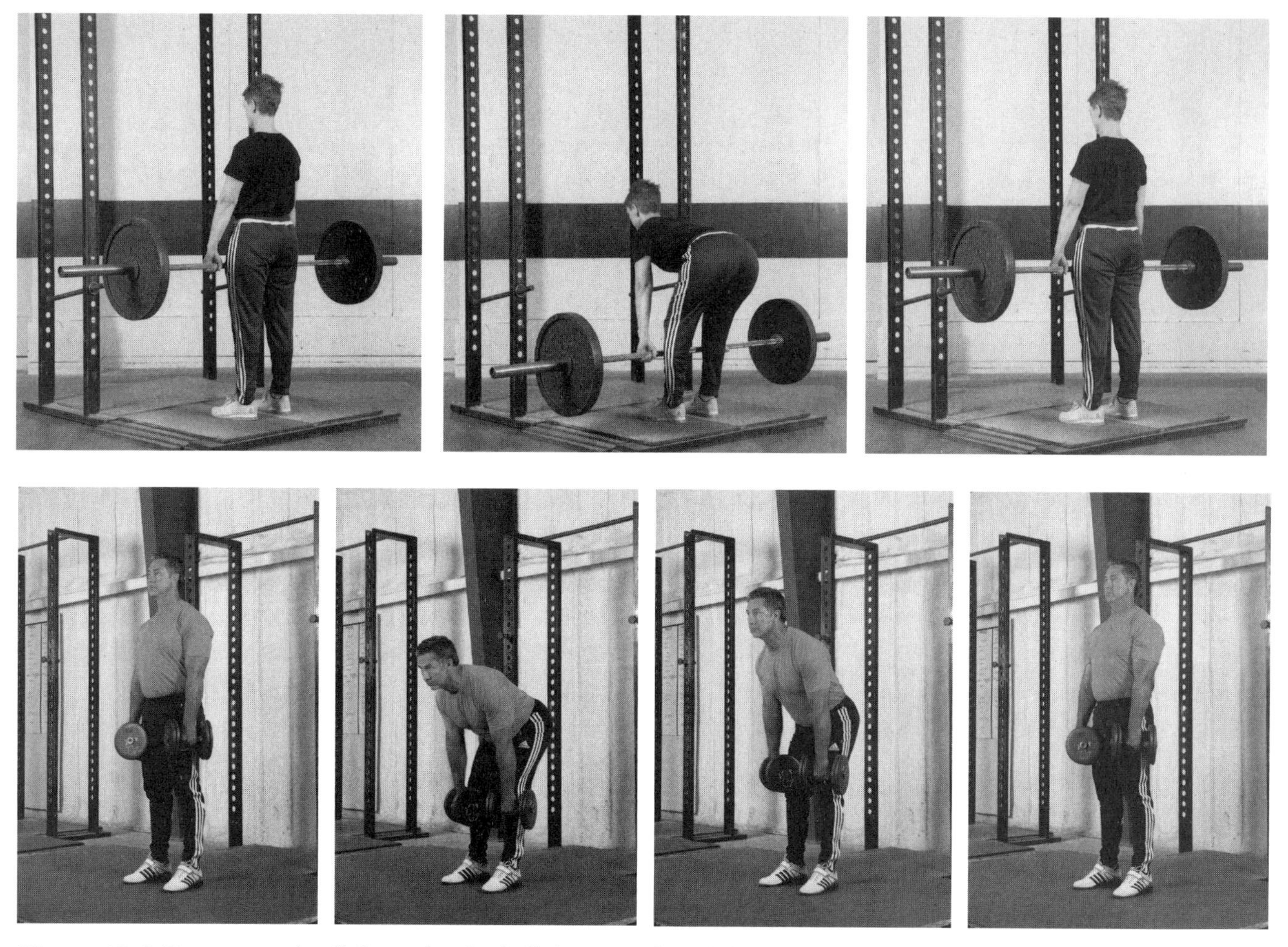

***Figure 13-8.*** Romanian deadlifts with a barbell (*top panel*) and dumbbells (*bottom panel*).

# Part III: HOW

## Programming for Strength and Conditioning

# 14

# Programming

Having established the central importance of strength for the aging adult and the superiority of barbell exercises for achieving this goal, we now consider how barbell *exercise* becomes barbell *training*. The progressive improvement of General Fitness Attributes can only be accomplished through the rational and systematic manipulation of training variables over time by way of an explicit plan of work, which we call *programming*. Programming is not constant variation for the sake of variety, nor is it endless repetition of the same exercise routine. The goals and methodology of programming are always explicit, and are based on coaching experience, data, and an appreciation of training biology.

In this chapter, the reader is given an introduction to programming concepts, an overview of Part III and how it should be used, and a preview of fundamental programming principles.

## The Program is the Prescription

In Part I, Sullivan made a meticulous, evidence-based, definitive argument for *Why* a progressive, barbell-based approach to strength training is not only appropriate, but *necessary* for older adults. In Part II, we gave you an overview of *What* is involved in barbell training – a brief introduction to the equipment, the gear, and some basic principles. We also gave you a preview of the exercises, what it's like to do them, and how they fit beautifully with the requirements of a General Exercise Prescription for the Masters Athlete.

The purpose of Part III is to translate the *Why* and *What* into *How*. Building strength is like building a house – it requires the right materials, the right tools, and the right plan. We've shown you *Why* you have to build strength and new tissue. We've shown you *What* is necessary to do this work, introducing you to the tools in your toolbox and explaining why they're the *right* tools. Squats, presses, and deadlifts are analogous to the hammer, the saw, and the drill. The gym is your workshop.

Now we will show you *How* to take those tools and start building. Part III is a detailed exploration of ***programming*** for strength training: a rational, long-term plan that manipulates training variables and specifies the structure of every workout and training period to achieve specific performance goals. Programming provides the blueprint for the house to be built. It tells us to pour the slab before we erect the walls and put on the roof. Programming gives our efforts in the gym a structure, an agenda, and a rationale. For each training session, each week, each month, and each year there is a step-by-step process to follow. Without the blueprint, the tools are useless.

Programming is what sets *training* apart from *exercise*. Programming is *the plan* that makes our time in the gym purposeful and effective. It's how we turn a 45-pound squat into a 200-pound squat. Programming tells us how to progress, how fast to progress – and what to do when we stop progressing. This is crucial. Like all good plans, effective programming provides for contingencies and difficulties. All trainees get *stuck* from time to time. Understanding how programming works is what gets you *unstuck*.

Sullivan has made the case that an exercise medicine should be prescribed like any other medicine, specifying the formulation, route of administration, dose, and frequency of that medicine. The formulation of the medicine is strength training. The route of administration is barbells. And the dose and frequency are all about the manipulation of training variables as part of a plan designed to produce targeted improvements in the General Fitness Attributes.

In a word: Programming.

*The program is the prescription.*

## What Programming is Not

Programming is often mistaken for the inclusion of constant variety – typically in the form of faddish, silly, even dangerous exercises. But the rational manipulation of training variables in a long-term program cannot be achieved by constant variation. Good programming is not variety for the sake of variety, or change for the sake of change. It is not about "shocking" or "confusing" our muscles with an exciting new routine each time we work out. Effective strength training uses a small set of powerful, comprehensive exercises that rarely change when we go to the gym, with the specific aim of progression on these exercises. Novice, intermediate, and advanced trainees all work from the same tool box: squats, deadlifts, bench presses, presses, and a few assistance exercises. The difference between novice and intermediate programs is not in exercise selection but in how they systematically manipulate training variables. The exercises don't change, the program is changed infrequently and only when necessary, and program complexity is always minimized to the extent possible. The most effective programming manipulates the *minimum number of variables* required to drive progress. Indeed, the novice athlete, who gets stronger faster than any other athlete, manipulates only one key variable in his entire program – the weight on the bar.

*Constant variation is the very antithesis of training.*

This means that incessantly fiddling with a program, or frequent switching from one program to another, will be entirely counterproductive. When the athlete is getting stronger, there's no need to make changes in the program. Ride the wave of progress until the program stalls before tinkering or switching.

## Programs are Formulas – Athletes are Individuals

Programming is both science and art. It demands a deep understanding of biological adaptation and how training stress and recovery drive that adaptation. Such understanding allows us to draw up ***program templates*** that are *generally* applicable in a given training situation, just as a particular medicine is understood to be useful in a range of clinical scenarios. A standard program template like the Rank Novice Program (1A, Chapter 19) or the Heavy-Light-Medium Program (6A, Chapter 24) works for almost all trainees in the appropriate training situation, because all trainees have the same fundamental biological attributes. We all share the same molecular components, have the same general anatomical plan and physiology, and burn the same fuels. As we shall see in the next chapter, we all respond to training stresses with the same ancient biological responses.

Nevertheless, each trainee is also unique. Each of us has enough genetic and phenotypic variation that programming must become more individualized as the trainee progresses over time. There is no such thing as a one-size-fits-all program that meets the specific needs of each individual athlete. Coaches and trainees must be familiar with the program templates and understand the principles that underlie them. But they must also be attuned to the athlete's unique needs, abilities, limitations, and potential. This allows a general program template to be applied to the situation of a particular athlete, just as medicine with a general application must be dosed to a particular patient. This is the *art* of programming, and it begins with the understanding that *training progress occurs on an individual time line.*

This important principle applies most particularly to the Masters Athlete. Decades of experiences, illnesses, injuries, nutrition, exercise patterns, and other time-dependent variables compound innate genetic differences. The Masters population is inherently heterogeneous. A hundred Masters Athletes will display more variability in their responses to a given training program than a hundred younger athletes, because they've had more time for their genetic differences and life experiences to have an impact on their biology and behavior.

In the chapters that follow, we will present a number of program templates suitable for particular stages of training and for particular indications. The temptation for the reader will be to select whatever training program sounds the most appealing and follow the program set-for-set, rep-for-rep, until he gets bored and then randomly selects another program to try. Instead, the reader should use the program templates, and the variations accompanying them, as examples of *how to apply the illustrated concepts* to their training programs – rather than blindly follow any one program exactly as we have it laid out.

# Overview of Part III

Part III begins with a few brief chapters introducing the reader to the fundamental principles of strength programming. In Chapter 15, we will look at the miracle of adaptation, the capacity of all organisms to respond to stress, and how that capacity is exploited by training to improve performance, strength, and health. In Chapter 16, we will focus on the most neglected component of the adaptive process: recovery. This will bring in considerations of training frequency, rest, sleep, hydration, diet, and stress reduction. In Chapter 17, we'll discuss the nuts and bolts of programming: sets, reps, rest, warm-ups, and so on. We will present the concept of programming categories in Chapter 18: the *novice*, the *intermediate*, and the *advanced*, and we'll show you why these words don't mean what most people think they mean.

The remaining chapters are devoted to description of specific program structures and examples of how they can be modified. In Chapters 19–21, we will present the basic structure of the novice program and show how it can be used, with or without modification, by almost any Master, regardless of age or other constraints. Program modifications will be broken down by age range, and various scheduling and remedial variants will be outlined.

In Chapters 22–24, we'll take a look at programs for the intermediate trainee, again broken down by age and in a variety of formulations. Few trainees over 50 will ever need to progress beyond an intermediate-level program, because such programs can produce slow, steady progress for many years in the Masters Athlete.

Nonetheless, in Chapter 25 we will provide sample programs for those rare, talented, and driven individuals who progress beyond the intermediate, to the advanced level. *These programs go beyond the objectives of exercise medicine*, are rarely if ever applicable to trainees over 50, and are necessary only for those who wish to lift competitively at the Masters level.

Chapter 26 will address approaches to conditioning, emphasizing high-intensity protocols that drive adaptations across the bioenergetic spectrum and prepare the Master for the Arena of Life.

This text concludes with Chapter 27, a short chapter devoted to special considerations for the female Master. The position and brevity of this final chapter should not suggest that female Masters are an afterthought. Indeed, most coaches who work with Masters have more female than male clients, and there is every reason to believe that female Masters derive more benefit from training than their male counterparts. But training for the female Master is *almost* identical to that for men, and the vast majority of women will begin their training using the programs in this book without modification. Women adapt to training stress in the same way that men do, especially in the Masters age range. Nevertheless, there *are* differences in physiology and strength distribution that will frequently indicate minor programming modifications for the female Master as she advances in her training.

## This is not a cookbook: how to use Part III

Some readers will be tempted to jump ahead to a particular program that seems suited to their age and situation (or that of their client or patient). This is understandable, but not at all ideal, just as it is not ideal to start building a house – even with a good plan – without having a familiarity with the underlying principles of that plan, and the fundamentals of construction. When, after a few short chapters, you have learned what *really* constitutes the difference between a novice and an intermediate, and when you have acquired an understanding of adaptation, recovery, training variables, and the building blocks of a training program, the material in Chapters 19–27 will make far more sense. These foundations will promote wiser choices in the selection and modifications of programs that best suit the training needs of the athlete.

*This is not a cookbook.* Read *everything* before you try *anything.*

Always return to the idea that strength programming is an *evolution.* This means that progress is generally sustained through "tweaks" and gradual modifications rather than completely overhauling your entire program every six weeks. Treat your training like a science experiment. The introduction of too many variables at once violates the basic structure of the scientific method. Learn all of the methods and protocols and then apply them one at a time at the appropriate moments in your progression. This is the only way to find out what works for you and what does not. While the basic principles of programming are pretty much the same for everyone, each person's progression will chart a unique course. Factors such as age, genetics, training history, and mental attitude are all factors that play into your progression.

Each major program is presented first as a general template, followed by one or more illustrations of how the template is executed. These examples are laid out in snapshots of anywhere from 1–21 weeks. The example timelines for these programs are *not prescriptive.* They are *illustrations.* A 12-week snapshot of the Texas Method is not intended to prescribe a 12-week program. And the particular weights used in these examples are most emphatically not prescriptive either.

Again: *there is no such thing as the one-size-fits-all training program.* There are only *principles* and *concepts* that must be tailored to the individual athlete. In the chapters that follow, you will see that the same principles come up over and again. A short list of such principles follows. Some of them will make sense to you immediately, on the basis of what you've already read, or just common sense. Others will become more clear as we proceed. Be on the lookout for them.

## Principles of strength programming for the Masters athlete

1. The essence of all strength programming is an exploitation the Stress-Recovery-Adaptation cycle.

2. Training progresses on an individual timeline, and this is particularly true of the Masters Athlete.

3. If the program is working, don't change it.

4. Focus on what the athlete *can* do, rather than what he can't.

5. When adjustment to a program is necessary, change one training variable at a time.

6. Patience, care, and consistency win out over greed and hurry.

7. The Masters Athlete is *volume-sensitive* and *intensity-dependent.*

8. Programming becomes more complex, and improvements in strength become smaller over time, as the athlete gets ever closer to his performance potential.

9. Recovery variables are the most crucial and most frequently neglected. Without proper rest, sleep, nutrition, and hydration, progress cannot occur. This is doubly true of the Masters Athlete. When the athlete is having trouble progressing in a well-designed program, the first place to look for the problem is in *recovery*.

10. The Masters Athlete trains to live, not the other way around.

## A Final Note: Start Where You Are

Each individual has aged on an individual timeline. Life has taken more of a toll on some than others, and these things matter. For the Masters Athlete in particular, there is little to be gained by comparing one's own progress to that of others, other than to see what *might* be possible or detrimental. Train yourself to be the best *you* can be, beginning from your own unique starting line and progressing on your own unique journey.

# 15
# Adaptation

In this chapter, the reader is introduced to the concept of biological *adaptation*. We begin with a brief examination of *Selye's General Adaptation Syndrome*, a classic model of the organism's variable responses to stress. This in turn leads us to a distillation of the General Adaptation Syndrome relevant to athletic training – the concept of the *Stress-Recovery-Adaptation Cycle*. This cycle forms the basis of all strength training programs. Regardless of their training level or complexity, all programs work by imposing a training stress, promoting recovery, and reaching an adapted state in which increased strength permits the imposition of a greater training stress and the initiation of a new training cycle. If no additional training stress is applied to the adapted state, the athlete will *detrain* and will never get stronger. If training stress is too heavy or applied too frequently, the athlete will leave the Stress-Recovery-Adaptation cycle and enter Stage III of Selye's General Adaptation Syndrome, a state of *overtraining*. The chapter closes by emphasizing the central importance of recovery in all training programs.

## The General Adaptation Syndrome

To understand and apply the *art* of programming for strength, one must first understand the *science* of adaptation.

Any rational training program, whatever its modality, and whatever its training goals, is nothing more than a cycle of applying a physical stress, recovering and adapting to the stress, and then increasing the stress to drive progress.

In other words, programming is an exploitation of the ***General Adaptation Syndrome.***

First presented by Hans Selye in 1936[1] and later expanded by Selye and others,[2] the General Adaptation Syndrome is a classic model of the organism's variable responses to stress. Depending on the nature, periodicity, and intensity of the stress and the organism's capacity to respond, the General Adaptation Syndrome will culminate in either an adaptation to the stress, or exhaustion and collapse. Repeated exposure to a specific stressor drives an organism through a series of hormonal, cellular, and molecular responses aimed at immediate survival of the stressful event and the rapid deployment of structural and functional adaptations to render the organism more tolerant to those same stressors if applied later. Inadequate or maladaptive responses arise if the stressor is too intense or frequent.

Selye's model of biological response to a stress encompasses 3 stages:

***Stage I*** of the General Adaptation Syndrome is the *alarm* stage. It begins with the application of a stress which disrupts ***homeostasis***, or physiological balance. This stress can be emotional or physical – anything from bad news to the onset of illness to a confrontation with a hungry predator. Stage I produces a rapid change in the organism's metabolic and endocrine landscape, a coordinated physiological response aimed at surviving the immediate challenge. Classically, this stage is associated with the release of epinephrine and increases in blood pressure, heart rate, ventilation, attention, serum glucose, and neuromuscular efficiency. In short, this is the "fight or flight" stage.

Assuming the stressor is sufficiently intense to disrupt homeostasis (but insufficient to kill outright), the organism will be measurably weaker and less resistant to insult than it was prior to the initial stress. Homeostasis has been sufficiently disrupted to drive the organism into the next stage.

***Stage II*** of Selye's syndrome is *resistance.* If the stress is not immediately resolved, or if it has significantly disrupted homeostasis, the body undergoes well-characterized changes in hormone production, energy metabolism, and the synthesis of structural and metabolic proteins. These responses are geared toward repairing damage to cells and tissues, and a rapid increase in the organism's ability to withstand another exposure to the same stress (or, if the stress is ongoing, to resist and resolve the stress). Accordingly, stage II results not just in a return to the pre-stress condition, but a more resilient state in which the organism is actually better adapted to the stress than it was before.

In other words, recovery from and adaptation to the stress makes *the organism stronger.*

***Stage III***, or *Exhaustion*, is the alternate, unhappy ending of the General Adaptation Syndrome. If the stressor drives the organism too far from homeostasis, the physiological or structural disruption will overwhelm adaptive responses. Alternatively, if the stressor is within the organism's adaptive range, but is applied too often or for too long, the adaptive capacities of the organism will ultimately fail and it will become progressively weaker and less adapted to the stress.

Let's look at a couple of examples. Consider a fine Scotch whisky. Better yet, *drink* a fine Scotch whisky. You've been a teetotaler until now, but for whatever reason you decide to start drinking a glass or three every night after dinner. Metabolizing the alcohol in the whisky requires the activity of special enzymes, particularly in the liver. Before you start your Scotch habit, these enzymes are produced at very low levels, and the liquor hits you hard. There is a significant disruption in homeostasis. You get snookered. You might even feel a bit sick. This first drinking bout has triggered stage I, or Alarm.

You'll live. Tomorrow you won't quite be yourself, but you'll already be in stage II, adapting to the stress by increasing the production of an enzyme called alcohol dehydrogenase. After a week or two of this routine, you'll find that a couple of shots of whisky after dinner, while pleasant, won't make you drunk or sick. The stressor has not been removed, but you have *adapted* to it.

Of course, if you increase the intensity and frequency of the stressor, say by drinking five shots of whisky six or seven times a day every day, you can eventually drive your liver into exhaustion. An exhausted liver is bad news. Drink responsibly.

Or consider an acute viral illness. In stage I, you're sick. You've got a sore throat, sneezing, sniffling, muscle aches, the lot. You're a NyQuil commercial. You're certainly weaker than you were yesterday. The infection incites an inflammatory response that most people find unpleasant. But as you rally and enter stage II, your immune system begins to resist the invader, and by the time stage II has resolved you've elaborated an antibody response that will protect you the next time you're exposed to that particular strain of virus. Stage II has produced an adaptation to the stress. Of course,

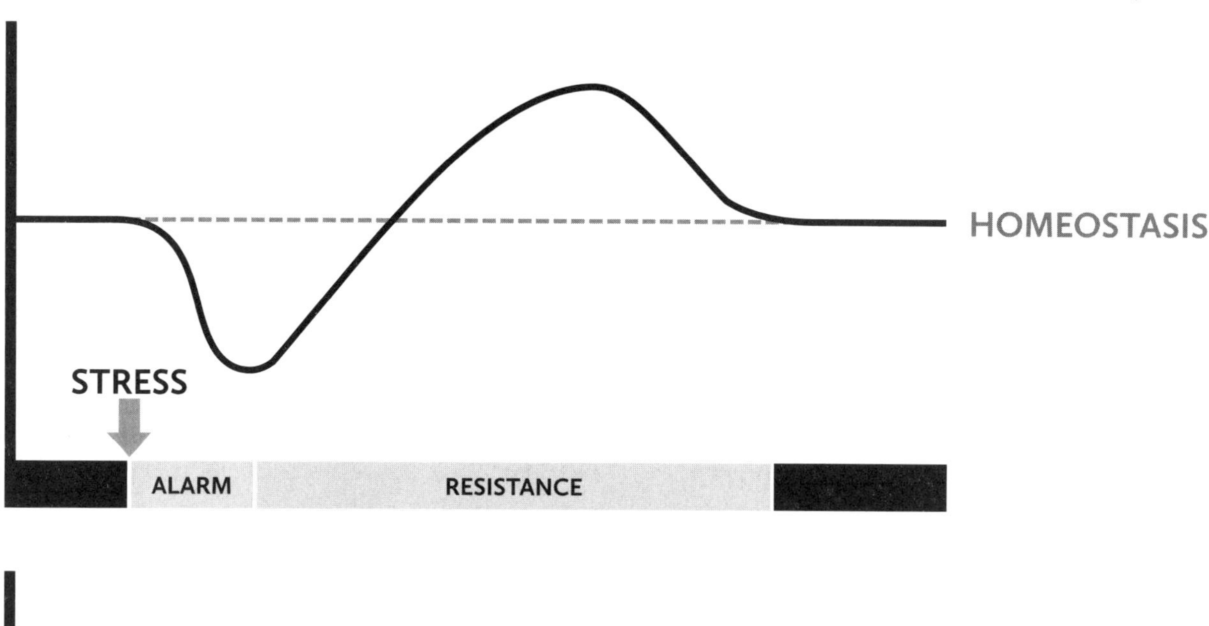


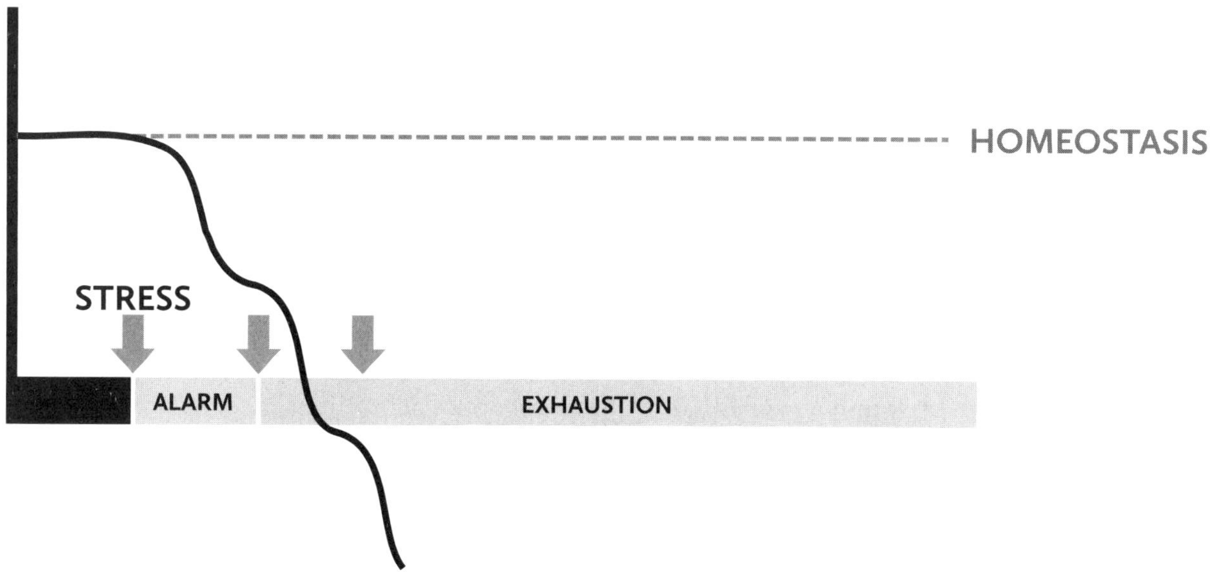


***Figure 15-1.*** Selye's original General Adaptation Syndrome. *Top*, Stage I, Alarm, progresses to Stage II, Resistance. *Bottom*, Repeated stresses overwhelm the adaptive response, leading to Stage III, Exhaustion.

if you're weak or immunocompromised, or if the infection is particularly virulent (Ebola or Spanish flu, say), the disruption of homeostasis may be too severe to permit recovery, and you'll enter stage III (exhaustion or collapse).

## The Stress-Recovery-Adaptation Cycle

Selye's model of adaptation has long since been appropriated by coaches and athletes,[3] although Selye did not present it in the context of exercise physiology or muscle adaptation, and its presumed relevance to training has not been without controversy.[4] Nevertheless, the application of Selye's overarching model of biological adaptation has been extraordinarily fruitful. For our purposes, it's easier to apply the General Adaptation Syndrome to training if we make some modifications to Selye's terminology. The biology will remain the same, but the vocabulary will be more suitable to our purposes, and it will delineate a 3-part training cycle that finds expression in all training programs.

Stage I, alarm, begins with a training stimulus powerful enough to disrupt homeostasis. We will call this part of the training cycle ***stress***. Stress in training is delivered in the form of an

***overload event***, the work necessary to disrupt homeostasis/equilibrium. The magnitude of the work necessary to constitute an overload event and its distribution over the training cycle varies with the training history, age, sex, nutritional status, and hormonal status of the athlete. Stage II, resistance, extends from the point at which the organism begins to recover from the stress to the point at which it has either returned to homeostasis or entered the downward slope to exhaustion. We shall consider that part of the training cycle during with the organism re-establishes homeostasis as ***recovery.*** If the stress has been of a sufficient but not excessive dose, and if recovery has been adequate, the organism will undergo ***adaptation*** during this period and not only attain its previous performance baseline, but will progress to a higher state, expressing its improved capacity to respond to a future stress. This is dependent on the correct application of the overload event.

This ***Stress-Recovery-Adaptation cycle*** is the underlying structure of all athletic programming.

Consider an example that is more directly relevant than our Scotch whisky and Ebola scenarios. As a novice, you walk into a gym and do a heavy barbell workout. It takes 60–90 minutes. This is the stress phase of your training cycle, corresponding to Selye's stage I, the alarm stage. *You* may not be alarmed, but your *body* is. Lifting heavy weight places an enormous demand on your energy metabolism, your cardiovascular system, and your musculoskeletal structures. The workout inflicts microscopic damage to muscle fibers, and bones and ligaments are under stress. Your epinephrine levels are elevated, you're splitting animal starch in the liver and the muscles to keep glucose levels high, you're ramping up your mitochondria to support your metabolism, your blood pressure is up, and your heart rate is elevated.

From a biological perspective, you're in combat.

This disruption of homeostasis persists well after the workout has been completed. A barbell training bout *really* shouldn't kill you[5]...but it will leave you tired, a little stiff, a bit sore, and rather less strong than you were when you got to the gym. Experienced lifters are familiar with post-workout fatigue, soreness, and "jelly legs."

This disruption of homeostasis and micro-trauma to tissues will drive you into recovery and adaptation (if you let it). Muscle and liver energy stores are restored and supplemented. Damage to muscle tissue and collagen fibers in tendons and ligaments is repaired. Muscle protein synthesis is stimulated.

During recovery, your body marshals its resources, repairs damage, and establishes a new baseline. These processes are facilitated by active rest, sleep, nutrition, and hydration, and will culminate in an adapted state. You'll be stronger than you were before the initial stress.

Now you have an opportunity to do something incredibly simple and incredibly powerful: *apply another training stress and start another training cycle.* If you time your training stresses correctly, you will be starting the new cycle at the new baseline, your new level of strength. This means that you're strong enough to tolerate a greater training stress than the first one. Then you recover and adapt again to produce a new level of performance, permitting an even greater training stress to be applied.

Understanding this repetitive application of the Stress-Recovery-Adaptation cycle is critical to understanding how programming works. Programming *at every level*, from novice to elite, hinges on the ability of the coach and the athlete to apply an appropriate overload event, realize adequate recovery and adaptation, and apply another training stress at an incrementally increased dose at precisely the time the athlete is strong enough to adapt to it. This Stress-Recovery-Adaptation cycle will grow longer as a trainee advances in strength and time under the barbell, and the components of the overload event will become more complex – changing from a single training stress to multiple stresses – and require more stringent attention to detail. But this underlying Stress-Recovery-Adaptation structure remains, no matter how strong the trainee or advanced his program.

Beginning trainees are best served by applying a small stress and allowing a short recovery

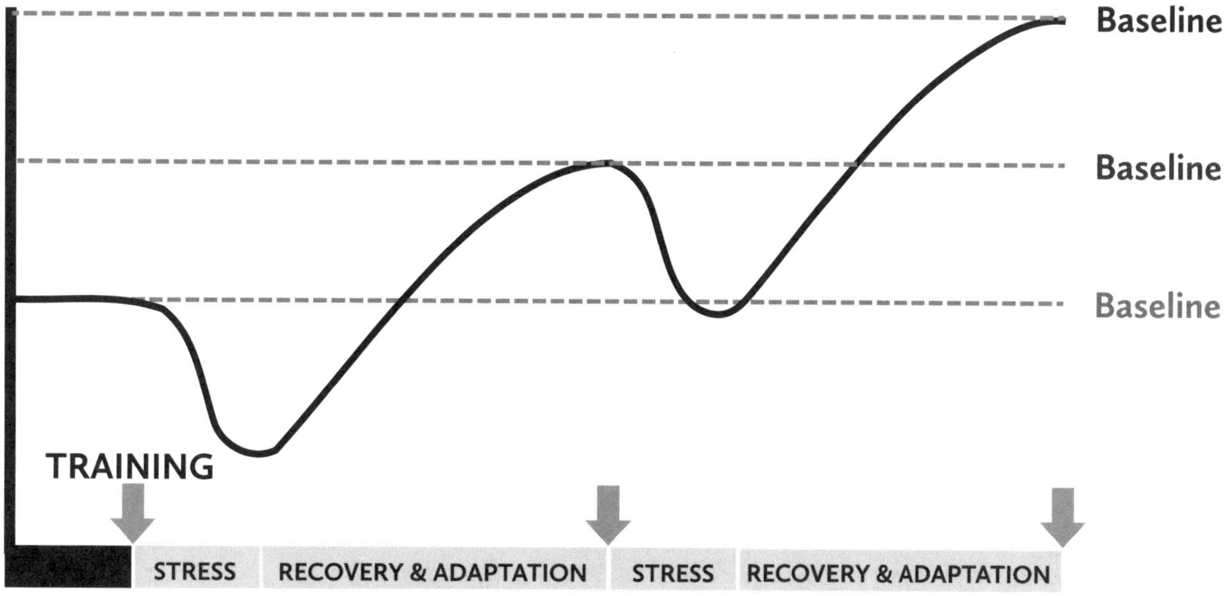

***Figure 15-2.*** The Stress-Recovery-Adaptation Cycle based on Selye's General Adaptation Syndrome. The ability to exploit cumulative recovery from stress into progressive adaptation is the basis of all correctly designed physical training.

period: *train a day, rest a day or two, repeat.* This is the simplest form of programming, in which a new Stress-Recovery-Adaptation cycle is initiated at every workout. Such training will ultimately result in an athlete who is strong enough to absorb a training stress too heavy to allow for recovery and adaptation before the next workout. The overload event will accumulate stress over a training period extended to a week or longer to permit completion of the cycle. As the athlete progresses even further, the overload event will be stretched out over several workouts, will include its own sub-phases of recovery and adaptation, and can require as long as a month (in some cases longer), with full recovery and adaptation taking about as long. Few athletes *of any age* will attain the advanced and elite levels of training where this degree of effort, commitment, and programming complexity is necessary. And a Masters Athlete who is just beginning his strength training cannot expect to *ever* require this level of training complexity. Most athletes, Masters included, will achieve and remain at a level where the complete Stress-Recovery-Adaptation cycle is between 1 week and 1 month. The crucial point to bear in mind is that, *regardless of the level of performance or the complexity of training, the underlying structure remains the same: Stress-Recovery-Adaptation.*

## Detraining and Overtraining

Of course, we know from Selye (and experience) that there are alternative outcomes. If the athlete fails to deliver a new training stress after adaptation has occurred, the body will not continue to expend the resources necessary to maintain this more robust level of adaptation. This will result in a return to a less adaptive baseline – a situation we call ***detraining***.

Alternatively, a poorly designed or implemented program can drive the athlete into Selye's stage III: exhaustion. If the stress applied during a training session is too great, or if recovery is short-changed by inadequate rest or nutrition, the trainee's adaptive capacities will be overwhelmed and full recovery and adaptation will not occur. This descent into Selye's stage III is what we call ***overtraining***. Overtraining is a spectrum of maladaptation ranging from mild performance detriments, requiring a short layoff, to chronic impairment that can ruin a professional athletic career, to complete collapse. All athletes must avoid entering into a state of overtraining, and increased vigilance is required as strength, program complexity, and age increase.

Young novices must be exceptionally misguided, reckless, or stupid to wander into an overtrained state. They simply don't have the strength or skill under the bar to apply crippling levels of stress just yet, and their recuperative abilities are in full gear. Anabolic hormone responses are still working well for the young novice. A young trainee needn't worry about overtraining until he has reached intermediate or advanced level status, when he has enough strength and stamina to apply sufficient stress, and with enough frequency, to enter Selye's stage III.

An older athlete, however, is much more susceptible to overtraining, even as a novice. Like the younger trainee, he is still not capable of producing huge amounts of stress early in his training program, but due to his decreased capacity for recovery, much smaller doses of stress can still exceed recuperative abilities, especially if they are applied too frequently. For the Masters Athlete, overtraining will at best result in a training plateau. The more likely scenario is actual regression in performance, and lost training time trying to get back to baseline.

Overtraining should always be a primary diagnostic consideration for an athlete who has begun to stall despite appropriate programming and assiduous attention to recovery. If overtraining appears to be the culprit, it must be attacked on both ends – stress should be reduced and recovery increased. This means decreased workloads during training sessions and reduced frequency of training. It also mandates an increase in high-quality protein, calories, hydration, and sleep – in other words, increased attention to recovery, the most neglected of all training variables, and the most critical for the Masters Athlete.

## Recovery and the Masters Athlete

During recovery we find a crucial difference between older and younger trainees, a difference with important implications for training. *The older the trainee, the less efficient he will be in recovery.* The Masters Athlete simply cannot tolerate training stresses of the same dose or frequency as his younger counterparts. It is this *relative* lack of efficiency in the recovery phase that partially explains why older adults can't productively train as often, or increase their strength as quickly.

During recovery, the release of a number of anabolic hormones such as testosterone, human growth hormone (HGH), insulin-like growth factor-1 (IGF-1), and others promote the repair of tissues, an increase in muscle protein synthesis, and an increase in muscle mass. Older adults simply do not express these anabolic hormones at the same levels as their younger counterparts. This means that recovery will be less efficient, and that adaptations to the stress will not be as dramatic. In very practical terms, a 25 year-old trainee might be able to add 10–20 pounds to his squat every 48 hours upon beginning a strength program. A 55 year-old trainee might only be able to add 5 pounds to the bar every 72 hours. But the Stress-Recovery-Adaptation cycle is operational in both trainees, and both can make progress.

Other factors affecting recovery from training stress in older adults include resistance to nutritional stimulation of muscle growth or ***anabolism***, the very common difficulties with sleep in older populations, competing and overlapping stresses from aging, disease, and medication, and the generally higher levels of stress found in older adults. Older adults will need more high-quality protein for the recovery process to take full effect. They will have to pay particular attention to sleep hygiene, attempt to minimize external and internal life stresses, work with their doctor to keep polypharmacy in check, and above all avoid the temptation to train too frequently.

It is in *recovery* that the Masters Athlete begins to adapt to training stress, it is in *recovery* that he gets stronger, and it is in *recovery* that training integrates with diet, sleep, and daily habits to generate a healthy way of life. So before we say one more word about the application of training stress, about warm-ups or work sets or reps, or when to squat and when to deadlift, we're going to devote the next chapter to this most crucial and most neglected training variable.

# 16

# Recovery: The Forgotten Training Variables

All elements of the Stress-Recovery-Adaptation cycle must be specifically addressed for training progress to occur. Because it does not take place in the gym, constitutes a complex set of behaviors, and is often not explicitly prescribed, recovery is the most frequently neglected program element. Careful attention to recovery completely integrates training into a healthy lifestyle and facilitates progress through the training cycle.

The principal components of effective recovery are *active rest*, adequate *nutrition*, quality *sleep*, *hydration,* and *stress reduction*. The Masters Athlete training for strength will usually require a caloric excess to promote anabolic adaptive processes, with increased consumption of high-quality protein. A very few nutritional supplements may be of some benefit, but most are unproven or even harmful.

Active rest between training bouts will incorporate light activity, which will promote energy utilization, preserve mobility and freshness, and promote good sleep. Adequate hydration is critical and easily addressed. Careful attention to sleep hygiene and stress reduction will allow the Master to get the most of out of training, and will concomitantly improve quality of life.

## The Central Importance of Recovery

> *"You don't get stronger by lifting weights. You get stronger by* ***recovering*** *from lifting weights."*
>
> —Mark Rippetoe

The quote above encapsulates the art and science of strength programming. It flows directly from a deep understanding of the General Adaptation Syndrome, and the emphasis on recovery is explicit. Burn it into your memory – it's strength programming in a nutshell.

Most trainees, and many coaches, focus on the obvious components of strength training –

volume and intensity, sets and reps, the load on the bar, interset rest, exercise selection and performance, how to split up routines, and so on. These are all important training variables, to be sure, but they are all useless without recovery. When a trainee is having trouble in a well-designed program, *the first place to look for the problem is recovery*, because recovery is the most frequently neglected training variable.

More correctly, recovery is an entire *set* of training variables. Recovery from training is more than just taking a day or two off from the gym, although such rest is certainly an essential component of the recuperative process. But in addition to taking a break from heavy training, recovery includes meticulous attention to nutrition, hydration, sleep, and physical activity between workouts. It is in attention to recovery that much of the health benefit of training is realized, because training – as opposed to exercise – integrates these multiple lifestyle variables as essential components of the program.

*Exercise* requires only that we engage in some sort of physical activity. *Training* demands not only the programmed physical activity, but also active rest, good nutrition, adequate sleep, stress reduction, and avoidance of bad food, excess drink, tobacco, and other toxins.

Exercise may be "part of a healthy lifestyle." But because of the central and encompassing role of recovery, training *is* a healthy lifestyle.

## Active Rest

The programs described in the chapters that follow all incorporate non-training days. These are crucial for adaptation to training stress, allowing for repair of microtrauma to muscle and collagen fibers, restoration of muscle energy stores (glycogen, fat, phosphocreatine, etc.), elimination of reaction products, re-establishment of homeostasis, and the generation of new tissue. Programs for the novice Master are typically 2–3 days/week, allowing plenty of time for recovery and adaptation. Advanced novice and intermediate programs that allow for more frequent training (e.g., 4-day programs) still permit a few days of rest in each training cycle, and tend to be of less volume on training days. Training for 5 or more days a week will be entirely counterproductive for the Masters Athlete.

This does not mean, however, that the athlete reverts to a state of torpor on rest days. Indeed, *we recommend that the Master exercise every day.*

By now it should be clear that this is explicitly not the same thing as *training* every day. Active rest is unprogrammed, *light* physical activity: a walk in the woods with the dog, a bike ride with a friend, cleaning out the garage, *T'ai Chi*, dancing, a game of golf, and the like.

This light exercise, or ***active rest***, can actually promote recovery by keeping muscle and connective tissues supple and perfused with blood and nutrients. Masters will find that active rest promotes better sleep, which is itself a powerful recovery factor, not to mention a major quality of life issue. Light activity signals the body that it needs to be ready to move even on non-training days, and maintains engagement with the life that the Master is training *for*.

The key is that *active rest must be low in intensity and volume*, especially during the novice phase. A ten-mile run or four hours of rock climbing doesn't make sense for a novice athlete, who is trying to exploit the once-in-a-lifetime potential of a complete linear progression, and needs his full recuperative capacities available. Such activities can be resumed, if desired, when the novice phase is complete. We also emphasize that active rest must not be in the form of a novel physical activity. If you do Highland Dancing or golf already, then fine. But this is no time to *take up* Highland Dancing or golf, or to engage in heavy home maintenance for the first time since the Clinton Administration. Active rest should be just what it says. Let common sense be your guide.

## Nutrition

A comprehensive treatment of nutrition for the Masters Athlete is beyond the scope of this text, but we can't talk about recovery without addressing diet.

Progressive increases in strength and muscle mass demand an adequate intake of energy and protein. The Masters Athlete will not make progress on a strength program unless he takes in more calories than he expends, and unless his daily protein intake is sufficient to support the construction of new tissue. Strength training will ultimately lead to improvements in body composition and reductions in visceral fat, but our exercise prescription is most emphatically *not* a weight loss program. The construction of new lean tissue simply cannot be achieved in the setting of a caloric deficit or even a perfect net energy balance (which, practically speaking, is a unicorn anyway).

There is no way around it: for strength training, *a caloric surplus must be present, and dietary protein will exceed the usual recommended daily allowance (RDA).*

We hasten to point out, however, that we are not talking about a *massive* caloric surplus. This is an excellent time to highlight one of the key differences between young athletes and Masters. For a 17-year-old kid engaged in barbell training for the first time, a *massive* caloric surplus can be extremely beneficial. Because his rate of growth is so rapid, he can actually *do something* with 8,000 calories a day. Young athletes are often advised to drink a gallon of whole milk a day (GOMAD) and visit the local buffet once or twice a week as a part of their nutritional strategy. Athletes in their teens and early twenties will immediately convert this mountain of food into strong contractile tissue, toxic serum concentrations of sex hormones, and all manner of ebullient adolescent depravity. Youth is wasted on the young.

*Masters do not benefit from such a massive caloric surplus.* Masters must contend with a state of ***anabolic resistance***,[1] the impairment of muscle tissue responses to training and feeding. They require extra calories in general and *extra protein* in particular to overcome this impairment and grow new muscle. But beyond a certain point, Masters simply cannot convert a *massive* caloric surplus into much of anything other than ear hair and bodyfat. At age 60 you can't eat your way out of a training plateau with mass quantities[2] of food, as a younger lifter can. For this reason, older athletes need to construct their nutritional plans more carefully and precisely.

## Caloric requirements for Masters

So...how much do you need to eat?

Calculating a general, one-size-fits-all formula for daily caloric needs is a perilous undertaking. Body composition, overall health, daily activity level (determined by lifestyle and profession), and training history are among the many factors that impact the athlete's nutritional requirements, and will vary considerably, particularly in the Masters population. That all being said, we can hazard some very rough daily guidelines: For every pound of bodyweight, the Master should consume about 1.25g of protein, 1g of carbohydrate, and just under 0.5g of fat.

So the "average" 200-pound, 55 year-old untrained male with ~25% bodyfat (the average Joe) can reasonably start at about 2600 calories/day, composed of about 250g protein, 200g of carbohydrate, and 90g of fat.

The "average" 125-pound, 55 year-old untrained female with ~ 30% bodyfat can reasonably start at 1740 calories/day, composed of about 150g protein, 130g of carbohydrate, and 70g of fat.

But neither of us have ever met an "average" Master, only individuals, and these numbers are *strictly ballpark*. Determining exactly how much is needed is a trial-and-error process that is part of each athlete's individual journey. These are guidelines, not prescriptions, and they are most emphatically starting points, not long-term mandates.

Monitoring the response to caloric intake is easily and simply accomplished by looking at the athlete's nutritional record (yes, he should have one), his bodyweight, and waist circumference at the navel. These metrics are simple but serviceable, and, along with performance in the gym, should give the athlete and coach a decent idea of the effectiveness of the nutrition plan. Weight gain with decrease or minimal increase in waist circumference is the ideal result. This is an indication that the majority of weight gained is lean mass and not bodyfat. The use of impedance bodyfat monitors, skin-fold calipers and other elaborate approaches to body composition analysis *are simply not necessary for most Masters.* They are unlikely to change management, unless there is a subjective change in body composition that is not acceptable to the athlete. Calipers, DEXA, hydrostatic weighing, and other body composition assays all require experienced practitioners and resources to extract data which will do no more to guide the program and diet than more simple investigations: waist measurement, bodyweight, before-and-after pictures, and how your pants fit.

*Body mass index* (BMI) is a particularly crude and unsuitable metric for the individual athlete, having been designed for the statistical analysis of *populations.* BMI correlates poorly with health and function, does not discriminate between weight due to fat and weight due to muscle, and is not appropriate for monitoring body composition in the Master training for strength.[3]

We don't need to make this complicated: The athlete who makes good progress in training and demonstrates healthy changes in bodyweight and waist circumference is doing a good job at the dinner table as well as the gym.

## Protein

The best nutritional plans start building out the diet with the protein sources first. There is compelling evidence that older athletes need more high-quality protein than their young counterparts to overcome the general anabolic resistance of aging.[4] A good estimate is about 1 g of protein per pound of bodyweight from high-quality animal sources.[5] Chicken, fish, beef, eggs, and milk are all excellent sources. Soy, nuts, and beans are of much lower quality. This protein recommendation is much higher than the RDA, but this level of protein intake, and particularly protein rich in certain amino acids (see below), is necessary to overcome the anabolic resistance of the Master. It sounds like a lot of protein to the average American, and it is. But the average American, sadly, is a couch potato, and certainly not engaged in vigorous barbell training.

Most athletes will more consistently attain their daily protein requirements through supplementation with whey-based protein shakes. Two scoops of most commercially available whey-protein supplements provide 40–50 grams of high-quality protein. A couple of protein shakes a day make the 1g/lb target much easier to hit. Whey is the preferred source for protein supplementation as it provides a very beneficial amino acid profile, one that is high in the critical *branched-chain amino acids* (BCAAs) – leucine, isoleucine, and valine. A couple of whey-based protein shakes per day should provide all the BCAAs the athlete needs.

Very overweight Masters will obviously not require a caloric surplus, and will usually make progress on a caloric deficit, increasing strength and muscle mass while decreasing waist circumference. Their protein requirements may also be more moderate at first. Around 0.75g per pound of bodyweight per day is a better prescription for most overweight trainees. Again, close monitoring of nutritional intake, performance, weight, and waist measurement will indicate any needed changes in the nutritional regimen.

Example 16-1 shows what a day might look like for a hypothetical 180-pound male with appropriate protein intake. This example incorporates *protein only*; other nutrient sources are not shown.

On the high end, this provides about 200g of protein per day, slightly in excess of what minimum protein requirements would be. It is critical to remember that muscle protein synthesis is vital to recovery. Adaptation and recovery occur in the time between training sessions, and many athletes make

**Example 16-1: Daily Protein Intake for a 180-pound Male Master**

**Breakfast**: 4 whole scrambled eggs (~25g)

**Midmorning**: Whey protein shake (~50g)

**Lunch**: Grilled chicken breast (~30–40g)

**Late Afternoon**: Whey protein shake (~50g)

**Dinner:** 6 oz sirloin steak (~40g)

the mistake of focusing on adequate nutrition only on workout days, and sometimes only the meal following the workout. For full recovery, adequate protein and calories must be ingested *daily*. If the final workout of the week falls on a Friday morning, the athlete may not be thinking about his nutrition on Sunday afternoon. The routine of training has been put on hold for the weekend, and time spent out of the gym can cause him to forget that he is still recovering from Friday's workout. Protein intake should be steady and consistent throughout the week.

## Carbohydrate

Fat and carbohydrate must also be present in the diet in order to drive muscle protein synthesis and fuel training. During exercise, particularly high-intensity exercise, glucose (and muscle ***glycogen*** – stored carbohydrate or "animal starch," which is split to yield glucose) is the body's preferred energy source. In other words, carbohydrate must be present in muscle to fuel hard training sessions. But too much dietary carbohydrate may promote fat accretion and possibly even the development of metabolic syndrome and insulin resistance. A good starting place for carbohydrate management is to consume most dietary starches and sugars around the training sessions. We call this ***bracketing***: eating starchy carbs like bread, potatoes, and rice just before and soon after training, while keeping ingestion of such carbohydrates lower at other times. Additionally, setting a "carb curfew" in the evening may mitigate some of the effects of over-consumption of carbohydrate in some trainees. The evening meal and any late-night snacks will be protein-based and rounded out with "fibrous carbs," such as green beans, spinach, asparagus, broccoli and the like.

Example 16-2 demonstrates bracketing carb intake around the training session using the same template from earlier in the text. The hypothetical example assumes a late morning workout.

In this example, the lifter splits up his normal mid-morning protein shake into pre- and post-workout servings. This ensures that adequate supplies of BCAAs are available to the muscle as soon as possible, even during the workout and in the minutes that follow. Some evidence suggests that a high concentration of BCAAs (as found in whey) along with a serving of simple carbohydrate is more effective for stimulating muscle protein synthesis, while other data suggests the impact of this strategy is marginal.[6] Notwithstanding the ambiguity of the data, our professional and personal experience suggests that this approach is beneficial.

**Example 16-2: Training Day Meal Plan for a 180-pound Male Master**

**Breakfast**: 4 whole eggs, ½ cup oatmeal (measured dry), 1 banana

**Pre-workout**: ½ protein shake (25g) mixed w/ ½ bottle of Gatorade

**Post-workout**: ½ protein shake (25g) mixed w/ ½ bottle of Gatorade

**Lunch**: Grilled chicken breast w/ 1 small potato

**Mid-afternoon**: Protein shake (50g)

**Dinner:** Sirloins steak, grilled asparagus or salad

On non-training days, and during meals that do not occur near the training session, athletes who want to minimize bodyfat accumulation should get their carbohydrate in the form of fibrous vegetables and fruits. Eating a wide variety of fruits and vegetables (as well as a variety of meat selections) is a good way to cover the micronutrient (vitamins and minerals) needs of the lifter. A clichéd but practical recommendation is to regularly consume lots of "color" when it comes to fruits and vegetables. Doing so greatly increases the amount of exposure one has to the micronutrients the body needs for health and performance.

## Fat

Fat is a key source of energy for the body at rest and during exercise. It is not an efficient source of fuel during any form of high-intensity, "anaerobic" training, including strength training, but it is

| | MONDAY (TRAINING) | TUESDAY (ACTIVE REST) | WEDNESDAY (ACTIVE REST) | THURSDAY (TRAINING) |
|---|---|---|---|---|
| **BREAKFAST** | Cheddar omelet, Canadian bacon, grilled tomato, black coffee | Scrambled eggs w/ cheese, sausage, bacon; cantaloupe, black tea | Greek yogurt w/ honey and pecans, ham steak, black coffee | Steak and eggs, goat cheese, black coffee |
| **SNACK** | Apple; Protein shake or bar | Carrot sticks, protein shake | Orange, protein shake | Nut-dried fruit mix |
| **LUNCH** | Chicken sandwich, raw green beans, orange, iced tea | Gazpacho, grilled salmon, mixed veg, salad, sparkling water | Sashimi, rice (½), Japanese pickles, miso soup, pot-stickers, yakitori skewers, green tea | Meatloaf, carrots, mashed potatoes, gravy, tea |
| **PRE-WORKOUT** | Protein shake w/ banana and granola | N/A | N/A | Protein shake w/ banana and granola |
| **POST-WORKOUT** | Protein shake, BCAA supplement | N/A | N/A | Protein shake, BCAA supplement |
| **DINNER** | Salad w/ dressing, sirloin steak, grilled asparagus, risotto, red wine | Roast chicken: thigh, breast, drumstick; broccoli in cheese sauce, fruit w/ crème fraiche | Lamb chops, grilled polenta w/ parmesan, grilled squash, peppers, asparagus, red wine | Pork chops, sweet potato, applesauce greens |
| **CALORIES (AVG: 2345)** | 2480 | 2208 | 2290 | 2522 |
| **PROTEIN g (AVG: 211)** | 236 | 207 | 186 | 235 |
| **CARB g (AVG: 145)** | 175 | 85 | 158 | 160 |
| **FAT g (AVG: 98)** | 130 | 105 | 68 | 108 |

critical for recovery (including supporting healthy hormonal levels), for low-intensity physical exercise, and for most daily activities. So *fat is not the enemy.* But the lingering perception that fat should be avoided is a stubborn one. For many decades the public has been told that "eating fat makes you fat." Yes, fat is higher in calories *per gram* than either protein or carbohydrate. But there is nothing inherently negative about the consumption of appropriate amounts of dietary fat. Egg yolks and red meat are not only outstanding sources of protein for the athlete, but also good supplies of dietary fat, not to mention rich in vitamins and minerals that support optimum health. Both are examples of beneficial foods demonized by many in the medical community, the food sciences, the food industry, and popular culture, despite flawed and conflicting evidence.[7]

Most Masters will do well with a daily fat intake of 0.5g per pound of bodyweight per day, which will put most of these athletes somewhere between 60–120g per day.

### Nutritional supplements and ergogenic Aids

As a general rule, nutritional supplements are valuable to those who make and market nutritional supplements, and just about nobody else. We have already discussed the usefulness of whey as a supplement and recommended it as a valuable approach to maintaining the necessary protein

| FRIDAY (ACTIVE REST) | SATURDAY (ACTIVE REST) | SUNDAY (ACTIVE REST) |
|---|---|---|
| Swiss and spinach omelet, bacon, black coffee | Sausage strata, canadian bacon | Protein bar |
| Greek yogurt, almonds; Protein shake or bar | Nut-dried fruit mix, protein shake | Raw green beans, carrots, and broccoli; protein shake |
| Tuna wrap, apple, soft drink | Pork enchilada, chicken mole, Spanish rice (½), salsa, beer (½) | Lamb kabobs, tabouli, hummus, falafel, Greek coffee |
| N/A | N/A | N/A |
| N/A | N/A | N/A |
| Dinner salad, New York strip, grilled shrimp, cheese flatbread, green beans almondine, red wine | Barbecued brisket, grilled vegetables, Texas toast, beer (½) | Sea bass, grilled vegetables, white wine |
| 2281 | 2333 | 2307 |
| 207 | 198 | 213 |
| 140 | 105 | 194 |
| 80 | 115 | 81 |

***Table 16-1.*** Sample weekly meal diary for a 56-year old novice engaged in a 2-day/week training program. This individual had been previously active, but had never engaged in strength training. He weighed approximately 190 pounds at the onset of training, and weighed approximately 212 pounds at the end of his 16-week novice progression, with the accumulation of considerable muscle and some fat. Note that caloric intake and protein intake are a little higher on training days. Note also that carbohydrate intake tends to increase on training days (with some allowance for Living Life). Caloric and macronutrient quantities will of course vary with portion sizes, brand selection, etc.

intake. In this section, we consider the very few other nutritional supplements that, based on limited data, *might* be beneficial for Masters Athletes engaged in strength training.

**Fish Oil.** Most Masters should consider supplementation with an essential fatty acid (EFA) product. The EFAs include the omega-3 fatty acids, which cannot be synthesized in the body, but must be obtained from dietary sources. Dietary and/or supplemental omega-3 fatty acids have a beneficial impact on the risk of cardiovascular disease.[8] Moreover, omega-3s are involved in the production of *eicosanoids*, many of which are involved in the body's regulation of systemic inflammation, which is of course a critical concern for the Masters Athlete. Omega-3 supplements such as fish oil seem to decrease muscle soreness after training,[9] although this data is decidedly mixed.[10] Omega-3 supplementation is not necessary if the athlete regularly consumes fatty cold-water fish such as salmon as part of the diet. If the lifter is not eating fish at least a couple of times every week, then an omega-3 supplement is worth the investment.

**Vitamin D and Calcium.** Vitamin D is not a single compound, but rather a group of molecules called *secosteroids* or, less properly, the *calciferols*. These compounds are fat-soluble, but their abundance in foodstuffs is low and adequate amounts of vitamin D are usually not found in the diet unless supplemented. The major source of vitamin D is synthesis in the skin when exposed to sunlight. The newly synthesized vitamin D must then be chemically modified in the liver to become active. The implications for this vital process of our modern way of life, which primarily takes place indoors, would seem to be obvious.

Vitamin D is critical for the absorption of minerals from dietary sources, particularly calcium, magnesium, iron, zinc, and phosphorous. Its central role in calcium absorption makes it essential for skeletal health. Deficiency is associated with osteoporosis and even rickets. Some recent data suggests that vitamin D deficiency may play a role in the development of Type 2 diabetes.[11] The prevalence of vitamin D deficiency in older adults has recently been recognized as a principal contributor to the morbidity of aging.[12] In one study, half of women being treated for osteoporosis were found to have insufficient levels of vitamin D.

Some research shows that supplementation with vitamin D and calcium is generally well-tolerated, and probably helps retard or even reverse bone loss.[13] This data is not unequivocal, and much work remains to be done. What does seem clear is that supplementation with vitamin D in the absence of exercise is far less effective.

In addition, vitamin D may be useful for those Masters who, on the advice (or insistence) of their physicians, take statins for their cholesterol. Setting aside the contentious issue of whether these drugs deliver as promised, there is legitimate concern that statins can cause muscle soreness and muscle damage, and may even exacerbate insulin resistance. Some researchers believe that vitamin D can soften these effects. In our judgment, the data is far from conclusive.

**Caffeine** is a *wonderful* molecule, and its very existence makes a strong case for the beneficent Grace of Providence – proof that God loves us and wants us to drink coffee and tea. The biomedical literature has yo-yoed for decades on the overall health impact of caffeine consumption and come up with *bupkis.*[14] At the date of this writing, the available evidence suggests that it neither causes horrible diseases, nor does it cure them.[15] It's neither healthy nor unhealthy.

It's just really, really *good.*

It may also be useful in training. The role of coffee as an *ergogenic aid*, a supplement to improve performance, has been extensively studied, although most of these trials are small and not particularly well-designed. On balance, however, they seem to show that caffeine can promote better performance during a workout,[16] probably due to its effects on neuromuscular function,[17] mood state,[18] calcium release during contraction, and an increase in plasma catecholamines (epinephrine and norepinephrine).[19]

The diuretic effect of coffee and tea is vastly overblown in the public consciousness. It won't make you pee much more than an equal volume of water, and it does not have a negative effect on hydration status in healthy humans.[20] In fact, we believe coffee and tea can serve double-duty, as both mild workout stimulants and hydration agents. Very elderly or caffeine-naive Masters, and those on certain medications, should take care with coffee and other caffeinated beverages, and may reasonably forego them altogether. The real downside to caffeinated beverages for the Master is their potential impact on sleep, an important recovery consideration.

**Creatine**. In Chapter 4, during our discussion of bioenergetics, we presented the phosphagen system, at the high-intensity end of the energy spectrum. Intense anaerobic effort (like a set of squats) draws heavily on the phosphagen system. This high-power/low-capacity anaerobic system consists of the ATP already present in the muscle, which will last only a few seconds, and phosphocreatine, a depot of high-energy phosphate that can be used to instantly recharge ADP back into ATP with no intervening metabolic steps. The participation of phosphocreatine extends the capacity of the phosphagen system, prolonging the brief period during which this system can operate at maximum effort.

Phosphocreatine is formed from dietary creatine imported into the muscle. It is particularly abundant in meat. Brains and Rocky Mountain oysters are also excellent sources, if you're into that sort of thing. Creatine supplements, available as powders, pills, liquids and chews, have been shown to be *moderately* useful for those engaged in anaerobic training.[21] Supplemental creatine is readily taken up by muscle and, in the trained state, can be converted to muscle phosphocreatine fully capable of participating in the phosphocreatine-ATP cycle.

*Creatine supplementation doesn't make you stronger.* Rather, it helps extend the capacity of the phosphagen system, which might allow you to make that last rep…so you can *get* stronger. There is also some evidence that creatine enhances muscle hypertrophy by promoting an increase in muscle cell nuclei and the activation of muscle satellite cells.[22]

Many coaches, trainers, and fitness gurus recommend that creatine be "loaded" during the first week or so of use, with intake of 15–20g per day, often in conjunction with sugar. After that, a maintenance dose of 5g per day appears to be sufficient to maintain the ergogenic effect. This common practice of front-loading creatine has never been demonstrated to be superior, however, and the athlete may reasonably elect to begin with the low daily maintenance regimen.[23] Special formulations of creatine, for example "buffered" preparations or those combined with other supplements, add nothing except cost and contamination, and are to be avoided. Plain old creatine monohydrate will do nicely.[24]

Contrary to what you may have heard, there is no conclusive evidence that creatine is effective in the prevention or treatment of neurodegenerative or other diseases. Likewise, there is no evidence that creatine inflicts any harm on the healthy kidney, and its use as a supplement appears to be very safe.[25] Its benefits to training appear to be both highly individual and also difficult to assess for any particular athlete.

## Hydration

Adequate hydration is critical for optimum performance and recovery. Hydration is mandatory for muscle protein synthesis and growth, even in the face of a caloric excess and adequate protein intake. Hydration is of course important for overall health as well, to maintain appropriate vascular and interstitial fluid volumes and promote the elimination of waste products. As with nutrition, it is difficult to provide a blanket prescription for hydration. Bigger individuals need more water than smaller individuals. Athletes need more water than those who are sedentary.

We can reasonably separate our hydration recommendations into two categories – maintenance and replacement. Maintenance hydration is just what it sounds like, maintaining good hydration for the athlete who is training or engaging in physical activity a few hours a day, and who does not display an increased tendency to *insensible fluid losses* – primarily by sweating and breathing heavily during exercise. For them, we recommend about 2–3 liters (0.5–0.8 gallons) per day. In the replacement category are the athletes who sweat very heavily and therefore have more pronounced insensible losses. These individuals may require a gallon or more per day.[26] The venerable recommendation of 8 glasses of water comes out to about a half-gallon of water per day (depending on the size of your glass), which is a not-unreasonable starting point for that mythical creature, the "average" Master.

During exercise, the athlete should have fluids at the ready, and use them liberally. If thirsty – drink. By the time you're actually craving water, you've already fallen behind. The consumption of drinks containing electrolytes and some carbohydrate ("sports drinks") during exercise is not unreasonable. The athlete should take care to account for the caloric content of these beverages in his nutritional plan.

## Analgesics and Anti-Inflammatory Agents

"No pain, no gain" goes the old saying, and like most old sayings it's a tiny little nugget of truth at the center of a big lump of excrement. The kernel of truth at the heart of this particular dung-ball is that hard training *will* produce some soreness, as well as the occasional tweak or sprain. Muscle soreness reflects the training-induced perturbations of muscle structure and chemistry that will produce adaptation and increased strength. But *soreness itself* contributes *nothing* to the realization of training goals. Athletes are often told to avoid nonsteroidal anti-inflammatory drugs (NSAIDs) like ibuprofen, or analgesics like acetaminophen, on the grounds that they will "stunt your gains." Such advice is based on ignorance at best, and on a puritanical, sadomasochistic, and deeply pathological world-view at worst. It has no foundation in the available clinical evidence.

There *is* a tenuous biological rationale for supposing that NSAIDs might suppress healing or the anabolic response to training, and opponents of their use often cite basic science studies, most of which involve muscle cells in Petri dishes,[27] mutilated mice,[28] or bizarre experiments conducted on exercise physiology students.[29] But when the issue is investigated in actual humans, with a view to their ability to make progress on a training program, it becomes clear that NSAID use has no practically significant effect on increases in strength. This appears to be most particularly true for older athletes, who actually seem to do *better* on a training program when they keep their soreness on a short leash.[30]

This issue has been treated in depth by Sullivan,[31] and readers who are interested in the biology and research details are referred to that article. The bottom line is that the *episodic* use of NSAIDs and non-narcotic analgesics (e.g., acetaminophen) does not appear to have any adverse effect on training progress, and probably has a positive impact, by allowing athletes to continue their training and active rest with minimal discomfort. These medicines do have some side effects, and they should be used as directed, and only intermittently, when needed. They may be contraindicated for some athletes who are on certain medications or who suffer from certain ailments. But in general, *Masters who have pain should treat it*, and be grateful they live in a world where effective analgesics and anti-inflammatories are available, cheap, and safe. Technological civilization has its perks.

## Sleep

Many of the anabolic processes that occur during recovery take place during sleep. The secretion of anabolic hormones is the most important of these processes for the recovering Master. Masters are struggling with optimal hormonal production as it is. When sleep is disrupted or in inadequate supply, production is limited even further.

Testosterone levels start to climb upon falling asleep, peaking during the critical REM cycles, which begin about 90 minutes later. Those levels remain elevated until one awakes. Human growth hormone (HGH), another anabolic hormone, is also elevated during sleep.[32] Among many other effects, HGH is important for the modulation of growth factor signaling and the effects of cortisol. Cortisol is a catabolic hormone released during periods of heavy physical stress like weight training. Continuously elevated levels of cortisol appear to promote entry into Selye's stage III – exhaustion or overtraining. So sleep has manifold impacts on recovery.

For a variety of reasons, many Masters will have trouble getting enough sleep, particularly REM sleep. Early awakening, or interruption of sleep every couple of hours through the night, shortens or prevents deep REM sleep and therefore limits the contributions available from longer periods of elevated anabolic hormone stimulation.

Eight hours of sleep is a reasonable target. That means eight hours of *sleep,* not two hours in bed watching *Letterman* and *Sports Center,* followed by 6 hours of actual sleep. Additionally, 8 hours of *continuous* sleep is not the same thing as 8 hours of sleep interrupted three or four times a night.

Many Masters will find that training markedly improves their sleep. But for many aging adults, interruption of regular continuous sleep is a recurring problem, even with exercise. This can come from a whole host of sources – emotional stress or anxiety, medications, joint pain, issues affecting urination (such as an enlarged prostate), and so on. Some of these may require medical investigation and treatment. But many Masters will benefit immensely from a few simple behavioral modifications: regulation of the amount and timing of food, caffeine, and alcohol intake, optimization of the sleep environment, and, when absolutely necessary, the episodic use of mild sleep aids.

### Caffeine, alcohol and food

Caffeine can keep the mind awake even when the body is exhausted. Regular consumers of caffeine products like coffee should make a note of their last serving on nights where sleep is a problem. With careful monitoring, it may be possible to discover useful patterns. If caffeine intake is stopped at a particular time of day, it may have no impact on sleep later.

Alcohol in the form of a "night cap" often has the pleasant perceived effect of easing one down, especially after a tiring, stressful day. A small glass of good bourbon in the evening may initially help ease you into sleep, but many report being wide awake just a few hours later. Alcohol disrupts the normal sleep cycle architecture, decreasing the amount of time in slow wave (stages 3 and 4) sleep. Again, looking for patterns can help the Master determine when, relative to bedtime, he needs to lock up the liquor cabinet.

Certain types of food can also interrupt the sleep pattern. Very spicy food in the evening is antagonistic to sleep for many, especially those in their sixth decade and beyond. Caffeine, nicotine, high-fat meals, chocolate, and alcohol all promote relaxation of the lower esophageal sphincter and can lead to reflux and heartburn, which will disrupt sleep and can cause other problems as well. The athlete should monitor his sleep quality in the context of his food and beverage intake, and then develop a composite evening meal-beverage-sleep routine once agreeable choices have been identified.

### The sleep environment

The sleep environment is crucial. Evidence, experience, and common sense dictate that the athlete's sleep environment should be comfortable, dark, and quiet. Most people find they sleep better in a room that is a bit on the cool side. Quiet is essential. Family, children, and pets must either respect the athlete's need for quiet, uninterrupted sleep, or go live elsewhere. Many find white noise helpful or even essential to sleep. Inexpensive white noise generators are available, but a little table fan may work just as well. Watching TV, eating, web-surfing, or working in bed are not acceptable for the Master looking to promote optimal recovery. Bedtime is for sex (an important recovery and lifestyle factor!), and for sleep, and that's it.

The key is consistency: the bed, the pillows, the temperature, the dark, the quiet, and the white noise should, like the time at which one retires, be the same from night to night. It all comes together to form a comprehensive sleep routine, a complex conditioned stimulus that sends a powerful signal to the nervous system and the body: *time to fall asleep now and grow some muscle.*

### Sleep aids

The *occasional* use of sleep aids may be helpful to those Masters who have difficulty falling asleep or staying asleep, but habitual use of such agents should be considered problematic in itself, and is to be avoided. This is especially true of powerful prescription sleep aids, which can have untoward side effects. Athletes with persistent insomnia despite attention to the previously noted sleep hygiene factors should discuss the issue with their doctor, and any pharmacologic sleep aids should be used by Masters only under the supervision of a physician.

Melatonin, valerian, and diphenhydramine, all available over the counter, may be helpful when used episodically. Melatonin has a mild impact and is generally well-tolerated. Valerian root is used by some to good effect. Diphenhydramine is often effective, but it can interact with other medications and has anticholinergic properties – meaning it's sort of a very mild form of deadly nightshade or jimson weed. It is usually quite safe, but will be contraindicated for some Masters. So we repeat: use pharmacologic sleep aids, even over-the-counter agents, only under a physician's supervision, and then only when other sleep hygiene factors have been adequately addressed.

## Stress Reduction

Chronic stress has an unwholesome effect on recovery at every level. An athlete who is mentally or emotionally overwhelmed by work, family, financial, or psychological stress will suffer at the physiological level as well, impacting not only recovery from training but also general health. Chronic stress suppresses anabolism and has unhealthy effects on cardiovascular parameters. A comprehensive treatment of stress reduction is far beyond the scope of this text. But the Master lives in an age of information, abundance, relative comfort, and medical knowledge that his ancestors could not have imagined in their most ecstatic dreams. There are resources available to assist the Master in identifying, minimizing, and neutralizing life stresses and putting them into context. Training itself can be a powerful tonic to stress. But stress that prevents or impairs productive training must be addressed, because its impacts are likely to go well beyond preventing gains in the gym. Overwhelming stress, worry, and despair are threats to health and even to life, and may indicate serious underlying endocrine or neuropsychiatric derangements. We implore the Master confronted by these difficulties to bring them promptly to the attention of medical or mental health professionals.

# 17

# Elements of Program Design and Execution

Training programs are built up from *training variables*, which are manipulated over the course of an overload event to produce a training stress, promote recovery, and permit the display of an adaptive response. The most prominent training variables in any given program will be volume and intensity. *Intensity* is the load relative to the athlete's maximum strength. *Volume* is a measure of the total number of times an exercise is performed, and is a function of sets and their constituent repetitions. Different set-repetition schemes allow for the training of different attributes and address different elements of the Stress-Recovery-Adaptation cycle. As such they constitute important components for the design of training programs. Masters Athletes respond differently to volume and intensity than their younger counterparts, and these variables require special considerations in the design of Masters programs. In this chapter, these components are examined in detail, followed by a description of the overall structure of a typical workout, and the method and importance of record-keeping.

## Intensity and Volume

A training program is constructed by manipulating training variables in such a way as to promote the realization of long-term improvement in physical performance. The resultant program will specify the structure of every workout, when each workout is to be performed, and how progress is to be assessed and tracked.

Numerous training variables are available for incorporation into program design, and programs that manipulate several variables simultaneously can become quite complex – usually unnecessarily, and sometimes to the point of being ridiculous. Masters will achieve excellent training results by engaging in programs that manipulate only a few training factors. The novice program – in which the athlete gets stronger faster than at any other time in his training career – makes significant manipulations in only *one* training variable.

Understanding training variables, how they address or correspond to the Stress-Recovery-

Adaptation cycle, and how they can be manipulated to achieve training goals, is fundamental to an understanding of programming for strength. An examination of these training variables will also introduce an elementary vocabulary that will be essential as we proceed.

By far the two most important training variables to understand *in the gym* are intensity and volume. The two are inversely related. As one goes up, the other must go down.

***Intensity*** is simply the load, or resistance, relative to the athlete's absolute strength.[1] Anything above 90% of a lifter's 1-repetition maximum (1RM) is considered *high intensity.* Work between 75–85% of 1RM is *medium intensity* – and is where much of the strength *building* is actually done. Loads between 60–70% are used for certain types of hypertrophy or power-based training protocols, and are considered *low intensity.*

In the weight room, there is nothing subjective about this variable. It has nothing to do with how "intense" the workout *felt,* how difficult the workout looked, how much you sweated, or how much you grunted and groaned. *Intensity* is not synonymous with *difficulty.* Squatting at 70% 1RM for 12 repetitions in a row is difficult. So is squatting 2 repetitions at 95%. Both are *hard,* but the former is considered low intensity, and the latter is high intensity.

It is important at this juncture to emphasize that the above discussion of relative intensities as a proportion of 1RM is only for the purposes of illustrating the concept of intensity itself. *Testing a novice athlete for a 1RM is* never *indicated.* Such a determination has no utility in novice programming, and offers nothing except a needless risk of injury. The true value of a 1RM has relevance only in the intermediate or advanced phases of training.

***Volume*** is simply the total number of times an exercise is performed. A workout in which the exercise is performed many times is a *high-volume* workout – regardless of its intensity. A *low-volume* workout is one in which the exercise is performed only a few times. It is easy to see how volume and intensity will be inversely related. For example, a workout at very high volume simply *cannot* be performed at very high intensity. Programs beyond the novice phase of training manipulate both variables, to generate training stress with both high-volume/moderate-intensity as well as low-volume/high-intensity work sets as part of the overload event. The latter are commonly used to demonstrate or test increased strength in a training period. Low-volume/low-intensity workouts are incorporated for recovery sessions.

The elements of volume are repetitions and sets. A ***repetition*** (or "rep") is simply a single execution of the exercise. A ***set*** is a prescribed number of repetitions, to be performed one immediately after the other. If a trainee lifts a barbell 5 times, racks it, rests a minute, and then does 5 more, he has performed 2 sets. Volume can be calculated daily, weekly, or monthly. Weekly and monthly volume calculations also take into account the ***frequency*** with which the exercises are performed in a given time frame. Frequency is an important variable for the design and modification of Masters training programs.

## Set Theory

Sets, and the rest between them, are the brick and mortar of a program, and of an individual workout. Several types of sets are used to achieve specific objectives in program design.

***Note: This text uses the following format when specifying training loads: Weight x reps x sets. Example: 45x5x2 = 45 pounds x 5 reps x 2 sets. Unless otherwise specified, weights are in pounds. For examples without weights specified, the format is: number of sets x number of reps. Example: 3x10 = 3 sets of 10 reps.***

***Work sets*** are the primary goal of the workout. A work set may be a single set of, say, 5 repetitions. But work sets are more commonly a "set of sets," as in a group of work sets consisting of 3 sets of 5 reps each (3x5). *It is through performance of the* *prescribed work sets that the objective of the training session is realized.* If the athlete is an intermediate trainee and the objective of today's workout is to produce a volume training stress, this objective may be achieved through the performance of 5 sets of 5 reps (5x5) at 85% 1RM – a high-volume/medium-intensity workout. If the goal of today's session is recovery, two work sets of 5 reps at 70% 1RM may be prescribed. If today training stress is also for displaying adaptation and demonstrating a new level of strength, the program might specify a low-volume/high-intensity workout with 1 set of 5 reps (1x5) at a new 5RM. If the trainee is a novice, his work sets do not manipulate volume or intensity but impose a new training stress and display adaptation each session as load is increased.

The work set is what the program tells the athlete to do *today*.

The programs in this book call for work sets to be performed as ***sets across.*** This means that all the work sets are performed with the same load for the same number of repetitions, and that all work sets for a particular exercise are performed in sequence. In other words, we don't mix up or stagger work sets for different exercises. We squat until our squat work sets are complete before we move on to the press or the deadlift.

***Warm-up sets*** are sets performed at lower intensity to prepare the lifter's tissues and nervous system for the heavier sets to come. Warm-up sets are not a specific goal of the workout, as they are not of sufficient volume or intensity to impose a training stress. Typically, warm-ups begin with an empty bar. Weight is then added for several sets of decreasing volume until the trainee is prepared to attack the work sets. We shall have more to say about this later in the chapter.

***Ascending sets*** are used in certain novice variants and some intermediate programs. These are work set variants in which the weight on the bar increases from one set to another, often (but not always) while decreasing the number of reps per set ("pyramid sets"). Examples are to be found in Chapters 21 and 22.

***Back-off sets*** are performed, if indicated, after the work sets, and at decreased intensity. Back-off sets are useful when a coach or an experienced trainee determines that the training situation requires more volume or technical work than is provided by the work set. For example, back-off sets can be used if a trainee is struggling with some element of technique during his work sets. It allows the coach to make corrections in real time with decreased weight on the bar rather than waiting until the next workout. Or perhaps the trainee has failed his last work set by a single rep. If in the coach's judgment the addition of a little more volume might drive sufficient adaptation before the next session and allow the trainee to achieve the target work set at that time, a back-off set at moderate intensity may be indicated. Specific examples of how and why back-off sets are used in program design will be found in relevant portions of the chapters ahead.

Not all exercises are created equal, and some obviously create more stress than others. Deadlifts in particular create a powerful training stress. This is a good thing, but the stress must be managed carefully. At work set weights, deadlifts are generally appropriate for just 1 set, whereas squats, presses, and bench presses typically use 3 sets. Exceptions to this rule might be in the initial stages of training (the first week or two), when the trainee is handling light weights, for the purposes of building exercise capacity and learning the proper techniques. During this time, the coach may ask the trainee to perform multiple deadlift sets (2–5) to practice form and provide the coach more opportunities to refine the athlete's technique. However, once the exercise is mastered and the weight on the bar grows truly heavy, deadlifts are limited to a single work set.

As a trainee progresses over time and grows in strength, he will start to tax his recovery capacity at his top work sets. Once this happens, athletes and coaches might consider a reduction in the number of work sets as a means of managing the stress in a way that recovery can still occur in a 48–72 hour window. We will see many examples of how this is done in the chapters ahead.

Most assistance exercises are not nearly as stressful to the system as a squat or a deadlift. More sets per exercise can be used for these movements when appropriate.

## Set-Repetition Schemes and Specific Training Goals

Sets and reps are fundamental components of program design because different set-rep schemes produce different forms of adaptation, and are therefore employed, in conjunction with appropriate intensity, in the pursuit of different training goals.[2] Sets of 1–3 reps at high intensity are classically associated with the production of raw strength and power. Sets of 8–12 reps at moderate intensity are used to increase muscle mass and size (hypertrophy). Such sets are important program elements for ***bodybuilding*** or athletes whose primary training goal is the rapid addition of muscular weight. Very high-repetition sets (between 15–20), necessarily performed at low intensity, are used to train muscular endurance, and so are effective tools for athletes who need to produce relatively low forces for long intervals while resisting extreme fatigue.

None of these set-rep ranges are optimal for the novice athlete. Even when power, hypertrophy, or endurance are the ultimate goals, using these set-rep schemes for a novice is premature and inefficient. Effective training for power, endurance, and muscle mass all require a foundation of strength. Power is simply strength displayed quickly, and power therefore increases as strength increases. Likewise, the lack of a foundation of whole body strength means the athlete will not be able to generate optimum stress for the training of hypertrophy or muscular endurance.

Although the ideal set-rep range has long been a matter of contention in the exercise science literature,[3] a tremendous amount of practical coaching experience has shown that general strength is very efficiently developed with multiple 5-repetition sets. In novice programming, the 5-rep set is the target for all primary barbell movements. Sets of 5 work in the optimal range for establishment of both strength and muscle mass – the two primary goals of the novice. Sets of 5 occupy the "metabolic middle" of the strength training spectrum. They produce a training stress powerful enough to drive adaptation, but which permits recovery within a 48–72 hour window.

Heavy sets of 1 and 2 are a very direct method of training for absolute strength, but are not as effective for hypertrophy as sets of 5, and in any case are not optimal or safe for novices who have not yet mastered the technical aspects of these exercises.

Sets of 3 or 4 repetitions are used in some novice program variants. These variants and their indications will be detailed in the training protocols to follow. Sets of more than 5 reps will be used in novice programming only for accessory or remedial exercises used to prepare for or replace the primary barbell movements due to individual physical limitations.

Training the primary barbell exercises with higher-rep schemes (e.g., sets of 8–20) is not a good idea for the Masters novice. The older the trainee, the more unwise such high-volume work is. It is common to assume that higher reps at lower loads will be safer for weak Masters novices, while still achieving training objectives. This assumption is reflected in some of the literature. We remind the reader that most of this literature is based on the use of machine-based resistance training, usually at low intensity, and we are forced to conclude that the authors of such recommendations have never witnessed the effects that a set of 10–15 barbell squats, even at low intensity, can have on a 60 year-old novice. *Masters Athletes are extremely volume-sensitive.* Barbell workouts at high volume in the Master are likely to result in a week or more of crippling muscle soreness, systemic inflammation, joint pain, fatigue – and the interruption or termination of training.

This is coaching malpractice. It should *never* happen. *The Masters novice must not be exposed to high-volume (>8 reps) barbell training at high- or moderately-high intensity*, and should keep repetitions for non-barbell accessory exercises such as chin-ups at 15 or less. Intermediate Masters who have built a foundation of strength and conditioning may require some modifications to their set-rep schemes, but these will usually tend toward less, not more volume.

## Rest Between Sets

Sitting down between sets in not being lazy. It is absolutely necessary to completely recover after a difficult work set. During this time, increased oxygen consumption (mitochondrial metabolism) supports the replenishment of muscle ATP, phosphocreatine, calcium gradients, and glucose.

Rest between sets can be manipulated like any other factor to elicit certain adaptations. For hypertrophy and muscular endurance, rest time is usually quite brief (30–120 seconds), and sets are often performed to failure, meaning the number of reps will vary. In strength training, however, the objective is to lift the prescribed work set weight for the prescribed volume. This cannot be done when fatigue is excessive and recovery from the previous set is incomplete. It is the *work* that causes the adaptation, not the rest between sets. For strength work, a minimum of 3–5 minutes should be taken between work sets at the onset of training. As strength increases and the weight on the bar gets heavier, rest intervals of 8–10 minutes will be needed.

We emphasize that rest between work sets is *complete* rest, not to be confused with the popular notion of active rest advocated by certain health and fitness organizations. Rest between sets does *not* include cardio intervals or other exercises. This is not a conditioning workout (although it will in fact promote conditioning adaptations). This is strength training. We aren't interested in maintaining a particular heart rate or constant activity for an hour. In fact, you should probably be prepared to do as much sitting as you will lifting during an hour of strength training. It's fine, and even beneficial, for the trainee to get up, walk around, and "shake it out" during the last minute or so of his timed rest interval. Anything more strenuous is entirely counterproductive. *The objective is to complete the work sets.* Failure to ensure adequate interset rest is one of the most common reasons we see for failure to progress on a strength program.

Later in the text, we will briefly discuss the concept of circuit training for selected, much older Masters who may have reached a point where maintenance of strength, or much slower progression, is now an appropriate goal. Circuit training for these *very uncommon* individuals involves the performance of multiple exercises, usually 2–4 back-to-back in a continuous circuit of movement with little to no rest between exercises. This type of training is popular, and may be tempting for some. But for the vast majority of Masters, who need to focus on the development of strength and lean tissue, it is relatively contraindicated.

## Volume-Intensity Dosing and Considerations for Masters

The most important consideration to remember when programming for Masters is that they are *volume-sensitive and intensity-dependent.* The quickest way to push a Master into a state of overtraining is through excessive volume. Too much work during the training session (excessive volume) or too many training sessions during the week (excessive frequency) can push the Master into exhaustion. On the other hand, Masters detrain very quickly in relation to their younger counterparts when the weight on the bar is decreased for any significant period of time.

When the athlete begins to stall on a well-designed program with well-managed recovery, the first adjustments should therefore come in the form of decreasing workout volume or workout frequency, not intensity. The wise programmer will eliminate sets or decrease the prescribed number of reps per set, eliminate an exercise, or even take a day out of the weekly training schedule before decreasing the weight on a Master's bar.

In the later stages of novice programming, Masters will begin using light days for the squat. This is not a contradiction of the volume-sensitive/intensity-dependent principle, but rather a harbinger of intermediate programming. Moreover, light days for Masters maintain higher intensity than light days for younger athletes.

# Structure of the Workout

## Preparation

It should go without saying that the athlete should begin the training session well-rested, well-nourished, free of competing obligations, reasonably sober, and so on. The athlete should have consumed a pre-workout meal, such as a protein shake with some carbohydrate, no sooner than an hour prior to beginning exercise. The athlete should appear in clean, appropriate attire. Trainees may understandably *get* smelly and dirty during a workout, but those who *show up* smelly and dirty are inconsiderate of others and may reasonably be dismissed. The athlete will have his training log at hand, and a clear idea of the day's work objectives: exercises to be performed and their corresponding work sets. A review of the last few workouts is a good idea. Many find it useful to write out the day's warm-up sets and work sets on a large whiteboard and place it where it can be referred to rapidly. This makes moving through the workout more efficient, especially when multiple athletes are sharing the coach, the gym, or even a single rack. Chalkboards, phone apps, and spreadsheets can also be used. Any system that assists the lifter in moving efficiently through the workout will do.

## Warm-up

The completion of each prescribed exercise in the workout will begin with a specific warm-up. The warm-up is essential for priming the movement pattern to be used, increasing muscle blood flow, temperature, and elasticity, and allowing the coach to make corrections to the movement while the weight is low. As the warm-ups get heavier, molecular, cellular, and systemic changes prepare the athlete to perform at work set weight.

It is useful to distinguish between *specific warm-up* and *general warm-up*. A general warm-up is any activity that causes the body's temperature to rise and increase blood flow to the entire system of muscles and joints. A general warm-up is not an absolute necessity, but it isn't a bad idea for an athlete over 50. A general warm-up can be any activity, lasting from 5–10 minutes, that gets the circulation going and loosens up sore muscles and stiff joints. A few minutes on a stationary bike, an elliptical machine, a rowing machine, or even a brisk walk around the block will do the trick. The coach should take great care not to exhaust a deconditioned trainee with the warm-up before the workout can even begin. High-intensity forms of aerobic activity such as rope-jumping and running should be avoided. The point is to increase blood flow, muscle temperature, and mobility without accumulating fatigue. If this can be done easily it should be.

The specific warm-up occurs after the completion of the general warm-up. It simply consists of one or two light sets (usually an empty bar) with whatever exercise the trainee is going to start with that day. He may do as little as one set of 5 reps or as many as 20 total reps if he is feeling particularly stiff or sore. Areas that have been affected by injury in the past will likely need additional warm-up. The first exercise of the day will also likely need more warm-up than the second and third exercises of the day. This is particularly true with the novice program, which begins every session with squats. The legs seem to start stiffer than the upper body and require more warm-up sets. However, once the squat portion of the workout is complete, the whole body is generally very warmed up and the second exercise of the day (press or bench) will warm up rather easily.

There is no set protocol for empty-bar warm-ups. Go by feel. Do enough work with the empty bar to get loose and pliable. That amount of work may vary from workout to workout based on how the trainee feels.

Moving the specific warm-up beyond the empty bar can be confusing for a new trainee who is trying to find the balance between preventing injury and not exhausting himself with excessive workloads. Warm-up mistakes are a frequent problem, and usually take one of the following forms.

**Too many warm-up sets.** This is a particularly common mistake, often caused by a lack of confidence by the trainee (or his coach). The athlete wants to "test the waters" as he moves up in weight, making smaller jumps as the warm-ups edge closer to the work set weight. This result is an excessive number of warm-up sets, and too many warm-up sets too close to work set weight.

Example 17-1 illustrates both flawed and appropriate warm-up plans for a prescribed work set of 305x5x3. In the incorrect warm-up (left), the athlete was either unsure of what he wanted to do that day, or was unsure of his ability to do what he had planned. Both are symptomatic of poor record keeping, poor planning, or no plan at all. An athlete with a good training plan and meticulous records shouldn't be unsure of what he can do on a particular day. His program should have *prepared* him to do the work sets. The warm-up sets at 290 and 300 should not have been done. A better warm-up protocol – shown on the right – is discussed below.

**Too many reps close to work set weight.** Unless the trainee's program explicitly prescribes ascending sets of multiple reps for the purposes of volume accumulation, there is no reason to do more than a single rep for the last several warm-up sets. In fact, any set done after the third warm-up set isn't so much for "warming" as it is for preparing the athlete's nervous system and muscle biochemistry for the heavy work sets to follow. This neural and biochemical preparation must be done incrementally, but it is not necessary to do multiple reps per set and accumulate excessive fatigue.

As an example, for a trainee working up to a 305-pound squat for five reps, the first three warm-ups will be about 10 reps with the bar (2x5), 5 reps with 135, and 3 reps with 185. After this the athlete is warm, well-perfused and limber…but he is obviously not ready to make the jump from 185x3 to 305x5. He must now incrementally prime his muscles and nervous system for the work set. This can be done with heavy singles. After 185x3, an excellent approach would be 225x1, then 255x1, and finally 285x1. More than that is not only a waste of energy, but will fatigue the athlete before the work sets even begin.

**Example 17-1: Warm-up**

| *Incorrect* Approach | Correct Approach |
|---|---|
| 45x5x2 | 45x5x2 |
| 135x5 | 135x5 |
| 185x3 | 185x3 |
| 225x1 | 225x1 |
| 255x1 | 255x1 |
| 275x1 | 285x1 |
| 285x1 | 305x5x3 |
| 290x1 | |
| 300x1 | |
| 305x5x3 | |

**Not enough warm-up sets – jumps too big.** This error is common among inexperienced, overzealous, *younger* lifters who haven't already made this mistake. This usually happens when an athlete feels invigorated by his initial warm-ups. He feels great – pliable and strong. So he arrogantly jumps from 185x3 to 305 for his 5RM attempt and gets quite thoroughly and deservedly stapled. It's tragic: He would have made 305x5, a new ***Personal Record*** (PR), had he conducted a proper warm-up. Perhaps he suffers from the common misconception that all the extra singles after 185x3 would only tire him out prior to his work set weights. If instead he takes adequate rest and the last several warm-ups are kept to just 1 rep, this heartbreak can be avoided.

**A general approach to warm-up set design.** There is no cookie-cutter formula that can be applied to every exercise for every trainee at every level of training. But we can apply the principles discussed above to come up with a good approach to designing warm-up sets.

1. **Establish last warm-up set first.** This will be for a single approximately 5–10% below the target work set weight.

2. **Plan the warm-up progression backwards** from the last warm-up single, using

approximately equal increments of 15–20% until you arrive at the empty bar.

3. **Do as many sets with the empty bar as it takes to feel loose and pliable**. This will vary day to day and lift to lift.

4. **The first warm-up set with weight added to the bar is done for 5 reps.**

5. **The next (and possibly one additional) warm-up set is done for a triple.**

6. **All other warm-up sets are done for singles.**

This approach can and must be individualized. Every athlete is different, and each day for each athlete is different, and conditions will influence the structure of the warm-up. Sometimes extra sets at the bottom end for sore and stiff joints are warranted, and sometimes an extra set at the top end is needed if the groove just doesn't feel right on a particular day. Athlete and coach should have rational approach to the *general* design of warm-up sets, but should learn to go by feel as well.

### Work sets and interset rest

After the last warm-up single, the athlete will rest for 3–5 minutes. The trainee then begins with the first work set, after which he will rest again, for 5, 8, or even 10 minutes.

Rest between work sets is essential. There is nothing to be gained by rushing from one work set to the next, except failure. Remember, *the work sets are the objective of the entire workout.* The athlete should rest long enough between work sets to ensure that they are completed with good form. Interset rest can be used for record-keeping, drinking, technical discussion with coach and training partners, and arguing over the music.

### Completing the workout

When the last work set is racked and the workout is over, the athlete still has some work to do. We believe it is good practice to take a protein shake or the equivalent as soon as possible after the workout is completed. Bars, plates and other materials should be returned to their proper place – this is not only respectful of the facility and the equipment, but also an important safety consideration. Debriefing with the coach or training partners and planning for the next workout are excellent ideas.

Finally, the athlete must ensure that his training log is complete, and record any observations or impressions that may be important to consider later. This brings us to the critical importance of record-keeping.

## The Training Log

People who just *exercise* don't need a log. They just need a calendar, or some sort of routine, a willingness to get up and move, and a cool-looking head band.

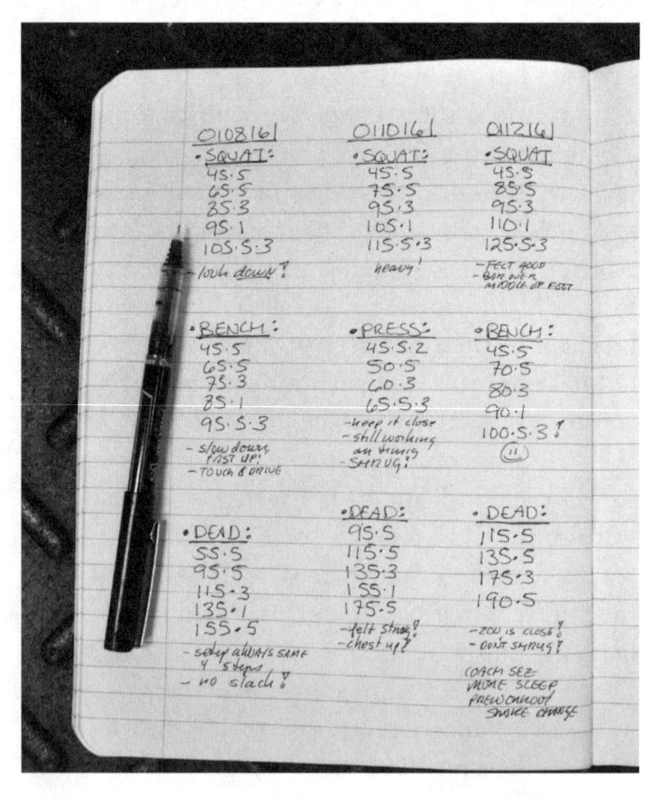


***Figure 17-1.*** The training log. The athlete records all sets and reps and includes notes on the workout. This example organizes the log into one column for each training session, but any format that works for both coach and athlete is acceptable.

But athletes don't exercise. They *train*. They're engaged in a program that manipulates one or more training variables to achieve improvements in the General Fitness Attributes, and as such they need to maintain a careful record of anything that might influence training progress.

In the Silicon Age, there are any number of options for "virtual" record-keeping. The athlete may have an app on his phone, a spreadsheet on his laptop, or a training log at lookhowstrongiam.com. That's all good, and you should do those things if you wish, but we're going to be fuddy-duddies here and insist that *a paper log is first priority.* The humble English composition book, available at any drugstore for about a dollar, is still the gold standard. It fits in your gym bag, it's simple, quick, and easy to use, it doesn't need a power cord, and nobody in their right mind is going to steal it. Spreadsheets and online training logs can be extremely useful. But paper logs don't have server crashes.

There are different formats for record-keeping in a paper log, but we're partial to the format illustrated in Figure 17-1. There's nothing magical about this approach: each workout logged in a column, one set per line, etc. It works. Athlete and coach should settle on a format that works for both and allows for rapid reference so that progress can be easily tracked and planned. Note that *every set is logged*, not just the work sets, and that the athlete has included ancillary notes and impressions. These can be crucial sources of information when the program stalls or a layoff is necessary.

We can't overemphasize the importance of recording your work. Training is a long-term, highly structured project in adjusting your physiology and performance to optimize your health. Think of that little book in your gym bag as a sort of treatment log or medical record, and maintain it accordingly.

# 18

# Athlete Program Categories: Novice, Intermediate, and Beyond

The structure of the training program for any particular athlete is governed by the rate at which that athlete progresses through the Stress-Recovery-Adaptation cycle. As an athlete gets stronger, he can impose a heavier training stress, requiring more time to recover and adapt and greater programming complexity. Program design and athlete classification therefore reflect and exploit the biology of adaptation.

Athletes and their appropriate training programs may be categorized as *novice*, *intermediate*, and *advanced*. This terminology explicitly identifies the capacity of an athlete to progress through an entire Stress-Recovery-Adaptation cycle, and the type of program appropriate to that athlete. The Master's adaptive capacity is a function of age, sex, genetic endowment, and other variables. The closer the athlete gets to his performance potential, the longer his training period will become, and the more complex the overload event will be. The athlete will always engage in the training program that produces strength at the fastest rate, utilizing the shortest possible training period and the minimum level of complexity. In this regard, the novice is the most enviable athlete of all.

## Program Design Reflects Adaptive Capacity

In this text we follow Rippetoe in classifying athletes and their training programs as *novice*, *intermediate*, and *advanced*. These categories have nothing to do with an athlete's absolute strength or their innate athletic abilities. In many areas of human endeavor, these terms denote a particular level of ability or experience. However, our use of this terminology explicitly identifies the *capacity of an athlete to progress through an entire Stress-Recovery-Adaptation cycle*, and the type of program appropriate to that athlete. A novice athlete may very well be much stronger than an intermediate or advanced athlete. The difference between these categories lies not in the absolute strength of the trainee, but in adaptive capacity.

Let us consider the example of a 63 year-old female Master who is just beginning a strength training program. She is healthy and not terribly deconditioned, and she is compliant with recovery factors such as active rest, nutrition and sleep. For the sake of simplicity, let us consider only her squat. On her first day of training, she achieves a work set weight of 50 pounds on the squat for 3 sets of five repetitions. She returns to the gym two days later, and finds that she can now squat 55 pounds for 3 sets of 5 reps. When she returns 3 days later, she is able to squat 60 pounds for her work sets.

This trainee is displaying the capacity to adapt to an increased training stress from one session to the next and each workout serves as an overload event. She can continue to exploit this pattern for quite some time, adding weight to the bar at every workout as her strength increases. Her program dictates that she do exactly that, thereby *fully exploiting her adaptive capacity.*

Put another way, this athlete is not yet strong enough to impose a training stress that exceeds her capacity to adapt before the next training session.

But she *is* getting stronger, and fast. Eventually, her progress will slow, and then stall. Certain techniques will allow her to jump-start her pattern of workout-to-workout increases, but they will only get her so far. This sort of progress simply cannot be maintained indefinitely. Sooner or later, our athlete gets strong enough to apply a training stress so heavy that she cannot recover and adapt before the next training session.

This does not mean our athlete has reached her maximum strength or the end of her strength training career. And it is most certainly *not* an indication to stop trying to get stronger, nor does it indicate some sort of "maintenance" program. Rather, it is simply a reflection of biological reality: The athlete now requires more time to recover from and adapt to a training stress, and a corresponding increase in the complexity of her training program design.

Since the athlete cannot recover and adapt from workout to workout, her program will now stretch the Stress-Recovery-Adaptation cycle over a longer period, encompassing multiple workouts. The overload event will impose training stress with one or more workouts of high-volume/moderate-intensity and/or low-volume/high-intensity. Sessions of low volume and intensity will allow her to train movements as she recovers, while further stimulating the cellular and hormonal systems that are supporting adaptation. Progress on the program will be determined by the display of a new level of strength adaptation, usually measured with a low-volume/high-intensity work set. This new level of strength will serve as the index for calculating new training stresses, and the cycle will begin again. The Stress-Recovery-Adaptation cycle, which could previously be completed within 48–72 hours and from one workout to the next, now takes a week, and multiple workouts. This new, longer, more elaborate program will allow the athlete to get stronger for a very long time, but at a slower rate, and at the cost of increased training complexity. As the level of strength increases, the athlete's adaptive capacity will be taxed further, and may eventually necessitate an even more complex program with a longer training period – a month or even longer.

*At each stage, the program reflects the adaptive capacity of the athlete and exploits it to the fullest.* We certainly *could* start her out with a longer, more complicated program, but to do so would simply be a waste of valuable training time. If our trainee *can* get stronger from workout to workout, then she *should*, and her program should reflect this adaptive capacity until the athlete's strength demands a change.

The adaptive capacity of any athlete is a function of many factors, the most important and fundamental of which is the athlete's ***genetic potential***, the theoretical upper limit of performance imposed by heritable characteristics – that is, the genotype. Anybody can get stronger, but some people are more "naturally strong" than others, by virtue of their genetic endowment. No matter how well-designed and exquisitely tailored the program, now matter how assiduously the athlete trains or attends to recovery factors, genetic endowment imposes a hard biological limit on strength (or power, mobility, endurance, or any other fitness attribute). Accordingly, the athlete's adaptive capacity depends not only on absolute strength, but how close the athlete approaches his genetically-determined athletic potential.

To illustrate, let's say our athlete in the above example has been training for four months, adding weight to the bar at every workout until she can no longer do so. A transition from this simple but incredibly powerful program to a more complex, more protracted program is now indicated. At this point, she has demonstrated the ability to squat 115 pounds for 5 repetitions. Another athlete of the same sex, age, body composition, weight, and commitment might achieve 145 pounds or more before requiring a change in her program. The *absolute* strength of the two athletes is very different, but both have achieved approximately the *same level of strength relative to their genetic potential* – the level of strength at which an increase in training period duration and program complexity is required for further progress.

## Training Period and Program Complexity Increase Over Time

Clearly, an increase in the duration of the training period corresponds to an increase in program complexity. When our athlete in the above example began her training program, she was working at the most fundamental level of program design. She performed the same number of sets and repetitions at each workout, holding the *volume* constant. The only variable manipulated was the *load*, the amount of weight on the bar, which increased at every training session. This situation is extraordinary, enviable, almost magical. It is the only rational starting point for training. Contrary to the conventional wisdom of the fitness industry, most personal trainers, and the vast majority of physicians, it seems self-evident to the authors that anybody who *can* get stronger with such a simple program...*should.*

Alas, nothing lasts forever, and as increasing strength mandates an increase in training period, the complexity of programming must also increase. Our athlete must now stretch the Stress-Recovery-Adaptation cycle over multiple workouts, and this in itself constitutes a primary increase in program complexity. As the athlete becomes more adapted to a strength training stress – as she becomes *stronger* – the nature of the overload event changes to accommodate the stress-recovery-adaptation cycle. As she gets stronger, she becomes capable of applying a higher intensity stress, which requires more time to recover from. But at the same time, her more adapted physiology requires more stress to cause an adaptation to occur.

These goals cannot be realized by simply adding weight to the bar, and so another layer of complexity will be required. Sets, reps, frequency, exercise selection, and intensity will *all* be manipulated so as to make each workout serve its purpose in the program.

A rank newcomer to training, who is working very far from his genetic potential, can get enormously stronger with the simplest program imaginable – one that substantively manipulates only a single training variable and where the Stress-Recovery-Adaptation cycle is completed from workout-to-workout. But as the athlete gets closer to his genetic potential, his rate of strength increase will slow, his training period will increase, and the complexity of his programming will grow. Advanced and elite athletes require training programs of a month, or many months, and their programs can become very complex indeed.

We point this out not because the Masters Athlete will ever require programming of such complexity (he will not), but rather to underscore two important principles.

The first is that *training period and complexity increase as the athlete works closer to his genetic potential.*

The second is that, regardless of their training period and complexity, *all rational programs exploit the Stress-Recovery-Adaptation cycle.* Underlying the elaborate structure of the most protracted and complex training programs of the strongest, most elite athletes, one *must* find the fundamental simplicity of Selye's adaptation syndrome.

Program period and complexity don't increase because we *want* them too. They increase because they *must.*

The athlete and coach who understand this will avoid the grievous error of jumping ahead into more advanced levels of programming prematurely, based on the faulty assumption that *intermediate* and *advanced* mean *better* or *faster.* In fact, the opposite is true. Intermediate and advanced level programming are slower, more complex, and less efficient than novice programming. There is no reason to go complex and slow, when simple and fast are available.

## The Novice

We define the ***novice*** as an individual who can recover from a training stress within 48–72 hours (up to 96 hours for some Masters) and increase the training stress at the next workout. A novice program reflects and exploits this adaptive capacity, increasing the weight on the bar for each exercise at every training session, while holding volume and other training variables constant.

Such an approach will allow a novice to gain strength rapidly. This is not because the program is particularly elaborate or fine-tuned – in fact, it is extremely simple and generalized. It works because just about *any* type of training program will work for a novice – for a while. Because the novice's strength is so far from his genetic potential, any resistance to force production is likely to constitute a training stress and result in an adaptation. A raw novice can make his squat stronger by riding a bike, doing some jumping jacks, cranking a ThighMaster, or even going for a walk every day. This approach will stop paying off very quickly – but it will persist long enough to promote the sale of useless exercise doodads or the publication of silly exercise physiology research. *Any* increase in physical activity virtually guarantees short-term increases in strength for the rank novice. This phenomenon is known as the ***novice effect:*** any physical activity that requires even the most minimal amount of effort and exertion will yield some positive effects for a completely untrained adult. The novice effect is responsible for much of the confusion about physical exercise that we find not only around the water cooler, but also in the exercise physiology literature.

The novice effect is nature's gift to the untrained. It's a free head start, a mulligan, a grant-in-aid. But if it's misunderstood or used improperly, it will be squandered. The novice effect can be exploited fully (if not for financial gain) by adopting the principle of *training specificity,* which tells us that the organism will mount a specific adaptation to the specific stress imposed upon it. When you use a shovel, you don't get calluses all over your hand. You get them where you need them. When you learn to juggle, you don't improve your golf swing. When you get the flu, you don't raise antibodies against leprosy.

So we don't use a bicycle to make the squat stronger. *We use the squat to make the squat stronger.* Both approaches will work at first, but only the specific training approach will allow the novice to extract the full benefit from the novice effect.

In practice, the novice program will take the form of a 3-day/week or 2-day/week program, in which the target number of repetitions and sets (volume) is held constant and the weight on the bar increases at every workout. During the novice phase, the athlete will engage in active rest (see Chapter 16) during non-training days, but will not engage in conditioning work or heavy physical activity outside the gym. *All of the novice's adaptive capacity is dedicated to maximizing the development of strength during this crucial phase of training.* Failure to do so will limit the rate at which strength can be increased or truncate the duration of the novice phase. Provided the addition of weight is judicious and the athlete attends properly to recovery factors, the novice program will produce rapid, steady increases in strength for many weeks, and in some cases for up to 6 months. For some Masters with age-delimited recovery capacity, modifications of the novice program can be used almost indefinitely, although obviously not with the same rate of long-term strength increase. Novice programs and their variants are explored in Chapters 19–21.

## The Intermediate

The novice program will rapidly bring the Masters Athlete closer to his genetic potential, and as the weight on the bar increases his capacity to recover and adapt to the training stress will be taxed further. We define the ***intermediate*** athlete as one who is no longer capable of demonstrating a strength increase from one workout to the next despite proper novice programming and attention to recovery.

Intermediate programs stretch the training period over a longer interval and introduce a new level of training complexity where stress is accumulated across the overload event. They also allow for greater variety of focus and flexibility, including the increased use of accessory exercises and other training elements. For example, once an athlete has entered the intermediate phase, he can begin to focus, as desired, on power, conditioning, hypertrophy, mobility, or balance, with the addition of appropriate exercises. Because of the longer training period, the increased time available for recovery, and the slower increases in strength, the addition of such elements, or the pursuit of a sport or other physical activity, will not have the same potential to interfere with training as it did for the novice progression.

Intermediate programs may incorporate training periods of 1–2 weeks, and include Heavy-Light-Medium approaches, Split Routines, the Texas Method and its variants, and others. In all of these programs, each set of each workout is directed at some aspect of the overload event, and both volume and intensity are manipulated, changing throughout the training period. Intermediate programs are discussed in detail in Chapters 22–24.

## The Advanced

Most Masters will never progress beyond some form of intermediate or "advanced intermediate" program. Training beyond the intermediate level requires extremely careful monitoring, complex programming, and grueling work. The ***advanced*** Master is training for strength competition, not for health. The potential for overtraining and injury becomes much more pronounced, because the athlete is working as close as possible to his genetic potential – "pushing the envelope." Working at the advanced level is not necessary to experience the optimal health benefits of strength training, and will not be well-tolerated by the vast majority of older athletes.

Advanced programs will not be treated in detail in this text, but we will give a brief overview of the general principles and architecture of such programming in Chapter 25.

# 19

# The Novice Master

No other time in the athlete's training career offers a greater potential for progress than the novice phase, during which weight is added to the bar 2–3 times/week. In this chapter, we examine the Starting Strength novice program and how to apply it to the Masters Athlete. These modifications will almost always take the form of reductions in volume or training frequency, while avoiding reductions in training intensity. Approaches to correct assessment and management of a "stuck" trainee who is stalling on the program are discussed. In the advanced phase of the novice program, the addition of light squat days and other modifications allow for maximal exploitation of the linear progression, but are unlikely to be as fruitful in the Master as in the younger athlete. At the end of the novice phase, useful progress is no longer possible from workout to workout, and intermediate training is indicated.

## Overview of Novice Programming

If you're wondering whether or not you're a novice, you're a novice. Recall from the previous chapter that a novice is a trainee who can recover from and adapt to a training stress before the next training bout and display a strength increase at every workout. So a novice might be someone who has been going to the gym a few times a week for 30 years, using the machines or working with free weights. A novice may even have a remote history of strength training or competition. An individual with such experience may have an advantage over somebody engaging in physical training for the first time ever – but he is still a novice.

The average guy in the gym is *exercising*, not *training*. He's focused on individual workouts rather than carefully exploiting the Stress-Recovery-Adaptation cycle to actually get stronger. He may engage in such unprogrammed and inefficient exercise for decades, wasting his time with an admirable but tragic dedication, never realizing that the Stress-Recovery-Adaptation cycle even exists.

Gains in strength and muscle mass are minimal and haphazard if they occur at all. This guy has never exploited the novice effect to get stronger to the degree permitted by his genetic potential and adaptive capacity. If we simply held his volume and exercise selection constant and made him add a little weight to the bar at each workout, he would display a strength increase every time he trained. So, despite his years in the gym, until he has fully exploited such a linear progression, *he is a novice.*

A ***linear progression*** occurs when the athlete is capable of sustaining repeated increases in workload in successive training sessions for a prolonged period of time. The novice athlete is engaged in just such a progression, adding weight to the bar at every workout. For most novices, this simply means "train a day, rest a day, repeat." For an older novice it might mean "train a day, rest 2–3 days, repeat."

Assuming appropriate workloads, novices are recovered and adapted to a training stress within a 48–72 hour window. For older trainees, this interval may have be a little longer. But a novice in his 20s, 30s, or 40s should be able to train on Monday, rest on Tuesday, and simultaneously impose another training stress and display a performance increase by Wednesday. Thursday is another day of recovery from the stress of Wednesday, and on Friday a third performance increase for the week can be displayed. This rapid progress is not due to some supernatural ability to recover. It's simply because *the novice is not strong enough to produce a training stress that exceeds his capacity to adapt over the next 48–72 hours.*

Three times a week is about as rapid a progression as a trainee of any age can expect to enjoy. With older trainees, this rate will likely be slower, but the principles remain the same. Progress for a novice is *by definition* from workout to workout, even if an age-related need for additional recovery limits progress to less than 3 times a week.

This is the Stress-Recovery-Adaptation cycle at its simplest and most effective. So simple is the general architecture of a novice program that it calls for the substantive manipulation of only a single training variable: *load.* Volume, recovery interval, and exercise selection are all "locked" while the weight on the bar is slowly dialed up from one workout to the next.

## The Starting Strength Model

Readers of this text may be familiar with the novice training model presented by Mark Rippetoe in *Starting Strength: Basic Barbell Training*[1] and *Practical Programming for Strength Training.*[2] This model has proven enormously successful, because it was explicitly constructed with a view to the novice trainee's ability to train and adapt from workout to workout. Our purpose in this section of the chapter is to present the Starting Strength model as it is *generally* applied. This program is suitable for training most novices under 50, although individual considerations are of course always important, and any particular athlete may require modifications of this approach. Later in this chapter, we will look at how this model is applied to the Masters Athlete over 50, and in future chapters how it is applied in the seventh and eighth decades.

We emphasize that modifications addressed to particular decades are inevitably arbitrary, and may not apply to a particular trainee. The physical differences between adults in any age range can be quite vast. Not everyone will be able to follow the programs exactly as presented, and some will require modifications early in the program. But the Starting Strength model provides a versatile foundation that can be modified as needed to accommodate a wide range of athlete ages and capabilities. The approach we will outline here has withstood the test of time, having been developed over the course of decades and applied productively in thousands of trainees.

### Basic Structure of the Starting Strength Novice Program

The Starting Strength model prescribes a 3-day/week program that traditionally occurs on Monday, Wednesday, and Friday. A Tuesday, Thursday, Saturday cycle accomplishes the same thing.

The ***rank novice,*** an athlete at the very start of training, begins with the simplest possible program (Program 1A), composed of two distinct

## PROGRAM 1A: RANK NOVICE PROGRAM

| WORKOUT A | WORKOUT B |
|---|---|
| SQUAT 3x5 | SQUAT 3x5 |
| BENCH 3x5 | PRESS 3x5 |
| DEADLIFT 1x5 | DEADLIFT 1x5 |

**PRESCRIPTION:** Workouts A and B are alternated in a M-W-F or equivalent pattern; e.g. week 1 = ABA; week 2 = BAB; week 3 = ABA, etc. Notation is sets x reps.

**INDICATIONS:** <40: Yes 40–49: Yes 50–59: Yes >60: Discretion

**PARAMETERS:** Initiated at the beginning of training; progress to Early Novice (1B) as deadlift weight surpasses squat weight and/or recovery limitations.

workouts, designated A and B. Trainees alternate between workouts, creating a rotation of ABA on Week 1, BAB on Week 2, ABA on week 3, and so on. The two workouts differ only in the pressing movements: the bench press is performed in workout A, and the press is performed in workout B. The squat and deadlift are performed at every session. Squats, bench presses, and presses are done for 3 work sets of 5 reps each, and deadlifts for a single set of 5.

Decades of trial and error and ongoing refinement have demonstrated that this balance of volume and intensity is just enough stress to drive adaptation, while still allowing the lifter to return in 48–72 hours and train again with more weight. More sets or more reps per set would likely still yield some progress, but the demands on recovery would be such that the lifter would not be able to display a performance improvement after 48–72 hours. More time would be required between workouts, and progress would therefore be unnecessarily slow for an athlete capable of progressing quickly.

Over the course of several workouts (1–3 weeks), the deadlift will progress in weight until it is significantly heavier than the squat. At this point, the power clean is introduced for 5 sets of 3 reps each, and the A and B workouts change. This is the Early Novice Program (1B).

In the Early Novice Program, the athlete continues to perform pulling movements (deadlifts and cleans) at every workout, but at this stage the clean is still light and allows for recovery from increasingly heavy deadlifts. Within 1–3 weeks, however, the clean will grow heavier and more stressful, and the program will change again to permit more recovery between heavy pulling sessions, and to permit the first incorporation of some limited assistance exercise work in the form of back extensions and chin-ups.

At this stage, the novice continues to alternate workouts A and B, but workout A itself alternates between the deadlift and the power clean. This means that deadlifts, which impose a very heavy training stress, are now performed only once every four workouts. This Novice Program (1C) will constitute the bulk of the novice progression for most trainees.

Example 19-1 illustrates 10 weeks of novice progression. Assume the trainee is a sedentary, deconditioned, but otherwise healthy 42-year-old male with no mobility or recovery issues. For the sake of clarity, we exclude back extensions; only chin-ups are shown for this progression.

This is a well-executed novice program. Notice the rate of progression for each exercise. Squats start with 10-pound jumps and quickly reduce to 5. Bench presses and presses get a few weeks' worth of 5-pound increases before slowing down to 2–3-pound increases. Notice also that on Week 1 the trainee starts his bench press off higher

### PROGRAM 1B: EARLY NOVICE PROGRAM

| WORKOUT A | WORKOUT B |
|---|---|
| SQUAT 3x5 | SQUAT 3x5 |
| BENCH 3x5 | PRESS 3x5 |
| DEADLIFT 1x5 | POWER CLEAN 5x3 |

**PRESCRIPTION:** Workouts A and B are alternated in a M-W-F or equivalent pattern; e.g. week 1 = ABA; week 2 = BAB; week 3 = ABA, etc. Notation is sets x reps.

**INDICATIONS:** <40: Yes 40–49: Yes 50–59: Discretion >60: Discretion

**PARAMETERS:** Initiated after the first 2–3 weeks of Program 1A, when deadlift strength has progressed well ahead of the squat. Usually progress to Novice Program (1C) after 1–3 weeks.

### PROGRAM 1C: NOVICE PROGRAM

| WORKOUT A | WORKOUT B |
|---|---|
| SQUAT 3x5 | SQUAT 3x5 |
| BENCH 3x5 | PRESS 3x5 |
| DEADLIFT 1x5 ***or*** | BACK EXTENSIONS |
| POWER CLEAN 5x3 | CHINS |

**PRESCRIPTION:** Workouts A and B are alternated in a M-W-F or equivalent pattern; e.g. week 1 = ABA; week 2 = BAB; week 3 = ABA, etc. Deadlift and power clean are alternated for Workout A. Notation is sets x reps.

**INDICATIONS:** <40: Yes 40–49: Yes 50–59: Discretion >60: Discretion

**PARAMETERS:** Initiated after 2–4 weeks of progress on Program 1B; progress to Program 1D as indicated.

than his squat and almost equal to his deadlift. This may be a common occurrence in younger men who have a history of training the upper body, in particular the bench press, while ignoring the lower body. Deadlifts go from 20-pound increases to 10-pound increases, but eventually slow to 5-pound increases as well. Because of the technical demands of the power clean, progress is never rushed. Jumps of 2–5 pounds are reasonable at the beginning of the program. *The point here is not to prescribe particular increases in weight,* but to illustrate that increases in loading will start out larger and then taper off. Progress will occur at a rate that is unique to each individual trainee.

This is a realistic progression for a male in his early 40s. In just a month he doubles his squat strength, something that probably won't ever happen again so quickly.

Of course, this can't go on forever. Progress could be expected for this trainee for several more months, but the jumps in weight will get smaller, and ultimately progress will stall.

**Example 19-1: A Well-Executed Novice Progression**

| (Program 1A) | Monday | Wednesday | Friday |
|---|---|---|---|
| **Week 1** | Squat 75x5x3 | Squat 85x5x3 | Squat 95x5x3 |
| | Bench 90x5x3 | Press 55x5x3 | Bench 95x5x3 |
| | Deadlift 95x5 | Deadlift 115x5 | Deadlift 135x5 |
| **Week 2** | Squat 105x5x3 | Squat 115x5x3 | Squat 125x5x3 |
| | Press 60x5x3 | Bench 100x5x3 | Press 65x5x3 |
| | Deadlift 155x5 | Deadlift 175x5 | Deadlift 190x5 |
| **(Program 1B)** | | | |
| **Week 3** | Squat 135x5x3 | Squat 145x5x3 | Squat 155x5x3 |
| | Bench 105x5x3 | Press 70x5x3 | Bench 110x5x3 |
| | Deadlift 205x5 | Power Clean 95x3x5 | Deadlift 215x5 |
| **Week 4** | Squat 160x5x3 | Squat 165x5x3 | Squat 170x5x3 |
| | Press 75x5x3 | Bench 115x5x3 | Press 80x5x3 |
| | Power Clean 100x3x5 | Deadlift 225x5 | Power Clean 105x3x5 |
| **Week 5** | Squat 175x5x3 | Squat 180x5x3 | Squat 185x5x3 |
| | Bench 120x5x3 | Press 82.5x5x3 | Bench 122.5x5x3 |
| | Deadlift 235x5 | Power Clean 110x3x5 | Deadlift 245x5 |
| **Week 6** | Squat 190x5x3 | Squat 195x5x3 | Squat 200x5x3 |
| | Press 85x5x3 | Bench 125x5x3 | Press 87.5x5x3 |
| | Power Clean 115x3x5 | Deadlift 255x5 | Power Clean 120x3x5 |
| **(Program 1C)** | | | |
| **Week 7** | Squat 205x5x3 | Squat 210x5x3 | Squat 215x5x3 |
| | Bench 127.5x5x3 | Press 90x5x3 | Bench 130x5x3 |
| | Deadlift 265x5 | Chins 5,3,3 | Power Clean 125x3x5 |
| **Week 8** | Squat 220x5x3 | Squat 225x5x3 | Squat 230x5x3 |
| | Press 92.5x5x3 | Bench 132.5x5x3 | Press 95x5x3 |
| | Chins 5,4,3 | Deadlift 270x5 | Chins 6,5,4 |
| **Week 9** | Squat 235x5x3 | Squat 240x5x3 | Squat 245x5x3 |
| | Bench 135x5x3 | Press 97.5x5x3 | Bench 137.5x5x3 |
| | Power Clean 127.5x3x5 | Chins 6,5,5 | Deadlift 275x5 |
| **Week 10** | Squat 250x5x3 | Squat 255x5x3 | Squat 260x5x3 |
| | Press 100x5x3 | Bench 140x5x3 | Press 102.5x5x3 |
| | Chins 7,5,5 | Power Clean 130x3x5 | Chins 7,6,5 |

## Getting unstuck: troubleshooting the novice program with back-off periods

Eventually all athletes who undertake a novice linear progression get stuck and will be unable to progress on one or more exercises in the program as it is written. The older the athlete, the sooner he will get stuck. Once the trainee's progress begins to slow or stall, modifications must be made. If the trainee has been using the Starting Strength model (or some very close variation), *the trainee will rarely if ever need to add additional work to the program in order to get progress going again.* If the trainee is struggling to progress on the standard novice program, it will be for 1 of 3 reasons:

1. **Excessive training *stress*** within the workout.

2. **Insufficient *recovery*** between sessions.

3. ***Greed.***

The first two scenarios are different faces of the same coin. Athlete and coach must decide whether to reduce the stress within each workout or increase the amount of rest between sessions. It is usually unnecessary and counterproductive to do both at the same time. Either approach should be adequate to give a boost to a tired trainee, provided it is the correct approach for the situation. In the case of a greed-induced stall, a more radical approach will be indicated.

To properly diagnose the situation and determine which approach to use, athlete and coach should review the last several weeks of training and search for the following trends. (Here we see just one of the many ways in which careful record-keeping is essential for successful training).

**Scenario 1: Running Out of Gas.** The trainee is struggling to *complete* workouts at the prescribed volume. The final exercise of the day (usually the heavy deadlift or the demanding and stressful power clean) is starting to regress, or at least stagnate. The trainee is reporting that he feels "out of gas," and this may be accompanied by significant fatigue in the hips and low back. The athlete may also display a pattern of missing reps on his *last* set of squats or pressing movements, even with increases in rest time between sets. He may report increased soreness in the legs and low back on the day following the workout. Sleep patterns on the night of the workout may be disrupted, where previously sleep had actually improved with training.

In this scenario, the stress *within* the individual training sessions is beginning to overwhelm the athlete's capacity. *Assuming that all recovery factors have been correctly addressed,* a reduction in training volume is indicated. The 3x5 model has become too much for the trainee to handle at the loads he has achieved in training, and the likely culprit is the squat, rather than the pressing movements. Although the 3 sets of 5 approach may have worked well early in the program, it is now more than the athlete can handle as his strength and ability to focus and grind have all improved. Work set weights are now heavier, and total training volume is also increased by the addition of more warm-up sets.

The best approach here is *a reduction in training volume at the day's maximum weight for the squat.* It is critical to understand that the recommendation is *not* to take weight off of the bar. The problem is volume, not intensity. Strength can be maintained with a reduction in overall volume, but will regress if weight is stripped off of the bar. As long as the trainee is maintaining quality form, every effort should be made to advance work set weights.

We have had success with 3 simple approaches for reducing per-session squat volume.

*Eliminate a set.* This is the simplest approach. If 3 sets have proven to be just too much at this phase of training, then 2 sets of 5 reps at the work set goal may be sufficient to drive some progress to the end of the novice phase – 6 heavy squat sets for a 3-day training week.

*Reduce repetitions.* The second strategy is to keep 3 total sets, but reduce the number of repetitions to 3. Again, this strategy works best in the late novice phase and may squeeze an additional few weeks out of the linear progression. This approach will immediately produce improved recovery and renewed progress – but not for very long. Sets of 3 tend to run their course within a few weeks, and at that point it's probably time to move to advanced novice (Program 1D) or intermediate programming.

*One work set, two back-offs.* In this strategy, the Master completes one work set at target weight, followed by 2 back-off sets at about 5–10% decrease in load. For example, if the target weight for today is 200 pounds, the athlete will put up one set of five at 200, followed by two sets of 5 at 180. This is not technically a reduction in total volume (still 3 sets of 5 reps), but it is a reduction in volume at the highest load.

**Scenario 2: Starting on Empty.** In contrast to scenario 1 above, in which the athlete had trouble *completing* his work sets, here he is getting into trouble on the *front end* of the workout. Rather than "running out of gas" the trainee is "starting on empty." Warming up with the empty bar and a few light sets is no longer enough to work out the stiffness from the previous training session. Moreover, the trainee will notice a substantial decrease in bar speed and breakdown in form, even on warm-up weights. Weights that had previously felt light now feel heavy. Instead of missing on the final exercises and work sets, the athlete fails his *first* work set of the day, and the workout goes downhill from there.

The culprit here is inadequate recovery, and the solution is *more rest between training sessions.* On a Monday-Wednesday-Friday protocol there are 48–72 hours between each training session – likely plenty of rest for the first several weeks of training. Over time, however, most coaches who use the standard novice program with their clients and athletes will consistently report that the Monday of a Monday-Wednesday-Friday schedule is always the best training session – obviously due to the extra day of rest in from the weekend break. The simple solution for scenario 2 is to give the trainee "a weekend" after every training session – sometimes a 3-day weekend.

**Example 19-2: A One-On, Two-Off Novice Training Schedule**

| | | |
|---|---|---|
| **Monday**<br>Squat 3x5<br>Bench 3x5<br>Deadlift 1x5 | **Thursday**<br>Squat 3x5<br>Press 3x5<br>Lat Pulls 3x10 | **Sunday**<br>Squat 3x5<br>Bench 3x5<br>Power Clean 5x3 |
| **Wednesday**<br>Squat 3x5<br>Press 3x5<br>Lat Pulls 3x10 | **Saturday**<br>Squat 3x5<br>Bench 3x5<br>Deadlift 1x5 | **Tuesday**<br>Squat 3x5<br>Press 3x5<br>Lat Pulls 3x10 |
| **Friday**<br>Squat 3x5<br>Bench 3x5<br>Power Clean 5x3 | **Monday**<br>Squat 3x5<br>Press 3x5<br>Lat Pulls 3x10 | **Thursday**<br>Squat 3x5<br>Bench 3x5<br>Deadlift 1x5 |

Practical considerations will usually dictate how the trainee alters their training schedule. In order to increase the rest period by one day, the trainee would need to adopt a "one on, two off" training schedule that is irregular throughout the week. This program is discussed in more detail in the next chapter, but would look like Example 19-2.

Notice the increased time between training sessions compared to the standard program. Due to work and career obligations, gym or coaching availability, family commitments, etc., such an irregular schedule may be impractical. If this is the case, setting a fixed 2-day/week schedule is an excellent choice. Monday/Thursday, Tuesday/Friday, Monday/Friday, or Wednesday/Saturday are all examples of schedules that evenly spread the workload across the week, allowing 2–3 full days of recovery between training sessions. A Tuesday/Thursday schedule, or something similar, would be less than ideal because of the lopsided workload and recovery time distribution across the week. Again, this type of reduced volume variation of the novice program is discussed in more detail in the next chapter (Program 3B).

Another scheduling alternative is to reduce the number of exercises done at each session. For example, we might take the 3-day program and make it a 4-day program. Even though the trainee is now actually in the gym more often, the time between the same exercises extends to 3–4 days, and there is less to do at each individual training session. A number of variations on the 4-day approach are examined in Chapter 20.

The same underlying principles and approach will apply to a 2- or 4-day program just as they would the standard 3-day program. The trainee is still progressing linearly, albeit with an extended break between sessions. These simple alterations to the training schedule will almost always provide the trainee with a tremendous surge in performance, provided *all other recovery factors are in place.* Without adequate rest, nutrition, sleep, and hydration, other manipulations of the program will be for naught.

**Scenario 3: Greed**. The gym offers no asylum from the Third Deadly Sin.[3] In this scenario, the addition of weight to the bar has been too aggressive. Rapid early success with the linear progression has emboldened the athlete (and possibly the coach) and created unrealistic expectations. Early gains are driven by improvements in form, confidence, neuromuscular efficiency, and the addition of some muscle tissue. Later gains are dependent on increases in strength and muscle mass, and inevitably come more slowly, even at the novice level. The athlete who adds 10 pounds to his squat every training session for the first couple of weeks must not hope to continue at this rate. Any attempt to do so will inevitably get him stuck, needlessly squandering valuable training time.

This situation is easily diagnosed by conducting a clear-eyed, realistic review of the training log. This investigation will reveal that, prior to the stall, there was no moderation of the incremental addition of weight to the bar, or (horrors!) an actual *increase* in the amount added from workout to workout.

This scenario is one of the few indications for an actual reduction in intensity. Most Masters who find themselves mired in this situation will require a reduction of *at least* 10% in their work set weight. The program will then resume as before, but with appropriate reductions in loading increments from workout to workout. The athlete will soon overtake the weight at which his greed caused him to stall and progress beyond it – stronger, and hopefully wiser.

## The Advanced Novice Program

An ***advanced novice*** has been training consistently on linear progression (Program 1C) for many weeks without interruption, but has now required at least one adjustment to correct for excessive workout volume or inadequate recovery as described above. Incremental additions to the bar have been judicious (greed is not an indication for advanced novice progression). Progress is now limited to small jumps in weight (e.g., 5 pounds or less for the squat, 10 pounds or less for the deadlift, 2.5 pounds or less for the pressing movements, depending on the athlete). At this stage, advanced novice programming is indicated. The Starting Strength model addresses this need by reducing the frequency of heavy pulls from the floor, and institutes a light squat day in the middle of the standard 3-day training week.

Any novice, regardless of age, will eventually struggle to maintain steady progress on 3 days/week of heavy squats. A simple solution is to decrease intensity on the middle squat day of the program by 5–20%. The exact percentage offset to use is an individual calculation. There is no fixed offset that will work for every trainee. With Masters, it is critical to remember that a drop in intensity allows detraining to creep in very quickly. The older the trainee, the lower the percentage offset will be. For some it will be better to keep only a 5% offset, and drop volume down to just a single set on the light day. This simple strategy will often yield several more consecutive weeks of progress and provide some physical and mental relief to an athlete who has been working very hard and gaining strength quickly. Many advanced novice trainees will be down to 1 day/week of heavy deadlifting at this time

**PROGRAM 1D: ADVANCED NOVICE PROGRAM**

**WEEK 1:**

| MONDAY | WEDNESDAY | FRIDAY |
|---|---|---|
| SQUAT 3x5 | LIGHT SQUAT 3x5 (80–95%) | SQUAT 3x5 |
| BENCH 3x5 | PRESS 3x5 | BENCH 3x5 |
| BACK EXTENSIONS | DEADLIFT 1x5 | BACK EXTENSIONS |
| CHINS | | CHINS |

**WEEK 2:**

| MONDAY | WEDNESDAY | FRIDAY |
|---|---|---|
| SQUAT 3x5 | LIGHT SQUAT 3x5 (80–95%) | SQUAT 3x5 |
| PRESS 3x5 | BENCH 3x5 | PRESS 3x5 |
| POWER CLEAN 5x3 | BACK EXTENSIONS | DEADLIFT 1x5 |
| | CHINS | |

**PRESCRIPTION:** Weeks 1 and 2 are alternated. Light squats are at 80–95% of Monday's work set weight. Notation is sets x reps.

**INDICATIONS:** <40: Yes 40–49: Yes 50–59: Discretion >60: Discretion

**PARAMETERS:** Initiated when progress stalls after initial adjustments to Program 1C, or at discretion of the coach. Terminate when intermediate programming is indicated.

in their training careers, and may prefer to move their heavy deadlifts to the light squat day to avoid the stress of squatting and pulling heavy in the same workout. This is an excellent strategy if the trainee's deadlift is beginning to stagnate.

## Novice Programs for Masters

The same programming principles that apply to young novice athletes also apply to the Masters novice. Everything that happens when the trainee is young happens when they are older – it just happens more slowly, and on a smaller scale. But a Masters novice, like any other novice, can add weight to the bar from workout to workout, in a linear progression, with about 48–96 hours of recovery between training sessions. So *most* novice Masters under 60 can add weight to the bar 2–3 times/week, at least to start.

This may sound unrealistic. But keep in mind that performance increases may be very small – 1 pound on the press, 2 pounds on the bench press, maybe 5 pounds on the squat and deadlift. As a general rule, the older the athlete, the smaller the appropriate increment of added weight, and the longer the recovery period needed between sessions. Females and lighter males will also need smaller increments of weight increase at each training session.

Progress for the Masters Athlete, even the novice, will be careful and conservative, but it is still progress. The Masters novice and his coach will focus on *relatively* small, judicious increases from workout to workout – increases that will produce impressive improvements in strength over the course of many weeks and months of consistent training. And that is what matters – constantly pushing the body forward, while age is trying to pull it back. Standing still is not an option.

## Novice masters aged 40–49

Trainees their 40s should begin with the standard *Starting Strength* novice model as just described, and make adjustments only as indicated. Three days a week and 3 primary exercises a day are manageable, assuming that loading increments are judicious and adequate attention is paid to recovery factors. The major difference between an athlete in his 40s and an athlete in his 20s is the amount of time he will be able to realize linear progress in this program. A hard-training 20-year old novice *may* be able to sustain 6–9 months of linear progression. A trainee in his 40s might only achieve 3–6 months of linear progression before major adjustments are indicated, the advanced novice progression is exhausted, and longer recovery periods are needed between stressful training sessions. At this point, he will transition into intermediate programming.

## Novice masters aged 50–59

Masters in their 50s will display age-related declines in their ability to recover from very difficult training – especially high-volume training. It is for individuals in this age range that significant adjustments to the novice model start to become necessary. Much will depend on the individual athlete: his experience, previous physical activity, health, and genetics.

Assume that our next hypothetical trainee is 55 years of age, and has no background with exercise or strength training. We will assume that this trainee has been sedentary for multiple decades and is extremely deconditioned, but able to perform the barbell movements. It is safe to begin this athlete with the Masters Rank Novice Program (2A).

The astute reader will immediately note that *this program is identical to the standard Rank Novice Program (1A)*. Again, the difference will be in the starting loads and increments of progression, with the Masters novice making smaller, more judicious jumps than his younger, less deserving counterparts.

As with the standard novice progression, the rank Masters novice continues this pattern until the deadlift grows stale and is relegated to every other workout. At this stage, he will transition to a Master's variation of the standard Starting Strength program that eliminates the power clean.

At age 55, with no training background, the trainee's ability use the clean to safely and productively to develop explosive power may well have passed him by. Much of the elasticity in his connective tissue has been lost to age and injury. Receiving heavy power cleans imposes enormous training stress that we'd rather save for squats and heavy deadlifts. And attaining proficiency in the power clean, which is a more technical exercise, requires the imposition of heavy training volume, which will tax recovery resources that we want to save for the production of muscle mass and raw strength. Power is still a trainable quality, and will improve to a degree sufficient for most Masters Athletes simply by increasing strength.[4]

In the Master's Early Novice Program (2B) the power clean is therefore replaced by an upper back exercise. Chins and pull-ups are the best options if they can be done. If they cannot, a lat pull-down machine or bodyweight rows on a pair of straps or rings or a bar are effective ways to add work to the back (Chapter 13). Either option is suitable, and the athlete might prefer to alternate between the two from workout to workout.

After 1–3 weeks, it will become necessary to decrease deadlift frequency further. The Masters Novice Program (1C), which will constitute the main phase of novice programming, therefore alternates the A-Workout between deadlifts and lat pulls or another upper back exercise that the Master can perform and tolerate.

Example 19-3 illustrates how these templates are put into training practice for a well-executed Masters novice progression. As with all the examples used in this text, this timeline is for illustrative purposes only, and the actual evolution of any particular athlete's pulling program will always occur at an individual rate. We note that this trainee was probably capable of squatting more than 45 pounds and deadlifting more than 95 pounds on day 1. To prevent severe delayed onset muscle soreness (DOMS) it is wise to begin the lower body training for the Master at a *slightly* lower intensity relative to his apparent capability, and progress from

## PROGRAM 2A: MASTERS RANK NOVICE PROGRAM

| WORKOUT A | WORKOUT B |
|---|---|
| SQUAT 3x5 | SQUAT 3x5 |
| BENCH 3x5 | PRESS 3x5 |
| DEADLIFT 1x5 | DEADLIFT 1x5 |

**PRESCRIPTION:** Workouts A and B are alternated in a M-W-F or equivalent pattern; e.g. week 1 = ABA; week 2 = BAB; week 3 =ABA, etc. Notation is sets x reps.

**INDICATIONS:** <40: Yes 40–49: Yes 50–59: Yes >60: Discretion

**PARAMETERS:** Initiated at the beginning of training; progress to Masters Early Novice (2B) as deadlift weight surpasses squat weight and/or recovery limitations.

## PROGRAM 2B: MASTERS EARLY NOVICE PROGRAM

| WORKOUT A | WORKOUT B |
|---|---|
| SQUAT 3x5 | SQUAT 3x5 |
| BENCH 3x5 | PRESS 3x5 |
| DEADLIFT 1x5 | LAT PULLS 3x8–10 ***or*** BODYWEIGHT ROWS 3x10 ***or*** CHINS |

**PRESCRIPTION:** Workouts A and B are alternated in a M-W-F or equivalent pattern; e.g. week 1 = ABA; week 2 = BAB; week 3 =ABA, etc. Workout B incorporates *one* of the back exercises indicated, chosen based on the athlete's ability. Notation is sets x reps.

**INDICATIONS:** <40: Discretion 40–49: Discretion 50–59: Yes >60: Discretion

**PARAMETERS:** Usually initiated after the first few workouts of Program 1A, when deadlift strength has progressed well ahead of the squat. Usually progress to Masters Novice Program (1C) after 1–3 weeks.

## PROGRAM 2C: MASTERS NOVICE PROGRAM

| WORKOUT A | WORKOUT B |
|---|---|
| SQUAT 3x5 | SQUAT 3x5 |
| BENCH 3x5 | PRESS 3x5 |
| DEADLIFT 1x5 ***or*** LAT PULLS 3x8–10 | BODYWEIGHT ROWS 3x10 ***or*** CHINS |

**PRESCRIPTION:** Workouts A and B are alternated in a M-W-F or equivalent pattern; e.g. week 1 = ABA; week 2 = BAB; week 3 =ABA, etc. Deadlift and lat pulls are alternated for Workout A. Notation is sets x reps.

**INDICATIONS:** <40: Discretion 40–49: Discretion 50–59: Yes >60: Discretion

**PARAMETERS:** Initiated after 1–3 weeks of Program 2B; progress to Masters Advanced Novice (2D) when progress slows despite indicated adjustments or resets.

there. We would also point out that this example illustrates the program's evolution from high-to-low deadlift frequency.

In the Masters population, the press is a frequent obstacle to conducting the program as written. Many rank novice Masters, especially females, have profound upper body weakness, and many others, especially males, have significant shoulder mobility issues. We find that most Masters can train the press using a novice program, but many require initial adjustments to the program to get them started.

A gym set up for Masters training should be equipped with very light barbells. For smaller or deconditioned athletes, barbells as light as 10–15 pounds may be necessary to begin training the overhead press. In the absence of light barbells, or in the case of profound upper body weakness that will not permit even a 10–15-pound press, the trainee should bench press at every training session for 3 days/week until the chest, deltoids, and triceps become strong enough that the trainee can overhead press with the facility's lightest available barbell. Once the trainee is capable of training the overhead press, then an AB rotation of press/bench should begin.

The 6-week snapshot in Example 19-4 shows how a trainee uses the bench press to get strong enough to press. Here, the trainee's second attempt with the 15-pound bar did not yield the ideal 3 sets of 5 reps. The trainee continued to press at alternate workouts with the 15-pound bar and simply added reps at each training session until all 3 sets of 5 reps were finally achieved in the middle of week 5. This ***repetition progression*** approach is very useful and versatile at all stages of training, and we will encounter it again in future chapters.

With careful attention to recovery and judicious increases in bar loading, progress on the Masters Novice Program (2C) will continue for many weeks, sometimes for 3–5 months or more. Slowed or stalled gains will be addressed by the same diagnostic and programming approach described for the standard novice model. These adjustments will restore progress for only so long before the introduction of a light squat day is needed, and the athlete will move to the Advanced Masters Novice Program (2D).

## PROGRAM 2D: ADVANCED MASTERS NOVICE PROGRAM

| | MONDAY | WEDNESDAY | FRIDAY |
|---|---|---|---|
| **WEEK 1:** | SQUAT 3x5 | LIGHT SQUAT 3x5 (80–95%) | SQUAT 3x5 |
| | BENCH 3x5 | PRESS 3x5 | BENCH 3x5 |
| | LAT PULLS 3x8–10 | DEADLIFT 1x5 | BW ROWS 3x10 ***or*** CHINS |
| **WEEK 2:** | **MONDAY** | **WEDNESDAY** | **FRIDAY** |
| | SQUAT 3x5 | LIGHT SQUAT 3x5 (80–95%) | SQUAT 3x5 |
| | PRESS 3x5 | BENCH 3x5 | PRESS 3x5 |
| | LAT PULLS 3x8–10 | DEADLIFT 1x5 | BW ROWS 3x10 ***or*** CHINS |

**PRESCRIPTION:** Weeks 1 and 2 are alternated. Light squats are at 80–95% of Monday's work set weight. Notation is sets x reps.

**INDICATIONS:** <40: Yes 40–49: Yes 50–59: Discretion >60: Discretion

**PARAMETERS:** Initiated when progress on Program 2C begins to stall or at discretion of coach. Terminate when Intermediate programming is indicated.

**Example 19-3: A Well-Executed Masters Novice Progression**

| | Monday | Wednesday | Friday |
|---|---|---|---|
| **(Program 2A)** | | | |
| **Week 1** | Squat 45x5x3 | Squat 55x5x3 | Squat 65x5x3 |
| | Bench 85x5x3 | Press 55x5x3 | Bench 90x5x3 |
| | Deadlift 95x5 | Deadlift 105x3x5 | Deadlift 115x5 |
| **Week 2** | Squat 75x5x3 | Squat 85x5x3 | Squat 95x5x3 |
| | Press 60x5x3 | Bench 95x5x3 | Press 65x5x3 |
| | Deadlift 125x5 | Deadlift 135x5 | Deadlift 145x5 |
| **Week 3** | Squat 105x5x3 | Squat 115x5x3 | Squat 125x5x3 |
| | Bench 100x5x3 | Press 67x5x3 | Bench 105x5x3 |
| | Deadlift 155x5 | Deadlift 165x5 | Deadlift 175x5 |
| **(Program 2B)** | | | |
| **Week 4** | Squat 130x5x3 | Squat 135x5x3 | Squat 140x5x3 |
| | Press 70x5x3 | Bench 108x5x3 | Press 72x5x3 |
| | Deadlift 185x5 | Lat Pulls 3x8–10 | Deadlift 190x5 |
| **Week 5** | Squat 145x5x3 | Squat 150x5x3 | Squat 155x5x3 |
| | Bench 112x5x3 | Press 75x5x3 | Bench 115x5x3 |
| | Lat Pulls 3x8–10 | Deadlift 195x5 | Lat Pulls 3x8–10 |
| **Week 6** | Squat 160x5x3 | Squat 165x5x3 | Squat 170x5x3 |
| | Press 78x5x3 | Bench 118x5x3 | Press 80x5x3 |
| | Deadlift 200x5 | Lat Pulls 3x8–10 | Deadlift 205x5 |
| **(Program 2C)** | | | |
| **Week 7** | Squat 175x5x3 | Squat 180x5x3 | Squat 185x5x3 |
| | Bench 122x5x3 | Press 82x5x3 | Bench 125x5x3 |
| | Chins | Deadlift 210x5 | Chins |

**Example 19-4: Accommodating a Weak Press in the Novice Master**

The trainee has profound upper body weakness. The press is attempted on day 1 but she cannot press a 15-pound barbell.

| Week | Monday | Wednesday | Friday |
|---|---|---|---|
| **1** | Bench 15x5x3 | Bench 18x5x3 | Bench 20x5x3 |
| **2** | Bench 22x5x3 | Bench 24x5x3 | Bench 26x5x3 |
| **3** | Bench 28x5x3 | Bench 30x5x3 | Bench 32x5x3 |
| **4** | Press 15x3x3 | Bench 34x5x3 | Press 15x4x3 |
| **5** | Bench 36x5x3 | Press 15x5x3 | Bench 38x5x3 |
| **6** | Press 16x5x3 | Bench 40x5x3 | Press 17x5x3 |

## Terminating the Novice Program

Inevitably, the novice's capacity to display adaptation from one workout to the next will be overwhelmed by his capacity to impose a training stress too heavy to permit recovery during this interval. As noted, this will occur more quickly for Masters Athletes than younger athletes. Moreover, once this stage has been reached, the very fine manipulations of volume, intensity and rest that may squeeze a few additional weeks out of a younger athlete (see Rippetoe, *Practical Programming for Strength Training, 3rd edition*, Chapter 6) are less likely to be effective for Masters, especially those over 50. If progress slows markedly early in training, athlete and coach should consider the three scenarios identified above (out of gas, starting on empty, greed), determine which situation applies to the present circumstance, and rectify it with the methods described in that section. When progress stalls in the advanced novice phase (Program 2D), two or at most three attempts may be made to modify the program and drive progress a bit further. *Any such interventions should focus on increasing time for recovery or reducing volume, rather than decreasing intensity.* But all such interventions will produce short-term results at best for the Master. At this stage, a longer training period is indicated, stretching the Stress-Recovery-Adaptation cycle over several workouts. The Masters Athlete will then transition to intermediate training, as described in Chapters 22–24.

# 20

# The Novice Over 60 and Common Novice Variants

Masters Athletes in their 60s often require extensive revisions of the novice program to accommodate blunted recovery capacity. Many can begin with the standard 3-day novice model presented in the previous chapter, but will soon transition to either a modified 3-day approach or a reduced frequency model to sustain progress. Reduced frequency models are highly versatile and can be tailored to suit the needs of almost any athlete in the seventh decade. Several variations are presented and discussed in detail. This chapter also presents 4-day novice variants and 2-day models for those few Masters who choose to incorporate the Olympic lifts into their training.

## The Seventh-Decade Novice

By the seventh decade, most novice Masters will demonstrate significant attenuation of their recovery capacity, despite careful attention to active rest, sleep, nutrition, and hydration. While some athletes in their 50s will have similar limitations, most under 60 will be able to follow a 3-day novice progression, albeit with judicious increases in weight and careful monitoring and individualized program adjustment as outlined in the last chapter. An athlete in his sixties, however, will be far more likely to require recovery intervals that extend beyond 72 hours and/or reductions in training volume, to make progress beyond the rank novice phase.

*Incorporation of a longer recovery phase and reduction in volume are the most powerful and appropriate program modifications for this population,* making it possible for athletes in their 60s and beyond to enjoy the benefits of a linear novice progression. Program-wide reductions in intensity are rarely indicated for the Masters Athlete, and in general such reductions will be highly counterproductive. Remember, the Master is *volume-sensitive* but *intensity-dependent.* Reduction in volume and training frequency will promote better recovery and thus more complete adaptation to training loads. Reduction in intensity may be instituted on a very limited basis to promote recovery and maintain progress (as detailed below), but backing off intensity for any significant period of time will lead only to detraining and loss of strength. Once a Masters Athlete has achieved a certain level of strength on an exercise, he requires frequent exposure to that same level of intensity (or more) to maintain his gains.

With these principles in hand, we can construct modified novice programs for the Master over 60. We must bear in mind, however, that *training always occurs on an individual timeline.* So it is critical to re-emphasize that 60 (or any other age) is an arbitrary cutoff. Some trainees in their seventh decade are unusually fit, have genetic predispositions to rapid recovery and adaptation, have the time and other resources to be particularly diligent about recovery, and so on. Conversely, some trainees in their 50s, or even in their 40s or 30s, may require some of the novice modifications outlined here.

The purpose of this chapter (indeed, the purpose of Part III of this book) is not to lay down hard-and-fast age-specific prescriptions, but rather to show how an understanding of the Stress-Recovery-Adaptation cycle and programming principles can be tailored to fit the individual athlete and complement his capacity to absorb, recover from, and adapt to a training stress.

### Beginning with the Rank Novice Program

Most Masters in the seventh decade can begin training with the Masters Rank Novice Program (2A).

The Master over 60 who is able to follow this program should be encouraged to do so for as long as possible, moving on to Programs 2B and 2C (see Chapter 19) as indicated and as tolerated. This potential will be maximized by careful attention to recovery factors and a highly conservative, judicious approach to bar loading, with small increases in weight. For the Masters Athlete over 60, increases of no more than 5 pounds in the squat and deadlift and 2.5 pounds in the pressing movements represent rough but rational rules of thumb *at the start*, with smaller jumps following on soon after. Some athletes may require even smaller loading increments. A few gifted individuals may tolerate a little more. But coach and athlete should always err on the side of conservative addition of weight.

Even so, for most individuals in this population, a 3-day program will ultimately grow stale, and program modification will be indicated.

### Modifications of the 3-day model

If the trainee wishes to maintain a 3-day training schedule (e.g., Mon/Wed/Fri) but is not recovering well, he will be forced to make modifications within the workout itself in order to reduce the amount of stress created by each session and allow for recovery to take place in the traditional 48–72 hour window. It will be desirable to maintain the 3-day/week frequency if progress is possible on 1 or 2 of the exercises, but not on the others. Switching to a twice-weekly schedule can slow the progress of the unaffected lifts, and may not provide enough weekly volume to drive progress. We often see squats and deadlifts stall on a 3-day plan, while the press and the bench are moving along nicely on a 3-day AB rotation. Squats and deadlifts move heavier loads and there is significant overlap between the two exercises. The hips, legs, and low backs of older Masters can be sensitive to the stress of a 3-day squat and pull schedule. The press and bench overlap as well, of course, but less so than squats and deadlifts, and the lighter nature of these exercises makes them inherently less stressful and easier on recovery. Here we present program modifications that allow the athlete to maintain a 3-day/week training schedule while reducing the overall stress produced by each workout.

**Modification of the Middle Squat Day.** For some Masters, a 3-day squat schedule is too much for recovery capacity, and better results are attained with less frequency. These individuals will benefit from the introduction of a light squat day, and may ultimately require elimination of the middle squat day completely.

Example 20-1 shows how a 60+ Masters novice who began with the standard 3-day/week program modifies the template as he grows stronger and develops greater training stress at each training session. This athlete is unable to use the low-bar squat, and has progressed using the high-bar variant. The 6-week time frame is for illustrative purposes. It is likely that each "phase" would be much longer than 2 weeks. The example begins with the last two weeks of the Master's Novice Program (2C).

## PROGRAM 2A: MASTERS RANK NOVICE PROGRAM

| WORKOUT A | WORKOUT B |
|---|---|
| SQUAT 3x5 | SQUAT 3x5 |
| BENCH 3x5 | PRESS 3x5 |
| DEADLIFT 1x5 | DEADLIFT 1x5 |

**PRESCRIPTION:** Workouts A and B are alternated; e.g. week 1 = ABA; week 2 = BAB; week 3 =ABA, etc. Notation is sets x reps.

**INDICATIONS:** <40: Yes 40–49: Yes 50–59: Yes >60: Discretion

**PARAMETERS:** Initiated at the beginning of training; progress to Masters Early Novice (2B) as deadlift weight surpasses squat weight and/or recovery limitations.

**Example 20-1: Modifying the Middle Squat Day**

| Week | Monday | Wednesday | Friday |
|---|---|---|---|
| 9 | Squat 82.5x5x3<br>Bench 40x5x3<br>Deadlift 110x5 | Squat 85x5x3<br>Press 33x5x3<br>Chins | Squat 87.5x5x3<br>Bench 42x5x3<br>Lat pulls 3x10 |
| 10 | Squat 90x5x3<br>Press 34x5x3<br>Chins | Squat ***92.5x4,3,3!***<br>Bench 44x5x3<br>Deadlift ***115x4!*** | Squat ***92.5x4,4,4!***<br>Press 35x5x3<br>Chins |

*After several weeks of progress in the novice program, the trainee is recovering poorly and squat progress is starting to stagnate. The fatigue from 3 heavy squat sessions per week is also bleeding over into his deadlifts and presses. The first modification to this 3-day program is a switch to a light squat day in the middle of the week.*

| Week | Monday | Wednesday | Friday |
|---|---|---|---|
| 11 | Squat ***92.5x5,4,4!***<br>Bench 46x5x3<br>Lat pulls 3x10 | Light Squat 80x5x3<br>Press 36x5x3<br>Chins | Squat 92.5x5x3<br>Bench 48x5x3<br>Deadlift 115x5 |
| 12 | Squat 95x5x3<br>Press 37x5x3<br>Chins | Squat 82.5x5x3<br>Bench 50x5x3<br>Lat pulls 3x10 | Squat 97.5x5x3<br>Press 38x5x3<br>Chins |

*The athlete is now feeling the accumulated stress of 9 sets per week of high-bar squats. Even with the addition of the light day, and even though he is now completing all his work sets again, the squat volume is producing fatigue in his knees and back, so we eliminate the middle squat day altogether.*

| Week | Monday | Wednesday | Friday |
|---|---|---|---|
| 13 | Squat 100x5x3<br>Bench 52x5x3<br>Deadlift 120x5 | Press 39x5x3<br>Chins | Squat 102.5x5x3<br>Bench 54x5x3<br>Lat pulls 3x10 |
| 14 | Squat 105x5x3<br>Press 40x5x3<br>Chins | Bench 56x5x3<br>Deadlift 125x5 | Squat 107.5x5x3<br>Press 41x5x3<br>Chins |

Depending on the athlete, this 3-day progression may continue, with any other needed modifications, to the termination of the novice phase, when intermediate programming is indicated.

### Reduced frequency models

Many Masters in their seventh decade will find that continuing on a 3-day program, even with the addition of light or eliminated squat days, overwhelms their recovery capacity. Alternatively, many Masters will have practical limitations in their ability to train 3 days per week, due to scheduling or other conflicts. In such cases, the introduction of a ***reduced frequency model*** of novice training is indicated. Such models offer both increased recovery time for adaptation to training stress and practical advantages in scheduling for both trainee and coach.

Consider the example of a female Master in her 60s with no significant limitations. She has dabbled off and on with some machine-based weight training programs, and has some background with the bench press, but she starts as a complete beginner on the squat, press, and deadlift. This is a common scenario for a lifetime recreational *exerciser*. She begins *training* to improve her strength and muscle mass for general health and function. She begins with the standard 3-day Masters Rank Novice Program (2A) and progresses through the Masters Early Novice Program (2B) to the standard Masters Novice Program (2C). After a couple of months of steady gains, her progress begins to stagnate and slow. Her recovery parameters are dialed in, but a review of her log reveals an interesting pattern: our athlete always completes her work sets on Monday, but struggles to hit her targets on Wednesday and Friday. Clearly, the 48-hour window has become insufficient for recovery from the stress she can now generate at each training session. The answer is not to decrease intensity, but to increase recovery. This athlete needs reduced-frequency programming.

**One-On, Two-Off Novice Programming.** The One-On, Two-Off training schedule is known in some circles as "The Old Guy's Novice Program." The effectiveness of this approach and its simplicity of implementation make it a favorite for those who coach Masters Athletes. The addition of an extra day of recovery after a training session is often sufficient to restore progress for a novice Master stalled on a 3-day/week plan. Not only does this simple modification usually get an athlete un-stuck, but it can also sustain new progress for many weeks or even months. Indeed, many Masters and coaches choose to start with this schedule rather than the traditional 3-day plan, depending on the athlete's capacities, scheduling restrictions, and so on.

In the One-On, Two-Off model (Program 3A), we recapitulate the Master's Novice Program (2C), with its alternating A and B workouts. The difference is that instead of alternating on a fixed weekly schedule, we give the tired athlete a "weekend" to recover after every workout. This results in a variable, staggered training schedule.

We emphasize that when transitioning to this program, the only change will be the frequency of training. The One-On, Two-Off model makes no changes to the workouts themselves. As a novice, the trainee should always err on the side of making the simplest change possible when running into programming challenges. The potential for programming errors increases when multiple changes are made simultaneously. This program differs from the standard novice approach by a single variable, *frequency*, while keeping everything else the same. Athlete and coach should observe the response carefully and change other variables only as needed.

**Fixed Two-Day Novice Program.** The One-On, Two-Off approach to reduced frequency modification of the novice program is highly effective, but increases the complexity of the training schedule. Many Masters and coaches will opt instead for a fixed 2-day approach to reduced frequency training. As with Program 3A, the Fixed 2-Day Novice Program (3B) can either be introduced after training in the 3-day model, or instituted at the very beginning of training if the athlete or his coach so decide. Again, neither the structure of the workout nor the AB-rotation is adjusted. The only change is to the amount of rest between training sessions – in

### PROGRAM 3A: ONE-ON, TWO-OFF (*PRACTICAL PROGRAMMING* MODEL 1)

| WORKOUT A | WORKOUT B |
|---|---|
| SQUAT 3x5 | SQUAT 3x5 |
| BENCH 3x5 | PRESS 3x5 |
| DEADLIFT 1x5 ***or*** | BODYWEIGHT ROWS 3x10 |
| LAT PULLS 3x8–10 | ***or*** CHINS |

**PRESCRIPTION:** Alternate workouts A and B with 2 days of rest between sessions, e.g.: Mon-A, Thu-B, Sun-A, Wed-B, Sat-A, etc. Notation is sets x reps.

**INDICATIONS:** <40: Discretion 40–49: Discretion 50–59: Discretion >60: Yes

For athletes who cannot engage in 3-day programs due to recovery or scheduling considerations.

**PARAMETERS:** May be instituted at the beginning of training or at any point in the novice progression, if indicated.

### PROGRAM 3B: FIXED 2-DAY RANK NOVICE

| WORKOUT A | WORKOUT B |
|---|---|
| SQUAT 3x5 | SQUAT 3x5 |
| BENCH 3x5 | PRESS 3x5 |
| DEADLIFT 1x5 | DEADLIFT 1x5 |

**PRESCRIPTION:** Alternate workouts A and B on 2 fixed days of the week, with at least 2 days between each session, e.g.: Mon-Thu, Mon-Fri, Tue-Fri, Wed-Sat. Notation is sets x reps.

**INDICATIONS:** <40: Discretion 40–49: Discretion 50–59: Discretion >60: Yes

For athletes who cannot engage in 3-day programs due to recovery or scheduling considerations, and when a fixed schedule is required.

**PARAMETERS:** May be instituted at the beginning of training or at any point in the novice progression, as indicated.

this case, 2 or 3 full days are taken between each workout. Many Masters in their 60s or 70s won't sustain more than a few weeks of training the whole body for 3 days a week, and in some cases it may be wise to avoid overreaching at the start. Patience will always win out over greed. In our experience, a fixed 2-day program is safe, effective, and practical for the vast majority of trainees in the seventh decade.

As with the standard (3-day) Rank Novice Program (1A, 2A), the 2-day variant (3B) begins with conservative weight and judicious increases in bar loading. The weights used for deadlifts start out light, so the risk of overtraining the pull is low, and the twice-weekly pulling schedule at the front end of the program will promote mastery of deadlift form. Soon, however, the deadlift will become

## PROGRAM 3C: 2-DAY EARLY NOVICE

| WORKOUT A | WORKOUT B |
| --- | --- |
| SQUAT 3x5 | SQUAT 3x5 |
| BENCH 3x5 | PRESS 3x5 |
| DEADLIFT 1x5 | LAT PULLS 3x8 ***or*** BODYWEIGHT ROWS 3x8–10 |

**PRESCRIPTION:** Alternate workouts A and B on 2 fixed days of the week, with at least 2 days between each session, e.g.: Mon-Thu, Mon-Fri, Tue-Fri, Wed-Sat. Notation is sets x reps.

**INDICATIONS:** <40: Discretion 40–49: Discretion 50–59: Discretion >60: Yes

For athletes who cannot engage in 3-day programs due to recovery or scheduling considerations, and when a fixed schedule is required.

**PARAMETERS:** Instituted after Phase I (3B) when deadlift becomes too heavy for twice-weekly training.

heavy enough to require reduction to once-weekly training. The athlete is then transitioned to the 2-Day Early Novice Program (3C). The deadlift on day 2 is replaced with another back exercise, such as lat pulls or bodyweight rows.

After some progress on 3C, the athlete will begin to struggle or stall on his second squat session of the week. Accumulated fatigue from heavy squats and deadlifts is bleeding over into the second day's session. Performance increases on day 2 are now harder to come by, with increases in fatigue and soreness. Progression to a 2-day variant of the 3-day Novice Program 1C is now indicated.

In the 2-Day Novice Program (3D), the second session becomes a light squat day. We are at pains to point out that this does *not* violate our principle of intensity-dependence. The light day serves the important function of maintaining the motor pathways necessary for this somewhat complex movement pattern, and also facilitates recovery without adding too much new stress. Reductions in training load should be between 5% and 10% at most. In general, the stronger and younger the trainee the more reduction will be required. A bit of trial and error may be required in order to find the right balance. Reducing intensity too far with a Master can allow a detraining effect to creep in. However, insufficient reduction does not facilitate recovery, but adds stress. A good idea is to start at about a 5% reduction and then manipulate the volume of the workout from there. If 3 sets of 5 at a 5% reduction are still difficult to complete, the athlete should reduce volume to just 1–2 sets of 5, or continue with 3 sets across but drop the reps to doubles or triples. If this is still difficult, then the athlete should increase the percentage offload by a small margin. The light day squat should not feel "easy." It's light for a reason – the trainee is not fully recovered from day 1. But if the trainee is struggling to complete reps the weight is too heavy.

In Program 3D, the deadlift has been moved to day 2. Many Masters prefer to place the heavy deadlift exercise on the light squat day. The light squat does an excellent job of warming up the athlete's legs and hips without creating the same level of fatigue as heavy squats. A performance increase on the deadlift often occurs when this adjustment is made. Training the deadlift in a less fatiguing situation can promote several weeks' worth of continued progression.

However, some will prefer to keep the deadlift on the same day as heavy squats (Program 3E). This makes day 1 the "heavy day" (squats,

## PROGRAM 3D: 2-DAY NOVICE

| WORKOUT A | WORKOUT B |
|---|---|
| SQUAT 3x5 | LIGHT SQUAT 3x5 |
| BENCH 3x5 | PRESS 3x5 |
| LAT PULLS 3x8–10 ***or*** BODYWEIGHT ROWS 3x8–10 | DEADLIFT 1x5 |

**PRESCRIPTION:** Alternate workouts A and B on 2 fixed days of the week, with at least 2 days between each session, e.g.: Mon-Thu, Mon-Fri, Tue-Fri, Wed-Sat. Alternate between lat pulls and bodyweight rows at each A Workout. Notation is sets x reps.

**INDICATIONS:** <40: Discretion 40–49: Discretion 50–59: Discretion >60: Yes

For athletes who cannot engage in 3-day programs due to recovery or scheduling considerations, and when a fixed schedule is required.

**PARAMETERS:** Initiated when progress in Phase 2 stagnates and the introduction of a light squat day is necessary.

## PROGRAM 3E: 2-DAY NOVICE (HARD-EASY)

| WORKOUT A | WORKOUT B |
|---|---|
| SQUAT 3x5 | LIGHT SQUAT 3x5 |
| BENCH 3x5 | PRESS 3x5 |
| DEADLIFT 1x5 | LAT PULLS 3x8–10 ***or*** BODYWEIGHT ROWS 3x8–10 |

**PRESCRIPTION:** Alternate workouts A and B on 2 fixed days of the week, with at least 2 days between each session, e.g.: Mon-Thu, Mon-Fri, Tue-Fri, Wed-Sat. Alternate between lat pulls and bodyweight rows at each B ("easy") Workout. Notation is sets x reps.

**INDICATIONS:** <40: Discretion 40–49: Discretion 50–59: Discretion >60: Yes

For athletes who cannot engage in 3-day programs due to recovery or scheduling considerations, when a fixed schedule is required, and when athlete and coach elect to alternate heavy and light workouts.

**PARAMETERS:** Initiated when progress in Phase 2 stagnates and the introduction of a light squat day is necessary; and when athlete and coach prefer a hard-easy configuration.

bench press, deadlift) and creates a situation where day 2 is a "light day" (light squats, press, lat pulls or bodyweight rows). Some athletes will prefer the systemic variation in having one easy day and one hard day. Each athlete and coach can and should experiment with both setups.

Example 20-2 is a detailed illustration of a Master transitioning through all 3 phases of the 2-day novice model. *For illustrative purposes only* it will be shown that each phase lasts 3 weeks. In reality, each phase would likely last much longer. *It is in no way suggested that this program be artificially programmed into 3-week phases.*

We direct the reader's attention to two important features of the following example. First, the trainee's deadlift slows at the end of 3B as fatigue begins to accumulate from pulling twice a week. After a reduction in deadlift frequency the trainee is able to return to 10-pound jumps at each deadlift session. This is a common scenario.

Second, the lat pull-down exercise illustrates the trainee's first experience using *rep progressions.* Machine-based exercises, especially when performed for higher repetitions, rarely display steady linear gains. The best approach with lat pulls is to use the same weight for 2–3 weeks in a row, increasing the volume performed with that weight. The use of rep progressions will be discussed in greater detail in the chapters on intermediate training.

## Other Common Variants of the Novice Program

By now it should be clear that novice programming can be tailored to the individual needs and limitations of virtually any athlete, given a fundamental understanding of what novice programming really *is,* and how the Stress-Recovery-Adaptation cycle is manipulated in this phase of training. Armed with a grasp of these fundamentals, age, strength, and scheduling constraints are no obstacles to the design of a program that allows any Master to pursue a linear progression, adding weight to the bar from workout to workout. Creatively and effectively exploiting these principles to meet the needs of the individual athlete is the *art* of programming.

With all this in mind, we now consider additional variations of the novice model. The programs explored below are not specific to athletes of any particular age group, and they do not

**Example 20-2: Using the Fixed 2-Day Novice Model**

| Week | Monday | Thursday |
|---|---|---|
| **3B (Rank Novice)** | | |
| **1** | Squat 45x5x3 | Squat 50x5x3 |
| | Bench 75x5x3 | Press 50x5x3 |
| | Deadlift 85x5 | Deadlift 95x5 |
| **2** | Squat 55x5x3 | Squat 60x5x3 |
| | Bench 80x5x3 | Press 55x5x3 |
| | Deadlift 105x5 | Deadlift 115x5 |
| **3** | Squat 65x5x3 | Squat 70x5x3 |
| | Bench 85x5x3 | Press 60x5x3 |
| | Deadlift 120x5 | Deadlift 125x5 |
| **3C (Early Novice)** | | |
| **4** | Squat 75x5x3 | Squat 80x5x3 |
| | Bench 90x5x3 | Press 62x5x3 |
| | **Deadlift 130x5** | **Lat Pulls 100x8x3** |
| **5** | Squat 85x5x3 | Squat 90x5x3 |
| | Bench 92x5x3 | Press 64x5x3 |
| | Deadlift 140x5 | Lat Pulls 100x10x3 |
| **6** | Squat 95x5x3 | Squat 100x5x3 |
| | Bench 94x5x3 | Press 66x5x3 |
| | Deadlift 150x5 | Lat Pulls 105x8x3 |
| **3D (Novice)** | | |
| **7** | Squat 105x5x3 | **Light Squat 95x3x3** |
| | Bench 96x5x3 | Press 68x5x3 |
| | **Lat Pulls 105x10x3** | **Deadlift 160x5** |
| **8** | Squat 110x5x3 | Light Squat 100x3x3 |
| | Bench 98x5x3 | Press 70x5x3 |
| | Lat Pulls 110x8x3 | Deadlift 170x5 |
| **9** | Squat 115x5x3 | Light Squat 105x3x3 |
| | Bench 100x5x3 | Press 72x5x3 |
| | Lat Pulls 110x10x3 | Deadlift 180x5 |

**(Bold = emphasized change during each phase)**

**Example 20-3: 4-Day Novice Type 1 Model**

| Monday | Tuesday | Thursday | Friday |
|---|---|---|---|
| Squat 3x5 | Deadlift 1x5 | Squat 3x5 | Deadlift 1x5 |
| Press 3x5 | Lat Pulls 3x10 | Bench 3x5 | Bodyweight Rows 3x10 |

**Example 20-4: 4-Day Novice Type 1 with Olympic Lifts**

| Monday | Tuesday | Thursday | Friday |
|---|---|---|---|
| Squat 3x5 | Power Clean 5x3 | Light Squat 3x5 | Deadlift 1x5 |
| Press 3x5 | Lat Pulls 3x10 ***or*** Chins | Bench 3x5 | Bodyweight Rows 3x10 ***or*** Chins |

exhaust the possibilities for modification of the novice progression. They are presented not just as additional options for program prescription, but more importantly as a wider exploration of how programming *principles* are put into *practice* to meet the needs of the individual athlete. Because the programs that follow are more individualized than the novice models presented previously, they are not presented as program templates.

### Four-day novice programs

These programs spread out the novice program over a 4-day period. This is an excellent way to reduce the workload of each individual training session for a Master struggling with recovery. And even though the athlete will be in the gym more often than with a 3-day plan, there are actually more days of rest between *each individual exercise* with a 4-day plan.

Total gym time for each training session should be reduced by 25–50% for a athlete following any of these plans. This is a good way to balance the training schedule on top of very busy personal and professional lives. Athletes should be able to get in and out of the gym in around an hour. Each of the 3 options below has some benefits and some drawbacks.

**4-Day Novice Type 1 Variants**. This option divides the workload into squats and presses on two of the training days, and all pulling and/or back exercises on the other two days. Because pulls from the floor work the back quite hard, it makes sense to put supplemental upper back and lat work such as chins, pulls, or bodyweight rows on this day. This setup has the benefit of creating some space between the squats and deadlifts, the two most stressful exercises in the program. The potential drawback is that pulling heavy from the floor *one day* after squats can be more difficult than pulling *one hour* after squats. Once the soreness and stiffness from the squats starts to set in the day after the exercise is performed, deadlifts or cleans may be out of the question. However, if the trainee is not experiencing much soreness from his squat training, then he may appreciate using a training template that allows for him to deadlift first at training sessions. Individual recovery capacity will dictate whether this is an appropriate training schedule.

This basic structure allows for many permutations. Example 20-3 assumes the trainee is still fairly early into his linear progression and is recovering at a rate that allows him to deadlift twice per week. Alternatively, a trainee in his 40s or early 50s who wishes to train the power clean might set up his program as in Example 20-4.

Observe that the deadlift workout is performed at the end of the week. This will be especially beneficial if the trainee is performing a light squat workout on Thursday. The legs will feel fresher than they would on Tuesday after heavy squats. The lighter pulling variant in Example 20-4 is reserved for the day after heavy squats. Deadlifting on Friday also has the added benefit of allowing 2 days of rest over the weekend for the low back to recover before Monday's heavy squats.

On a 4-day plan, Masters novices should aim for no more than a 5–10% reduction in bar weight for the light day. *Masters are intensity-dependent.* If intensity is decreased too much for too long, detraining will occur. If the athlete is only going to squat twice a week, and one of those days is light, that leaves one high-intensity squat session per week. Although this approach may be necessary for optimal recovery due to age, the frequency is still low for any novice, and intensity should be kept high. This may require the athlete to reduce the total volume of his light squat day. If 3 sets of 5 with a 5% reduction is not enough of an offload, then good options for the light day would be just a single set of 5 reps, or 2–3 sets of 3 reps. Both options are illustrated in Example 20-5 (only squats are shown).

If the athlete has not implemented a light squat day and is performing heavy squats on Thursday, the Friday workout could even be moved to Saturday morning to create a little more space between sessions. If this were the scenario, then the athlete could actually set up a training schedule that allowed him to use a 3-day/week AB rotation for his pressing exercises (Monday/Thursday /Saturday schedule), while maintaining 2-day/week frequency for squats and pulls, as in Example 20-6.

**Example 20-5: 4-Day Novice Type 1 with Light Squat Day Options**

| Monday | Thursday (Light Squat Day) |
|---|---|
| Squat 225x5x3 | Squat 210x5 |
| | ***or*** |
| | Squat 210x3x2 |

**Four-Day Novice Type 2 (Split) Variants.** This model places all the lower body work on one day and all the upper body work on another day. This option allows for longest recovery for each area of the body, as there is minimal overlap between muscle groups on consecutive training days. A potential drawback is that training the two pressing movements on the same day forces the second exercise performed during the training session to progress a little slower due to the fatigue created by the first exercise. In the grand scheme of the training program, this is not a huge issue. We recommend that the press be the second exercise of the day and the athlete begin upper body sessions with the bench. We find that bench presses affect presses less than presses affect bench presses, probably because presses exhaust the triceps more than bench presses. And once the reserves in the triceps are gone, all hope for effective benching during that session evaporates. For this reason alone, it makes sense to bench first and press second. Moreover, after heavy benches, the nervous system will be "primed" for a lighter pressing variation after dealing with the heavier weight of the bench at the beginning of the workout. The lighter weights on the press should move well even though the deltoids and triceps may be a bit fatigued.

Training day order is interchangeable. Some may find that the overall systemic fatigue created by squats and deadlifts has negative carryover to the upper body exercises in the next day even though there is no direct overlap. In this case, it is completely acceptable to do upper body on Monday /Thursday

**Example 20-6: 4-Day Novice Type 1 with 3-Day Pressing Rotation**

| Week | Monday | Tuesday | Thursday | Saturday |
|---|---|---|---|---|
| **1** | Squat 3x5 | Power Clean 5x3 | Squat 3x5 | Deadlift 1x5 |
| | Bench 3x5 | Lat Pulls 3x10 ***or*** Chins | Press 3x5 | Bench Press 3x5 |
| **2** | Squat 3x5 | Power Clean 5x3 | Squat 3x5 | Deadlift 1x5 |
| | Press 3x5 | Lat Pulls 3x10 ***or*** Chins | Bench Press 3x5 | Press 3x5 |

**Example 20-7: Basic 4-Day Novice Type 2 Model**

| Monday | Tuesday | Thursday | Friday |
|---|---|---|---|
| Squat 3x5 | Bench 3x5 | Squat 3x5 | Bench 3x5 |
| Deadlift 1x5 | Press 3x5 | Deadlift 1x5 | Press 3x5 |

**Example 20-8: 4-Day Novice Type 2 with Light Squat Days and Power Clean**

| Monday | Tuesday | Thursday | Friday |
|---|---|---|---|
| Squat 3x5 | Bench 3x5 | Light Squat 2x3 | Bench 3x5 |
| Power Clean 5x3 | Press 3x5 | Deadlift 1x5 | Press 3x5 |

and lower body on Tuesday/Friday. If the trainee has the time and energy, upper back exercises such as chins, lat pulls, or bodyweight rows could be added to the end of the upper body or lower body training days.

Above are two different examples of the Type 2 4-day model. Example 20-7 would be suitable for a relatively new novice Master who will not be training the power clean and can recover well enough to train all 4 primary exercises twice per week for the prescribed sets and reps. This is the simplest of all 4-day novice programs to operate.

Example 20-8 illustrates an appropriate approach for a novice athlete in his 40s who has gained enough strength and experience to warrant a light squat day on Thursday and is actively training the power clean. As before, if the athlete is using a light squat day, it makes sense to train the deadlift on the same day.

**Four-Day Novice Type 3 Variants.** For most Masters Athletes the sets-across approach is one of the most difficult elements of the entire program, particularly with regard to squats. Squats take time to warm up, need long rest times between work sets, and the fatigue from heavy sets across almost always bleeds over into the second and third exercises of the day. Type 3 4-day variants allow the athlete to focus entirely on the squat on 2 of the 4 training days. It has the added benefit of saving time in the gym. Trainees should be able to warm up and execute all 3 work sets for the squat in under an hour. That makes the squat day quite short, and significantly reduces the time in the gym for the pressing/pulling day.

This is not only convenient for many, but shorter training sessions make systemic recovery easier – always an important consideration for the Masters Athlete. The drawback is the same as for the Type 1 variant. Soreness and stiffness from the previous day's squats may make pulling the day after harder than pulling the same day as the squat.

Several variants of the Type 3 structure are illustrated below. Example 20-9 is the simplest approach.

**Example 20-9: Basic 4-Day Novice Type 3 Model**

| Monday | Tuesday | Thursday | Friday |
|---|---|---|---|
| Squat 3x5 | Bench 3x5 | Squat 3x5 | Press 3x5 |
| | Deadlift 1x5 | | Deadlift 1x5 |

**Example 20-10: Basic 4-Day Novice Type 3 with Light Squats**

| Week | Monday | Tuesday | Thursday | Saturday |
|---|---|---|---|---|
| 1 | Squat 3x5 | Bench 3x5 | Light Squat 2x3 | Bench 3x5 |
| | | Deadlift 1x5 | Press 3x5 | Deadlift 1x5 |
| 2 | Squat 3x5 | Press 3x5 | Light Squat 2x3 | Press 3x5 |
| | | Deadlift 1x5 | Bench 3x5 | Deadlift 1x5 |

Example 20-10 illustrates two modifications to the Type 3 structure. First, a light squat day, at a 5% reduction, is implemented on Thursday. Because this reduces training time it allows the athlete to introduce an extra press or bench session into the week. The Friday workout will be moved to Saturday to set up a Tuesday/Thursday/Saturday pressing schedule. The independence of the heavy sets-across squat workout is left on Monday so the athlete can thoroughly warm up and take as much rest time as needed between sets.

Trainees can experiment with all 3 models if a 4-day plan is to be implemented. The right choice will be the model that matches up best with the trainee's individual recovery capacities – primarily his individual response to the heavy squat training. Other factors include the trainee's preference on press and bench frequency (2 or 3 days per week) and the compatibility of the training schedule with the rest of his personal and professional life. Gym time is at a premium for many. If an hour or so is all that can be allocated on a given day for training, then a 4-day/week plan is an excellent time-saving alternative to the standard 3-day model.

## Two-day models with Olympic lifts

With a certain hesitance and trepidation, we present here an approach to incorporating the Olympic lifts in a reduced-frequency model of training. Such approaches can be used by Masters who are willing and able to train and tolerate the Olympic variants, but we are compelled to reiterate, *again*, that such Masters *are few and far between*. The Olympic variants must be used *with great caution* in any athlete over 40, and that sense of caution must increase exponentially with each passing year. Some Masters derive great joy and confidence from training the Olympic variants, and an even smaller number may actually make impressive progress in these exercises. But athlete and coach must be clear-headed about the probability of benefit from adding these lifts to their regimen relative to the risk of harm.

**Example 20-11: 2-Day Model with Olympic Lifts**

| Week | Monday | Thursday |
|---|---|---|
| 1 | Squat 3x5 | Squat 3x5 |
| | Bench 3x5 | Press 3x5 |
| | Deadlift 1x5 | Power Clean 5x3 |
| 2 | Squat 3x5 | Squat 3x5 |
| | Bench 3x5 | Press 3x5 |
| | Deadlift 1x5 | Power Snatch 5x2 |

*The Olympic lifts are not necessary components of a General Exercise Prescription for health, and their inclusion in a Masters' life constitutes the pursuit of a sport or hobby, like tennis, rock climbing, or judo.* Do them if (like Sullivan) you just can't live without them, in the certain knowledge that you actually *could* live without them.

With the caveats out of the way, below are 3 different example models for a more fit and athletic trainee, likely (but not necessarily) under 60 years of age, who wishes to experiment with the Olympic power variants on the 2-day plan. We assume the trainee has demonstrated proficiency in the safe performance of light power cleans and light power snatches, and wishes to train *both* exercises.

In Example 20-11 the trainee continues to pull heavy once a week, to keep building his absolute pulling strength. Power cleans and power snatches are simply alternated every other week as the light pulling variant. Some Masters will decide to concentrate on only one Olympic variant. Perhaps arthritic shoulders do not allow for properly receiving a snatch. In this case, the trainee would simply perform his one Olympic lift of choice each Thursday.

As the trainee grows in strength and the deadlift becomes more taxing to his recovery capacity, he may decide to switch from pulling heavy once a week to once every 3 workouts. If he wishes to continue learning and practicing both Olympic lifts, he could set up a simple 3-day rotation of pulling variants spread across a 2-day training week as shown in Example 20-12.

In Example 20-13, the trainee's hips and low back will only tolerate pulling from the floor (deadlifts *or* Olympic variants) once a week, yet he still wishes to train the clean or snatch. *This scenario mandates a serious re-appraisal of the trainee's priorities.* But if he remains passionately dedicated to training the Olympic variants, this model may prove suitable. The athlete will deadlift heavy every other week, and train the clean and/or snatch on alternate weeks. If both lifts are to be done, no more than 2–3 work sets of each exercise (triples for the clean, doubles for the snatch) should be performed.

## Terminating the Novice Program (Redux)

As noted at the end of the previous chapter, the effective execution of any novice program will eventually produce a level of strength that will permit the athlete to impose a training stress that overwhelms his capacity to recover before the next workout. In the Master over 60, reductions in training volume and increases in recovery time can be used to stretch the novice program out a bit longer after this point is reached, but will not be as effective as they are for younger athletes. After at most 3–6 months of novice training, most Masters will require a longer training period, stretching the overload event and Stress-Recovery Adaptation cycle over multiple workouts. The Masters Athlete has become an intermediate, and his programming is discussed in Chapters 22–24.

**Example 20-12: 2-Day Model with Olympic Lifts, Decreased Deadlift Frequency**

| Week | Monday | Thursday |
|---|---|---|
| 1 | Squat 3x5 | Squat 3x5 |
| | Bench 3x5 | Press 3x5 |
| | Deadlift 1x5 | Power Clean 5x3 |
| 2 | Squat 3x5 | Squat 3x5 |
| | Bench 3x5 | Press 3x5 |
| | Power Snatch 5x2 | Deadlift 1x5 |
| 3 | Squat 3x5 | Squat 3x5 |
| | Bench 3x5 | Press 3x5 |
| | Power Clean 5x3 | Power Snatch 5x2 |

**Example 20-13: 2-Day Model with Olympic Lifts, Decreased Pulling Frequency**

| Week | Monday | Thursday |
|---|---|---|
| 1 | Squat 3x5 | Squat 3x5 |
| | Bench 3x5 | Press 3x5 |
| | Deadlift 1x5 | Lat Pulls 3x8 |
| 2 | Squat 3x5 | Squat 3x5 |
| | Bench 3x5 | Press 3x5 |
| | Power Clean 5x3 *or* Power Snatch 5x2 | Lat Pulls 3x8 |
| | ***or*** | |
| | Power Clean 3x3 *and* Power Snatch 3x2 | |

# 21

# The Novice Over 70 and Remedial Variants

Novice programs for athletes over 70, and for particularly weak or deconditioned individuals, are necessarily the most conservative of all. Such programs will use less overall volume and decreased exercise frequency, while aiming to keep intensity high. This chapter explores the 3-in-2 and 1-day/week reduced frequency models of training. This chapter also presents remedial programming options for individuals who are unable to squat to depth due to weakness, and for those with shoulder mobility limitations that preclude barbell squats and presses.

## The Eighth Decade Novice

Athletes in the eighth decade and beyond are critically dependent on careful, conservative programming, with assiduous attention to recovery factors and prevention of overtraining and injury. Their recovery capacity is blunted by an advanced multifactorial anabolic resistance, a greater tendency to counterproductive inflammatory responses, and the manifold stresses attendant upon living life in one's 70s, 80s, or 90s – suppressed appetite, fitful sleep, and anxiety about the past, present and future.

Being 70 years old is *hard,* but it's *usually* better than the alternative.

Being a 70-year old athlete is *damn* hard, but it's *always* better than the alternative.

As always, modifications for athletes in their eighth decade and beyond, and for those who are similarly deconditioned or physically challenged, will be focused on moderation of volume, maintenance of intensity, optimization of recovery, extremely judicious and conservative increases in loading, and an emphasis on what the athlete *can* do, rather than what he can't. With appropriate programming, careful exercise selection, and careful, attentive coaching, athletes in these populations can safely realize and maintain optimum gains in strength and muscle mass and profoundly improve their physical function and quality of life.

We again acknowledge that categorizing athletes by decade is inherently arbitrary, and that training always occurs on an individual timeline. It is entirely possible that an athlete over 70 can start with the standard 3-day rank novice progression (Program 2A). However, most of these Masters will require more recovery time than such a schedule

## PROGRAM 4A: 3-IN-2 NOVICE

| WORKOUT A | WORKOUT B |
| --- | --- |
| SQUAT 3x5 | SQUAT 3x5 |
| BENCH 3x5 | PRESS (OR BENCH) 3x5 |
| DEADLIFT 1x5 | DEADLIFT 1x5 |

**PRESCRIPTION:** Alternate workouts A and B, such that the trainee works out three times in a two-week period, e.g. Week 1=AB, Week 2=A, Week 3=BA, Week 4=B, etc. Notation is sets x reps.

**INDICATIONS:** <50: Discretion 50–59: Discretion 60–69: Yes >70: Yes

For athletes who cannot engage in 3-day programs due to recovery or scheduling considerations, and when a fixed schedule is required.

**PARAMETERS:** May be instituted at the beginning of training or at any point in the novice progression, as indicated.

permits, and even if they are able to tolerate a 3-day program to start, they are likely to get stale quickly. A reduced frequency program (Chapter 20) is more likely to be well-tolerated and sustain progress from the start, and is a very rational choice for the rank novice in his 70s or early 80s. Movement to a program which relegates deadlifts to once a week or less will be indicated sooner rather than later, as will the transition to light squat days or a reduction in the number of squat days.

Even so, many of these athletes will soon find they are strong enough to impose a training stress that surpasses their recovery capacity on a 2-day program, and a more conservative reduced frequency model will be required. The *3-in-2 Model* is more conservative than a 2-day approach, and can be used in athletes who have tolerated a 2-day program but are beginning to have difficulty adapting from workout to workout. One-day models are the most conservative of all, and can be used to produce and/or maintain strength in very aged athletes.

### 3-IN-2 NOVICE MODELS

A 3-in-2 program structure may be used at the initiation of training, but is more often used to sustain progress after the trainee begins with another more aggressive approach. The 3-in-2 structure can also be used as a short-term solution for an athlete who is recovering from injury or fatigue. After a month or so of less frequent training, the trainee will recoup his energy, heal up, and get back to a more aggressive program.

The 3-in-2 model prescribes training each core barbell exercise 3 times within a 2-week time frame. There are 2 major variations. The first is a series of 3 full-body workouts, and the athlete is only in the gym once about every 4–5 days, as shown in Program 4A. This approach is particularly useful when an athlete is limited to training fewer movements. For instance, when a trainee is physically unable to perform a press because of limited shoulder mobility, there is no pressing exercise to alternate with the bench press. Sustaining progress on the bench is more easily managed with the prolonged rest between workouts of the 3-in-2 template than in programs training it 2–3 times per week (Example 21-1).

Program 4B is a recently developed variant of the 3-in-2 template is an upper body/lower body (split) structure that maintains the same frequency of training an exercise 3 times in a 2-week period, but puts the athlete in the gym a little more often, albeit with much shorter training sessions. This is a good option for those who simply don't want to be out of the gym for a 4- or 5-day stretch (it might be too tempting to not come back!). It's also a fine choice for those who struggle with full-body workouts for recovery or logistical reasons.

In week 1, the lower body will be trained twice and the upper body once. In week 2, the pattern will switch.

Upper back work, such as lat pulls or bodyweight rows, could be added 1–2 days/week on either upper- or lower-body training days.

### One-day training plans

The majority of novice Masters, regardless of age or condition, can tolerate training more than once a week, provided bar loading is appropriate and recovery factors are dialed in properly. In the ideal circumstance, a 3-in-2 structure would be the minimum frequency for long-term Masters training. However, there are reasons to train less frequently. Some athletes of very advanced

**Example 21-1: 3-In-2 Program, No Presses**

**Week 1**

| Monday | Wednesday | Friday |
|---|---|---|
| Squat 3x5 | — | Squat 3x5 |
| Bench 3x5 | | Bench 3x5 |
| Deadlift 1x5 | | Deadlift 1x5 |
| Lat Pulls 3x10 | | Lat Pulls 3x10 |

**Week 2**

| Monday | Wednesday | Friday |
|---|---|---|
| — | Squat 3x5 | — |
| | Bench 3x5 | |
| | Deadlifts 1x5 | |
| | Lat Pulls 3x10 | |

**Week 3**

| Monday | Wednesday | Friday |
|---|---|---|
| Squat 3x5 | — | Squat 3x5 |
| Bench 3x5 | | Bench 3x5 |
| Deadlifts 1x5 | | Deadlift 1x5 |
| Lat Pulls 3x10 | | Lat Pulls 3x10 |

### PROGRAM 4B: 3-IN-2 NOVICE SPLIT

**WEEK 1:**

| MONDAY | WEDNESDAY | FRIDAY |
|---|---|---|
| SQUAT 3x5 | BENCH 3x5 | SQUAT 3x5 |
| DEADLIFT 1x5 | PRESS 3x5 | DEADLIFT 1x5 |

**WEEK 2:**

| MONDAY | WEDNESDAY | FRIDAY |
|---|---|---|
| BENCH 3x5 | SQUAT 3x5 | BENCH 3x5 |
| PRESS 3x5 | DEADLIFT 1x5 | PRESS 3x5 |

**PRESCRIPTION**: Alternate weeks 1 and 2. Notation is sets x reps.

**INDICATIONS**: <50: Discretion 50–59: Discretion 60–69: Yes >70: Yes

For athletes who cannot engage in 3-day full-body programs, or to accommodate recovery or scheduling considerations, and when a fixed schedule is required.

**PARAMETERS**: May be instituted at the beginning of training or at any point in the novice progression, as indicated.

## PROGRAM 4C: 1 DAY/WEEK

**FIXED WORKOUT**

SQUAT 6x5 (Ascending sets)
BENCH 3x5
DEADLIFT 1x5, 1x5 (Back-off)
PRESS 2x8
LAT PULLS 2–3x8–10

**PRESCRIPTION:** Perform the fixed workout once weekly, focusing on those movements the trainee can tolerate and do well, to the exclusion of those he cannot. Notation is sets x reps.

**INDICATIONS:** <50: No 50–59: No 60–69: Discretion >70: Discretion
For very aged or deconditioned athletes who cannot participate in 3-day or other reduced frequency programs.

**PARAMETERS:** May be instituted at the beginning of training or at any point thereafter, as indicated.

age or deconditioning may not tolerate training more frequently than once a week. In other cases, practical considerations predominate: scheduling, transportation, availability of coaching, and so on.

Once per week training programs assume the hypothetical trainee is weak and deconditioned, and probably has some age-related limitations to their mobility, recovery capacity, and exercise tolerance. The guiding principle in this circumstance is that *each weekly training session must yield the highest return possible on limited training time*. This demands an unswerving focus on *what the trainee can do well*. A 1-day/week program doesn't allow us to waste time trying to remediate exercises the trainee is never going to master anyway. Coach and athlete must identify the big, multi-joint exercises the trainee can perform well, and dedicate training time and effort there.

If possible, emphasis should be on the squat, bench press, and deadlift. Of the principal exercises, these are the heaviest, and will stress the largest volume of muscle mass. Olympic movements are obviously excluded. If a weak, deconditioned trainee is only going to pull once a week, it should be a deadlift. Presses are of course extremely useful for an older Master and should be included – but only if the athlete can do them well. Many in this population cannot press properly or even safely. For these trainees, faster progress (and therefore greater returns) will be generated by a program focused on the bench press. Upper body "pulling" exercises like lat pulls are useful to include if there is time in the session, but often 3–4 compound lifts are all that time and energy will allow. Deadlifts generate ample lat and back work for aged or deconditioned Masters, so if lat pulls must be skipped it is of no great consequence.

Note the use of ascending sets (see Chapter 17) to accumulate volume for the squat portion of the workout in Program 4C. The first 4 sets are light to medium in intensity and the final two sets of the workout are work sets across. Bench presses are still effective here for the standard 3 sets of 5 across. Deadlifts are done for one work set of 5 reps, followed by 1 back-off set at a 5–10% offload. This added back-off set makes up for the overall lack of volume in the program. Program 4C is built on the assumption that the trainee cannot press heavy due to shoulder mobility limitations. The weight is accordingly light and two sets of 8 are prescribed, with utmost attention paid to best possible form and technique. This the best possible ratio of bench and pressing volume under the circumstances, to promote shoulder strength and health. Reducing the press work to just two sets will also save a little time for a trainee who probably feels like hitting the showers at this point. If time and energy are available at the end of the 4 basic barbell movements, a few sets of lat pulls, bodyweight rows, or bicep curls are included to round out the session.

# Remedial Squat Programming

By now it will clear to the reader that the squat is the cornerstone of every program in this text. But what happens when a trainee cannot perform a single full range-of-motion bodyweight squat on day one, much less a loaded barbell squat? This is a common problem, encountered by every coach who works with Masters. Implementing a strength program based on the squat is difficult when the trainee can't squat.

Many trainees assume they are not *flexible* enough to squat down and stand back up without assistance. In fact, flexibility and mobility issues are *very rarely* the reason a trainee cannot achieve a full-depth bodyweight squat. The reason is almost always *strength*. The trainee is simply not strong enough to get down into the hole and come back under his own power. This is because many trainees simply have not asked their bodies to get down into a squat position for many years – perhaps decades. Getting in and out of chairs for most of their adult lives has involved using significant assistance from the arms to push or pull themselves onto their feet.

So how do we take a Master from not being able to do single bodyweight squat to multiple sets of barbell squats? Different approaches are available to address this scenario.

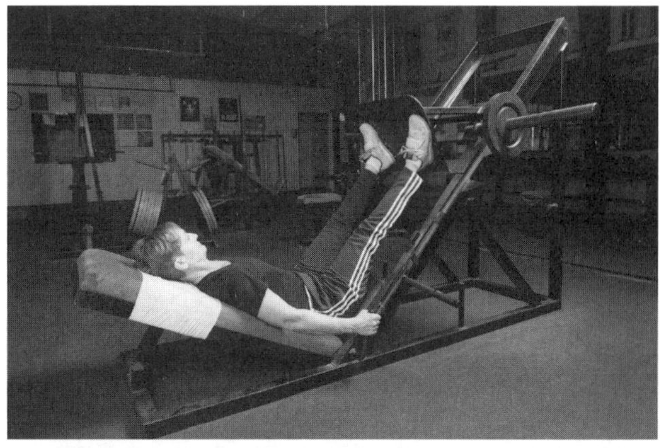

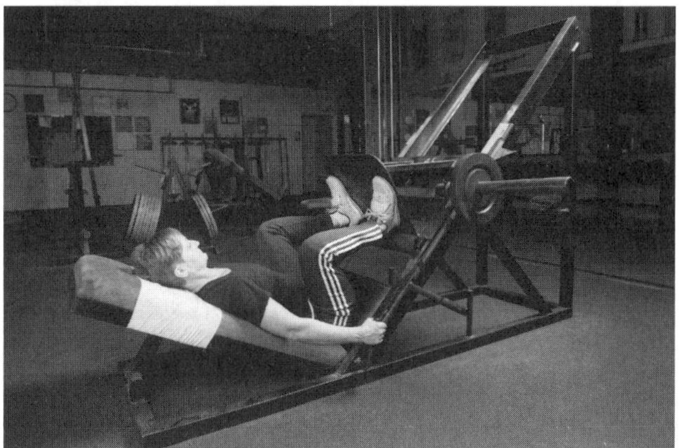

***Figure 21-1.*** Using the leg press.

### Method 1: the leg press

This approach assumes access to a leg press machine (Chapter 13). Most large commercial health club facilities will have one. Preferably the model should be one that is also commonly referred to as a "hip sled," or a leg press machine that allows the lifter to lay back at a 45 degree angle.

Leg presses will be done for sets of 10. The foot position and toe angle will mimic the squat as closely as possible (Figure 21-1). On day one, the trainee should leg press a light weight for 3 sets of 10. Each training session, weight will be added until the trainee can leg press the equivalent of their own bodyweight at this volume. It is usually possible to add about 10–20 pounds per session. This method only works when each and every rep is done as "deep" (hips as flexed) as the machine will safely allow, with no assistance from the hands. We find that once the trainee can leg press their bodyweight for 3x10, they will be able to squat a very light bar for a set of 5.

In a standard 2- or 3-day novice program, leg presses will simply take the place of squats as the first exercise of the day, with a goal of 3 sets of 10. Example 21-2 shows how the Rank Novice Program (2A) is modified for such an athlete.

**Example 21-2: Using the Leg Press for Squat Remediation**

| Monday | Wednesday | Friday |
|---|---|---|
| Leg Press 3x10 | Leg Press 3x10 | Leg Press 3x10 |
| Bench 3x5 | Press 3x5 | Bench 3x5 |
| Deadlift 1x5 | Deadlift 1x5 | Deadlift 1x5 |

## Method 2: partial range-of-motion squats

Many athletes will not have access to a leg press. In this case, partial range-of-motion (PROM) squats can be used to progressively train the athlete's range of motion and attain full depth. The trick here is to have a metric for progression. Simply "eyeballing" the depth and yelling at the trainee to "go deeper" will not work. There must be a mechanism for precisely measuring, tracking, and adjusting the depth of the squat from one session to the next.

**PROM Option 1: Box Squatting.** This approach uses plyometric boxes ranging from 12–18 inches in height. Other sturdy surfaces, such as a stack of thick bumper plates, can also be used, as long as they are sturdy and stable enough to support the trainee's bodyweight (Figure 21-2). A stack of ½ or ¾ inch squares of plywood or thick rubber matting will also be required. The dimensions should be large enough for the trainee to sit on them, but small enough that they stack neatly on top of the plyometric box.

On day 1, mats or boards are stacked on the box or other surface to create a stable platform that roughly replicates the height of a quarter-squat position for the trainee. The trainee will squat down to the box, lightly tap it with their buttocks, and come back up. This exercise will be repeated for a set of five. If this is easy, then one or two mats are removed and the trainee will do another set of five to the increased depth. This titration will be repeated until the trainee reaches a height where a set of 5 reps is difficult but achievable with good form. Three sets of five will be performed at this height. The following training session the trainee will return to the box and do 3 more work sets, this time at a slightly increased depth. Instead of adding weight to the bar of a full range-of-motion squat, we hold the load (bodyweight) constant and progress by adding depth, ½ or ¾ inch at a time. This may seem tedious (and it is), but adding a small increment of depth for each workout is real progress. Even the tiniest increment of increased depth makes the squat *much* more difficult. This approach permits the imposition of a quantifiable linear progression that is based on squat depth and not on added weight or reps. This process continues until the trainee achieves the strength to squat to just below parallel with good form for 3 sets of 5.

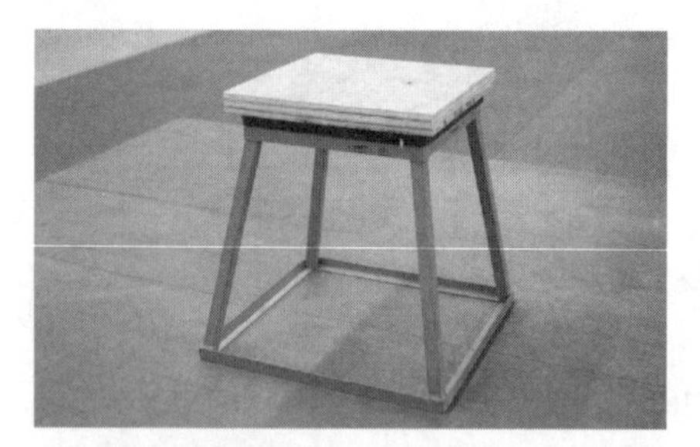

***Figure 21-2.*** PROM option 1: Box squats. *Left,* A sturdy plyometric box or other stable surface of stacked bumper plates, mats or boards allows for the titration and progression of squat depth and provides the trainee a measure of confidence and safety. *Below,* The athlete squats as deep as manageable on day 1. As the athlete grows strong at a particular depth, layers will be removed, until the she can squat below parallel.

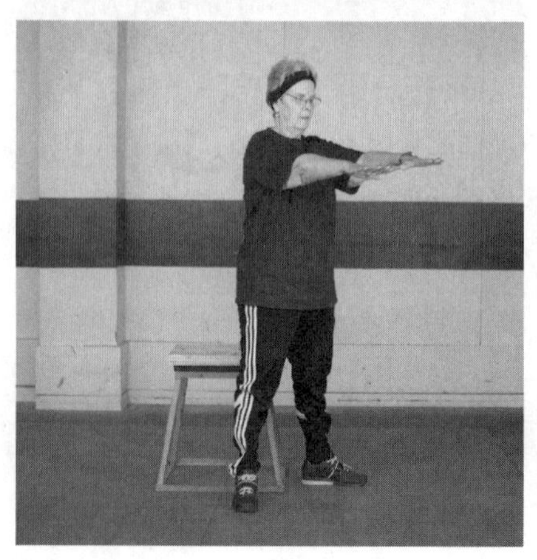

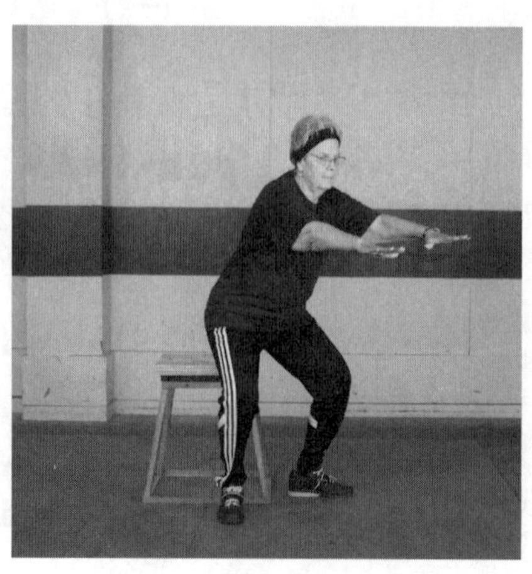

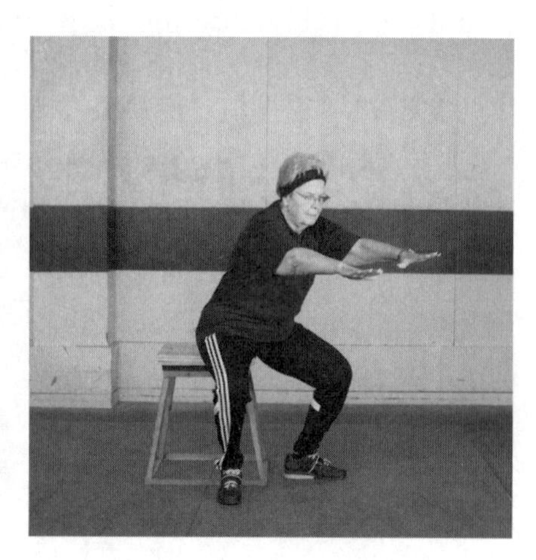

Extreme care must be taken with this method to ensure the athlete does not develop a dependence on the box. The trainee should never be allowed to sit or relax onto the box. They will be tempted to do this as depth increases. More importantly, trainees should not be allowed to pause, rock back and forward, and gather momentum for a rep. If a trainee has to sit and gather momentum to get off the box, the height should be lowered no further. Allowing trainees to do a "rocking box squat" virtually ensures that any progress with this method will not carry over to a regular squat with no box. To progress to regular training in the squat, the athlete must demonstrate the ability to lower themselves under complete control, very lightly touch the surface of the box and return to a standing position. *The box serves only as marker for depth.* All of this should be done while mimicking the mechanics of a back squat as closely as possible – stance, toe angle, back angle, knees out, hips back, and hip drive must be coached during this remedial exercise for the transition to a proper back squat to occur.

**PROM Option 2: Bungee Cord in a Power Rack.** The best way to avoid the potential problems and bad habits promoted by the box squat approach is a bungee cord strapped horizontally between the uprights of a power cage (Figure 21-3). The bungee cord will serve as a marker for depth, but it is not strong enough for the trainee to sit on it. (If they try they will end up on the floor. It's a good idea for coaches to remind their trainees of this!) Instead of using mats or boards to increase depth each workout, the bungee cord can be moved down the rack's uprights until proper depth is achieved. If the power rack has 1-inch hole spacing, then simply going down one hole per training session will work well. If the power rack has 3-inch hole spacing, splitting the difference and setting the bungee cord between holes every other workout works well – 3 inches is usually too large an increment for this method. Once the trainee can squat to depth using this method, it should be safe to add a very light bar and attempt the back squat.

We wish to emphasize that trainees who progress from either PROM option must begin with *very light bars.* Jumping from a difficult bodyweight squat to a 45-pound back squat is far too aggressive. Start with a 15–25-pound barbell for day one. If necessary, reduce the reps from 5 to 3 and build up

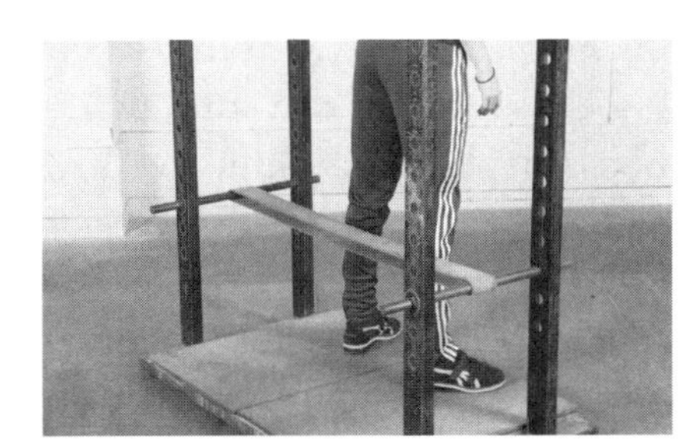

***Figure 21-3.*** PROM option 2: Bungee squats. A bungee cord is set between the uprights of a power rack (*left*) to allow for the titration and progression of squat depth, as in PROM Option 1, but without providing support for the trainee's weight. As the trainee grows strong at a particular depth, the bungee cord is lowered (*bottom panels*), forcing a deeper squat until the athlete can squat below parallel.

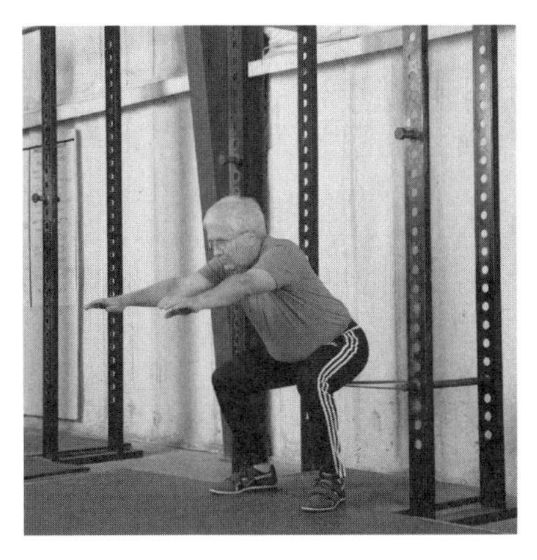

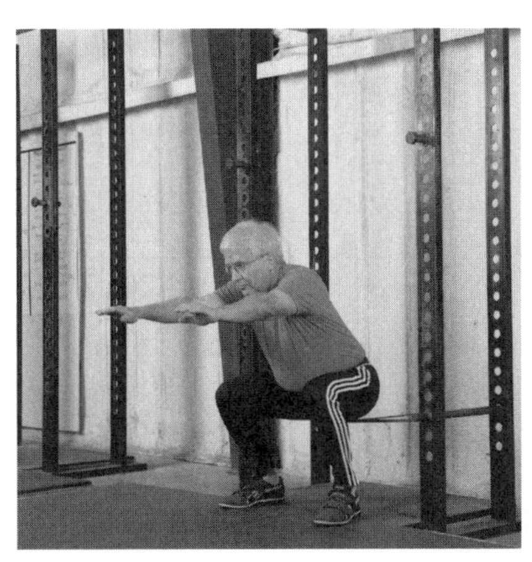

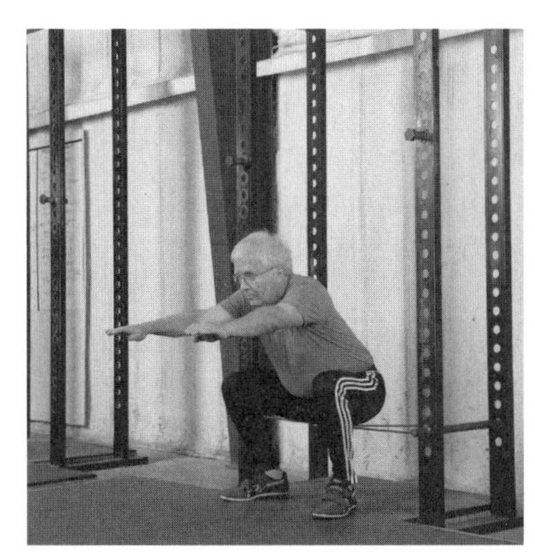

the reps over the course of 2–3 training sessions. After that it should be safe to add weight to the bar.

Given the choice between the PROM squat variations, we find the bungee cord method far more reliable. Both methods can work well, but the problems with learning to squat on a box are manifold, and the transition from the box is not always smooth. Dependence on the security of the box is not a problem that arises with the bungee cord method. On the other hand, the box method is portable. Many reading this book will be doing so not for their own sake, but for guidance on how to help an aging friend or family member. The reader may or may not be an experienced coach, and the aging friend or family member may not be willing or able to set foot in a fully equipped gym. The box squat approach can be brought to this person, and it can be "coached" by someone who isn't necessarily a professionally-trained strength coach. The box squat approach is most commonly used to prepare weak and deconditioned trainees for barbell squats. But they can also be used as an end in themselves.

Consider the example of an elderly lady confined to her home. She has trouble walking from room to room and spends most of her day sitting because it's just too hard to get up. Guiding this individual through the box squat protocol to the point where she can perform bodyweight squats below parallel *will transform this lady's life.* She may start barely able to perform a few high quarter squats – if that. But if we can get her to the point where can sit down to below parallel and drive her own bodyweight back up to standing for a few sets of five or even a set of 10, she will observe a profound improvement in her daily functioning and physical ability. And once she sees the power of progressive resistance training, she may be more inclined to reconsider coming to the gym. The potential rewards of this safe, simple approach are tremendous.

### The Importance of the Deadlift in Remedial Squat Programs

If a trainee is forced to use one of these remedial squat programs, the importance of the deadlift is amplified. Leg presses and PROM squats are very quadriceps-dominant. They lack the posterior chain involvement necessary for a full range-of-motion squat. Rapid progress on the deadlift assumes paramount importance in these scenarios. In the first few weeks of the novice progression, the trainee should try to deadlift at every training session. Increases in deadlift strength, with corresponding improvements in hamstring and spinal erector strength, will be just as important for remedial squat programming as any of the above-described approaches.

### Adding Reps to Remedial Squat Variants

For many aged or debilitated trainees, especially those with particularly poor shoulder mobility, the transition to any form of barbell squat may be out of reach. If this is the case, deadlifts can and should be made the priority of the program. For these athletes, deadlifts will be trained as the first exercise of the day, and the remedial squat variant or the leg press can be done later in the session.

For instance, an overweight female trainee in her 80s with extremely poor shoulder mobility will likely never progress to barbell squats. The best case scenario for her might be dumbbell (goblet) front squats to a below-parallel box. An important drawback of dumbbell squats is that the ability to hold the dumbbell in place will limit loading. As the dumbbell get heavier and larger, it gets awkward. Assume that this trainee hits a ceiling at the 15-pound dumbbell. Once she has achieved 3 sets of 5 with this weight, then the next step in the progression might be to simply add reps while maintaining weight. A conservative approach would be to add 1 rep to each set every 1–2 weeks. Over the course of weeks and months, the trainee could conceivably build up her capacity to do 15-rep sets with a 15-pound dumbbell off of the box. This sort of progress will pay enormous dividends in the trainee's daily life.

Example 21-3 illustrates this remedial squat program with rep progression. Assume the athlete trains twice per week, on Monday and Friday.

**Example 21-3: Remedial Squat Program with Rep Progression**

| Week | Monday | Friday |
|---|---|---|
| 1 | 24" Box Squat 3x5 | 23" Box Squat 3x5 |
| 2 | 22" Box Squat 3x5 | 21" Box Squat 3x5 |
| 3 | 20" Box Squat 3x5 | 19" Box Squat 3x5 |
| 4 | 18" Box Squat 3x5 | 17" Box Squat 3x5 |
| 5 | **16" Box Squat 3x5 (Represents a below-parallel Squat)** | 16" Box Squat 3x5 (+ 5 lb DB) |
| 6 | 16" Box Squat 3x5 (+ 8-lb DB) | 16" Box Squat 3x5 (+ 10 lb DB) |
| 7 | 16" Box Squat 3x5 (+ 12-lb DB) | 16" Box Squat 3x5 (+ 15-lb* DB) |
| 8 | 16" Box Squat 3x6 (+ 15-lb DB) | 16" Box Squat 3x6 (+ 15-lb DB) |
| 9 | 16" Box Squat 3x7 (+ 15-lb DB) | 16" Box Squat 3x7 (+ 15-lb DB) |
| 10 | 16" Box Squat 3x8 (+ 15-lb DB) | 16" Box Squat 3x8 (+ 15-lb DB) |
| 11 | 16" Box Squat 3x9 (+ 15-lb DB) | 16" Box Squat 3x9 (+ 15-lb DB) |
| 12 | 16" Box Squat 3x10 (+ 15-lb DB) | 16" Box Squat 3x10 (+ 15-lb DB) |

***Current dumbbell (DB) weight limit.**

# Other Remedial Plans

For some athletes over 60, certain barbell exercises will simply be inaccessible. In particular, many will not be able to perform squats and presses with barbells due to poor shoulder mobility. This common limitation will prevent the trainee from carrying a barbell anywhere on their back for squats, or effectively pressing a bar overhead. The same problem will usually impose severe restrictions on the usefulness of the front squat and pressing variants.

These trainees require a program focused on the deadlift and the bench press. Everything else in the program will be supplemental to these two exercises. A program based around just two major barbell movements will seem quite limited – and it is – but still represents a full-body workout with the potential to produce massive increases in strength and preserve muscle mass and function. Bench presses work the pectorals, triceps, and deltoids. Deadlifts effectively train the hamstrings, glutes, quads, low back, upper back, forearms, and abdominals. That's the lion's share of muscle mass. Improving the strength of a mobility-limited athlete on just these two exercises will be of tremendous value.

The Deadlift-Bench Specialist Program (4D) is indicated for these trainees, and supplements the two primary lifts with accessory exercises selected in accordance with the athlete's abilities.

Because the deadlift is the focus of this program, it should be trained first in the workout, while the legs are fresh. When the trainee begins the program, he may use up to 3 working sets for the deadlift because the weights will be low. As weight on the bar increases, volume will be reduced over time to a single set. Many trainees will be able to sustain a twice-weekly deadlift frequency for a longer period of time than if they were also training heavy barbell squats 2–3 times a week. In this scenario, the deadlift does not compete with the squat for recovery resources. Bench presses are second in the workout and can usually sustain 3 sets across twice a week. For the third exercise of the day, lat pulls are alternated with barbell curls.

**PROGRAM 4D: THE DEADLIFT-BENCH SPECIALIST**

| WORKOUT A | WORKOUT B |
|---|---|
| DEADLIFT 1–3x5 | DEADLIFT 1–3x5 |
| BENCH 3x5 | BENCH 3x5 |
| LAT PULLS 3x8–10 | BARBELL CURLS 3x8 |
| BODYWEIGHT SQUATS *or* DUMBBELL SQUATS *or* LEG PRESS 3x10 | BODYWEIGHT SQUATS *or* DUMBBELL SQUATS *or* LEG PRESS 3x10 |

**PRESCRIPTION:** Alternate A and B. Notation is sets x reps.

**INDICATIONS:** <50: Discretion 50–59: Discretion 60–69: Discretion >70: Discretion

For athletes with significant fixed shoulder mobility issues who cannot safely or productively use the barbell back squat or overhead press.

**PARAMETERS:** Initiated at the beginning of training for selected athletes.

At the conclusion of the workout, the trainee will engage in some additional lower body work if possible. Bodyweight squats, squats with dumbbells, or leg presses are good options. Because all these exercises will either start or progress to higher rep ranges, training them last is reasonable.

## Terminating the Novice Program (Second Redux)

Novices in their eighth decade and beyond using a 3-in-2 program *may* be able to progress to a highly individualized intermediate plan, usually with a longer training period.

Novice athletes on an *appropriate* once-per-week prescription will rarely have the ability or need to progress to a true intermediate program. For these athletes of advanced age and limited recovery capacity, the 1-day model, with increasingly individualized variation over time, will form the backbone of their entire training career. Beyond the initial period, when they gain strength like any other novice (albeit more slowly), the emphasis for these trainees will be on *maintenance* of strength – which, for an athlete in his late 70s, 80s, or 90s, is a remarkable accomplishment.

There will be times when training can be sustained, recovery factors are optimized, and the athlete is doing particularly well. These good times will present the athlete and coach with opportunities to sneak up the load and make small gains – every one of which will be a triumph, and every one of which will require dedication and training to retain. At other times, attenuated recovery due to poor appetite or new medications, interruptions in training caused by illness, and other vagaries of life will make maintenance of strength more difficult. Ground may be lost, and the athlete's challenge will be to make it up.

With commitment and luck, he *will* make it up, or at least not lose any more this year. *And that will be progress.* Every athlete, if he lives long enough, will reach a point where, to put it bluntly, he's running hard to stand still. He is the toughest, most courageous, most dedicated athlete of all.

# 22

# The Intermediate Master

The complete realization of novice training demands a longer training period and more complex manipulation of training variables for progress to continue. Intermediate training is characterized by continued use of the squat, press, deadlift, and bench, with more liberal use of assistance work only as indicated. Progress is slower but programming is more individualized and geared toward specific performance goals. Intermediate programming manipulates both intensity and volume to create workouts that extend the length and complexity of the overload event, with the structure of the Texas Method being a particularly good example. The use of the repetition progression technique, in which progress is maintained by increasing the number of reps performed at a given weight from one training period to another, is illustrated in depth.

## The Intermediate Transition

As the trainee approaches the end of a well-executed novice progression, he cannot continue to display performance increases on each exercise at every workout. Progress inevitably slows. This is not because the trainee loses his ability to recover, but rather because he increases his ability to produce stress. This forces longer and more carefully managed recovery intervals. Trainees at this stage can display performance increases about once per week at best. The program must reflect this new reality, modulating not only intensity but also volume in such a way as to produce a display of increased performance for each exercise after several workouts, rather than from session to session. "Heavy days," in which the trainee either absorbs a training stress or displays a strength increase, are alternated with "light days" that facilitate recovery and keep the trainee fresh during the longer intervals now required for recovery and adaptation. Such a structure, which limits the display of increased strength to about once a week, and which introduces fluctuations in volume as well as intensity, is by definition no longer a novice program. At this point, the athlete is an intermediate.

This transition will usually occur sooner for the Masters Athlete. The ceiling for strength and muscle gains is much higher for a young trainee, and therefore each phase of programming (novice, intermediate, advanced) is prolonged by the youthful athlete's enviable and undeserved capacity to grow stronger and add muscle fast. Moreover, the young athlete can literally force-feed new muscle mass onto his frame by bombarding himself with surplus calories. His body knows what to do with the extra food: build muscle and lots of it. His metabolism will vaporize any organic matter it encounters and turn it into contractile tissue. The metabolism of a Masters Athlete is not so avidly anabolic. He still needs a caloric surplus, but a trainee in his 50s or 60s who consumes as much extra food as the young athlete converts that excess into *some* muscle…and a lot of belly fat, nose hair, and ear cartilage. All strength and conditioning coaches have encountered the problem of the kid who won't eat like a kid should eat, usually out of a misguided desire for a "six-pack." This kid won't get nearly as strong as he could or should on any program. Unfortunately, older athletes have more in common with the skinny kid who refuses to eat enough to recover than with the 19 year-old hard-training athlete who's swimming in testosterone and eating like a garbage disposal. And this punk recovers better, sleeps better, and doesn't have a mortgage or a prostate to worry about. So the novice linear progression for a Master is going to be shorter with age.

We are constrained to point out that many Masters won't ever even *get* to the intermediate level of programming. Even if they do, they may not stay for long. Older trainees tend to miss more training time than their younger counterparts. Major illnesses, surgical procedures, chronic pain, familial and work obligations, vacations, travel, and other unavoidable or richly-deserved discontinuities are more common for older trainees. Such discontinuities inevitably result in performance declines. For many Masters, training therefore becomes a virtuous cycle of making progress followed by some sort of hiatus from training. Each time such an athlete resumes training, he returns to a form of novice programming, because he has detrained to a point where an appropriate training stress will no longer be heavy enough to exceed his adaptive capacities from one workout to the next. This "life cycle" prevents many Masters from ever establishing a true or lasting intermediate status. Even short breaks from training tend to be a more significant setback for older trainees. A week of missed training for the flu might mean 2–3 weeks of training just to get back to where he left off.

For some this will be frustrating, but it's important to keep things in perspective. A Masters Athlete who has exploited the novice progression has probably grown strong enough to shake off a serious illness, or go on a Grand Canyon hike with his grandkids, or take a trip to Spain with his wife. He is hardly a tragic figure, even if he does detrain during his time away from the platform and finds himself ever the novice. He can still get stronger over time, and *put his strength to use* when he's not in the gym. One trains to live, not the other way around.

Even so, many dedicated Masters *will* move on to intermediate status, and it is essential for athlete and coach to understand the principles of program design beyond the basic linear progression. This is where things begin to get complicated. At the novice level it was simple. Do a few sets of 5 on each exercise, rest a few days, and repeat the process with a little more weight. At the intermediate level, more complex manipulations of multiple training variables are necessary.

## Intermediate Programming Principles

The underlying structure of intermediate programming is exactly the same as that for novice programming: the Stress-Recovery-Adaptation cycle. Stretching this cycle out with a longer, more complex overload event allows for the development of a wide range of intermediate-level training programs suited to the specific needs of the athlete. Within this range, however, we will find certain constant features, discussed in the following section, which must be considered in the design of such programs.

The design of intermediate programs for Masters also demands that we bear in mind some of the principles that we touched upon in the novice chapters, because they become even more important at this stage:

1. **Masters need frequent breaks from very hard training.**

2. **Masters are volume-sensitive**. They will not benefit from or even tolerate very high-volume workouts, or volume work done at a high percentage of 1RM.

3. **Masters are intensity-dependent**. They will detrain very quickly when intensity is reduced.

4. **Masters require conservative progression in load**. Even more so than during the novice phase, addition of weight must be judicious and patient.

With all of this in mind, we now examine the salient features of intermediate programming in detail.

### Intermediate training builds on novice gains

When novice training doesn't work anymore, many trainees (young and old) are left scratching their heads, wondering what to do next. They are confronted by many options (some useful, some silly) for the next stage of their training. Most never set specific goals. In a whirlwind of confusion they contract the disease we call ***CPH: Chronic Program Hopping.*** This behavioral disorder affects trainees of all ages, and it almost always starts at the intermediate level. The disease is easily diagnosed by examining the athlete's log (if he has one). "Programs" are switched in and out willy-nilly every six to eight weeks or so. Athletes start a new program because it sounds good at the time they read about it (most likely on the Internet). They select a program because it proposes to exploit some fancy new idea (Muscle Confusion! Broad Domains! Selective Biphasic Quantum Interdimensional Myocyte Superposition!) or because it resonates with some particular emotion or difficulty they are experiencing with their current training program.

The novice is relatively immune to CPH, because this phase of training is self-limited, progress is rapid and exciting, and the novice program is relatively invariant in both its application and in its short-term objectives, which are the same from workout to workout. Boredom and frustration are major contributors to the pathogenesis of the CPH syndrome. The novelty of training has worn off. Progress is slower and more difficult. Every time it's the same old thing: squat, deadlift, press, bench. The gritty medicinal realities of *training* set the athlete up for the seductive allure of a shiny, gimmicky new approach promising new exercises, a new training schedule, and weird new set and rep schemes they have never tried before.

The intermediate is also more susceptible to CPH because at this level the number of program options begins to expand, and there's more room for experimentation and fine tuning. But there's a big difference between individualizing training and CPH, which is a killer. Months or even years can be wasted, and as a Master you don't have months or years to squander on unproductive training plans. Nor do you have the ability to recover from colossal programming mistakes.

The intermediate programs presented in this book allow for more goal-specific training and individuation than the novice program, as they must. But they all represent long-term, rational *continuation* of the novice phase. The primary goal of training is still *strength*, regardless of the specific goals of the individual athlete. Intermediate programs must allow the athlete to seamlessly progress with the strength built during the novice phase and continue its long-term development.

### Slower progress

It goes without saying that intermediate athletes are now stronger than they were as novices. They are now working at a level closer to their genetic potential and producing much higher levels of stress at each training session. They are therefore at an increased risk for overtraining if careful attention is not paid to all of the training variables. At the intermediate and advanced levels the margin for error is tighter than at the novice level, and the price of programming mistakes is more costly.

In the chapters on novice programming, we saw how more advanced novices could manipulate the program to sustain "linear" progress, with reductions in volume, increased recovery, and the introduction of light days. These were all harbingers of intermediate programming. So there's no bright line here. Trainees don't go to bed as a novices and wake up as intermediates. Moreover, not every exercise will progress at the same rate. It isn't uncommon to see squats and pulls moving to intermediate programming while press and bench training sustain linear progress for a few weeks longer, or vice-versa. As the intermediate transition draws near, coach and athlete are well-advised to program one lift at a time, one week at a time, and make small changes when things are not progressing.

## General vs. specific goals

Once novice gains have been exhausted, programming becomes more individualized. *As a novice, the purpose of training is entirely general.* Development of a base of general strength on a handful of extremely efficient exercises will provide carryover to any specific goal later on. The novice thus has an overarching long-term goal: get stronger on a handful of very basic, very comprehensive exercises. And he has a short-term goal: complete today's work sets at a weight just a bit heavier than the work sets from the last session.

At the intermediate level, the ultimate goal is the same: get strong on a handful of very basic exercises. But the intermediate lifter now has "intermediate" goals, and his immediate objectives change from workout to workout. Each training period will consist of several sessions designed to produce a display of increased strength, so that a new training period can begin. During the novice phase, an increase in strength from workout-to-workout is a matter of course. As an intermediate, the display of a strength increase is an event, requiring a week, maybe two, of training to achieve. It's more like training for a competition, with all the dedication, complexity, and care that such training demands.

This is why preparation for sports competitions, including sanctioned strength competitions (powerlifting and Olympic weightlifting) can be such a valuable experience for dedicated Masters. The authors are most emphatically *not* saying that all Masters should compete. But you should understand why doing so can be such a powerful tool. A competition on the horizon provides a little incentive, motivation, accountability, and consequence for your training. More importantly, it provides focus. Focus gives purpose and meaning to each and every training session. Focus allows you to more efficiently evolve the training program, because you know where you want to go. Other objectives also provide focus: setting specific weight-rep goals for this year's training, getting ready for a physically demanding vacation or sporting event, excelling at a particular physical pastime, meeting the requirements of a physically strenuous profession – all can provide motivation and drive the individuation and focus of an intermediate-level program.

## Exercise selection and assistance work

Novice, intermediate, and advanced trainees will all use the same core group of exercises. Squats, pressing movements and deadlifts are the beating heart of the training program at all levels. As a novice, it isn't necessary to utilize more than the 4 primary barbell exercises. Frequent performance of the lifts for a 5-rep set is all that is needed to drive continuous adaptation. As an intermediate, however, there will be reasons to add additional exercises and make substitutions for some of the primary exercises.

*The sole purpose of supplemental and assistance work is to drive progress on the primary exercises.* Serious strength training does not rely on silly concepts like "muscle confusion." When we rotate various exercises in or out of a program, we are not doing so to "confuse" a muscle. This type of work should always be thought of as a means to an end, and not an end in itself. The best assistance exercises are those that mimic the primary lifts as closely as possible – which means they are usually barbell-based, multi-joint exercises.

Exercises that isolate single joints or muscle groups, especially at high volumes, can be dangerous for an older lifter, and offer little in return. The potential to channel this type of "bodybuilding" work into actual muscular hypertrophy is lower with an older athlete. While the risk for a catastrophic muscle belly rupture is fairly low, it exists, and there is certainly a risk for inflammatory conditions such as tendonitis. High-repetition triceps cable press-downs can used for adding work to the triceps to help spur along progress on the bench and the press. However, any time isolation work is done, *all* the stress is delivered across just a single joint. This tends to create inflammation, even though loads are light. Distribution of the work load across multiple joints is the reason why multi-joint barbell exercises are superior to single-joint movements. If a single-joint isolation movement is to be used, then volume should be restricted to just two or at most three heavy work sets.

### Fluctuations in volume and intensity

Intermediate programming is characterized by explicit, targeted manipulation of sets and reps to the core group of primary lifts. The novice program "locked" volume and held it relatively constant while increasing load. At the intermediate stage, more complexity is required. Manipulation of volume and intensity allows for the construction of an overload event that can drive the Stress-Recovery-Adaptation cycle.

### Utilization of repetition progressions

Masters cannot operate at the red line day in and day out. *The best programs for Masters strike the critical balance between allowing some form of offload from extremely difficult training without allowing drastic decreases in intensity.*

One of the best ways to strike this balance is through the use of rep progressions. The rep progression is a programming element that does not require the addition of weight to the bar every week. When using this approach, the weight on the bar will remain static while repetitions are added over 2–3 weeks. Every second or third week, the weight on the bar is increased, balanced by a decrease in prescribed work set repetitions. This satisfies the intermediate criteria of weekly progression – but sometimes with load, and sometimes with volume. This type of progression allows the Master to "taste" the heavier weight for 2–3 weeks in a row before adding more. This addresses the principle that Masters are intensity-dependent, and has both physical and psychological benefits. Masters (and their coaches!) may be understandably apprehensive about piling on more weight every week. Knowing the weight on the bar has already been managed in previous sessions, the rep progression model allows both athlete and coach to approach training sessions with more confidence. This will pay off with greater adherence to the program, fewer setbacks, and more gains.

*Rep progression is not a program.* It is rather a programming *technique* which can be utilized with just about any intermediate or advanced program as an alternative to adding weight to the bar each week.

Example 22-1 below shows rep progressions using a twice-weekly full body routine. For the purposes of illustration, two different mechanisms for accumulating volume are presented. The squats will utilize ascending sets of 5. Ascending sets are an excellent method of volume accumulation (especially for an older Master) and recognize the principle that Masters are volume-sensitive. Ascending sets use about 4–6 light and medium sets before one heavy work set. Ascending sets can be adjusted to increase or decrease the amount of stress they provide. For the bench press and the press, back-off sets will be utilized after the main work set in order to accumulate volume. This rep progression model is an example of doing all the volume and intensity work for the lift, for that week, in a single session. Ascending sets use volume on the front end, and intensity on the back end. The back-off method does the intensity work on the front end, and the volume work on the back end. Warm-up sets are not shown here, but note that fewer warm-up sets will be required with ascending sets.

The hypothetical 8-week snapshot here shows what a training program might look like using a rep-progressions and the two different variations of conservative volume accumulation. The top-end set for each day (the last set for squats and the first set for bench, press, and deadlift) holds the same weight for 3 weeks in a row, while the trainee adds 1 rep every week with that weight. Every time the athlete sets a new 5RM, the weight is increased by 2–5 pounds for the following week, but the rep goal for that week is reduced to a set of 3. The following week is a set of 4, and the final week is a set of 5. Then the process repeats itself. This method allows the Master to build in frequent respite from very difficult training while keeping intensity high. The drop from 5 reps to 3 reps every time weight is increased provides enormous physical and mental relief for the athlete, *but he never takes weight off the bar*, which would invite a detraining effect.

**Example 22-1: Using Rep Progressions**

| Week | Monday (Heavy Day) | | | Thursday (Light Day) | | |
|---|---|---|---|---|---|---|
| 1 | **Squat** | **Bench** | **Deadlift** | **Squat** | **Press** | **Chins** |
| | 135x5 | **205x5** | **285x5** | 135x5 | **140x5** | 3 sets |
| | 165x5 | 190x5x4 | 255x5 | 165x5 | 130x5x4 | |
| | 195x5 | | | 195x5 | | |
| | 215x5 | | | 215x5x2 | | |
| | **235x5** | | | | | |
| 2 | **Squat** | **Bench** | **Deadlift** | **Squat** | **Press** | **Chins** |
| | 135x5 | **210x3** | **290x3** | 135x5 | **142x3** | 3 sets |
| | 165x5 | 192x5x4 | 260x5 | 165x5 | 132x5x4 | |
| | 195x5 | | | 195x5 | | |
| | 220x5 | | | 220x5x2 | | |
| | **240x3** | | | | | |
| 3 | **Squat** | **Bench** | **Deadlift** | **Squat** | **Press** | **Chins** |
| | 135x5 | **210x4** | **290x4** | 135x5 | **142x4** | 3 sets |
| | 165x5 | 195x5x4 | 260x5 | 165x5 | 132x5x4 | |
| | 195x4 | | | 195x5 | | |
| | 220x5 | | | 220x5x2 | | |
| | **240x4** | | | | | |
| 4 | **Squat** | **Bench** | **Deadlift** | **Squat** | **Press** | **Chins** |
| | 135x5 | **210x5** | **290x5** | 135x5 | **142x5** | 3 sets |
| | 165x5 | 197x5x4 | 260x5 | 165x5 | 132x5x4 | |
| | 195x5 | | | 195x5 | | |
| | 220x5 | | | 220x5x2 | | |
| | **240x5** | | | | | |

The exact volume and intensity for the back-off work is an individual decision for the athlete and coach. Four total sets were used in this example, but 2 or 3 might be sufficient. As a general rule, back-off sets will be 5–10% lower than the work set. This varies from athlete to athlete and lift to lift. Stronger athletes and more stressful exercises will use a larger offset. The same titrated process must occur for the ascending sets. The athlete will have to experiment and find the right balance of total sets, and the intensity level of each of those sets. Progression on the back-off work is also an individual decision made on a week-to-week basis between lifter and coach. If the back-off sets are very easy, there is no reason not to add a little weight the next week. If the back-off sets are very difficult, repeating the workout is acceptable.

**Higher-Volume Rep Progression**. Example 22-2 follows the same set of principles and progressions outlined in the previous example. The difference here is that the work sets for the day are at a higher volume – 3 to 5 sets are done with the top weight at each training session. Ascending sets and back-off

| Week | Monday (Heavy Day) | | | Thursday (Light Day) | | |
|---|---|---|---|---|---|---|
| 5 | **Squat** | **Bench** | **Deadlift** | **Squat** | **Press** | **Chins** |
| | 135x5 | **215x3** | **295x3** | 135x5 | **145x3** | 3 sets |
| | 175x5 | 200x5x4 | 265x5 | 165x5 | 135x5x4 | |
| | 200x5 | | | 195x5 | | |
| | 225x5 | | | 225x5x2 | | |
| | **245x3** | | | | | |
| 6 | **Squat** | **Bench** | **Deadlift** | **Squat** | **Press** | **Chins** |
| | 135x5 | **215x4** | **295x4** | 135x5 | **145x4** | 3 sets |
| | 175x5 | 202x5x4 | 265x5 | 165x5 | 135x5x4 | |
| | 200x5 | | | 195x5 | | |
| | 225x5 | | | 225x5x2 | | |
| | **245x4** | | | | | |
| 7 | **Squat** | **Bench** | **Deadlift** | **Squat** | **Press** | **Chins** |
| | 135x5 | **215x5** | **295x5** | 135x5 | **145x5** | 3 sets |
| | 175x5 | 205x5x4 | 265x5 | 165x5 | 135x5x4 | |
| | 200x5 | | | 195x5 | | |
| | 225x5 | | | 225x5x2 | | |
| | **245x5** | | | | | |
| 8 | **Squat** | **Bench** | **Deadlift** | **Squat** | **Press** | **Chins** |
| | 135x5 | **220x3** | **300x3** | 135x5 | **148x3** | 3 sets |
| | 175x5 | 207x5x4 | 270x5 | 165x5 | 137x5x4 | |
| | 200x5 | | | 195x5 | | |
| | 225x5 | | | 225x5x2 | | |
| | **250x3** | | | | | |

sets are not used. This program works with fewer variables, which makes it simpler than the first rep progression program. On the other hand, it's more taxing to recovery, due to the higher volume of work with top-end weights. Again, warm-up sets are not shown.

The rep progression illustrated in Example 22-2 seeks to maintain a training volume of about 15 total reps on the squat, bench, and press. For each cycle of 3 weeks the goal is to end by completing the target weight for 3 sets of 5 reps. Once this is achieved, 2–5 pounds are added to the bar for the next week, but the goal for the next week is not 3 sets of 5, it's 5 sets of 3 reps. The *total workload remains the same*, but doing triples at the new weight is easier than doing 5s at the new weight. Again, this keeps weight on the bar and maintains total volume, but allows the Master a bit of physical and mental respite after achieving a new 3 sets of 5 maximum. The second week, the weight on the bar stays the same, and 16 reps are done using 4 sets of 4 reps. This additional rep for each set will be slightly more difficult than the previous week and paves the way for a new 3x5 PR on the last week of the cycle. By

**Example 22-2: High-Volume Rep Progression**

| Week | Monday (Heavy Day) | | | Thursday (Light Day) | | |
|---|---|---|---|---|---|---|
| 1 | **Squat** | **Bench** | **Deadlift** | **Light Squat** | **Press** | **Chins** |
| | 275x5x3 | 225x5x3 | 325x5 | 245x5x3 | 145x5x3 | 3 sets to failure |
| 2 | **Squat** | **Bench** | **Deadlift** | **Light Squat** | **Press** | **Chins** |
| | 280x3x5 | 230x3x5 | 330x3 | 250x5x3 | 150x3x5 | 3 sets to failure |
| 3 | **Squat** | **Bench** | **Deadlift** | **Light Squat** | **Press** | **Chins** |
| | 280x4x4 | 230x4x4 | 330x4 | 250x5x3 | 150x4x4 | 3 sets to failure |
| 4 | **Squat** | **Bench** | **Deadlift** | **Light Squat** | **Press** | **Chins** |
| | 280x5x3 | 230x5x3 | 330x5 | 250x5x3 | 150x5x3 | 3 sets to failure |
| 5 | **Squat** | **Bench** | **Deadlift** | **Light Squat** | **Press** | **Chins** |
| | 285x3x5 | 235x3x5 | 335x3 | 255x5x3 | 155x3x5 | 3 sets to failure |
| 6 | **Squat** | **Bench** | **Deadlift** | **Light Squat** | **Press** | **Chins** |
| | 285x4x4 | 235x4x4 | 335x4 | 255x5x3 | 155x4x4 | 3 sets to failure |
| 7 | **Squat** | **Bench** | **Deadlift** | **Light Squat** | **Press** | **Chins** |
| | 285x5x3 | 235x5x3 | 335x5 | 255x5x3 | 155x5x3 | 3 sets to failure |
| 8 | **Squat** | **Bench** | **Deadlift** | **Light Squat** | **Press** | **Chins** |
| | 290x3x5 | 240x3x5 | 340x3 | 260x5x3 | 160x3x5 | 3 sets to failure |
| 9 | **Squat** | **Bench** | **Deadlift** | **Light Squat** | **Press** | **Chins** |
| | 290x4x4 | 240x4x4 | 340x4 | 260x5x3 | 160x4x4 | 3 sets to failure |
| 10 | **Squat** | **Bench** | **Deadlift** | **Light Squat** | **Press** | **Chins** |
| | 290x5x3 | 240x5x3 | 340x5 | 260x5x3 | 160x5x3 | 3 sets to failure |

this week, the trainee has handled this load on 2 previous occasions so he should be well-prepared, mentally and physically.

### Each intermediate workout is a component of a longer overload event

This is a definitive feature of intermediate programming. In the novice phase, every workout served two simultaneous functions: the imposition of a training stress, and the demonstration of adaptation to the previous workout as a performance increase. The entire Stress-Recovery-Adaptation cycle progressed from session to session, with each workout having the same structure and function.

In the intermediate phase, where a longer training period and cumulative stress in the overload event is mandated, we can for the purpose of illustration think of each workout as reflecting a particular phase of the cycle. This approach can take on many forms. Perhaps the most explicit and well-known such structure is the Texas Method, in which volume and intensity are carefully manipulated over the course of about one week to produce a workout that imposes a training stress, a workout that facilitates productive recovery, and a workout that displays the adaptation. The imposition of high volume at the beginning of the cycle creates a primary training stress. The recovery workout is constructed, as one might imagine, by using low-volume, low-intensity sets. Adaptation is displayed on the third day of the program with a low-volume workout at very high intensity. This means that, although "stress" and "adaptation" phases of the cycle are different, they are both hard, and in fact both *constitute a training stress.* Indeed, all components of the Stress-Recovery-Adaptation cycle are operant across the week. For example, the trainee's ability to handle higher loads at high volume on the first workout of the next cycle not only imposes a new training stress, but also displays a new level of adaptation from the previous cycle. For illustrative purposes, we can *think* of each workout in the Texas Method as corresponding loosely to a particular phase of the Stress-Recovery-Adaptation cycle, and this way of looking at the program underscores that the cycle forms the foundation of any program. But the reader should understand that this is only an expository model; the underlying biological reality is of course more complex.

So the Texas Method is demanding, and it's not for everybody. But it can be adapted for use by many Masters in their 40s and 50s. Moreover, an examination of the Texas Method's structure and application is highly instructive, illustrating many principles of intermediate programming. It is to this program and its variants that we therefore turn our attention in the next chapter.

# 23
# The Texas Method

The Texas Method is a classic intermediate program with a 1-week period encompassing 3 workouts. A *volume day* workout imposes the primary training stress with high volume at moderately heavy weight, the *recovery day* workout is performed at light weights and low volume, and on *intensity day* a strength increase is displayed at low volume. This approach is suitable for intermediate Masters who have made strength acquisition their primary athletic focus (as opposed to some other sport- or profession-specific goals), and who are willing and able to train on a fairly grueling program. Other intermediates are referred to programs discussed in Chapter 24. The Texas Method is extremely flexible, permitting a wide range of variations to extend progress, accommodate different training schedules, and allow for the diminished recovery capacities of the Masters Athlete. After a discussion of the overall structure of the Texas Method and its initialization, this chapter will explore how it can be modified for older trainees, and how stalled progress is addressed. The use of rotating rep ranges, dynamic effort sets, and supplemental exercises will be discussed in detail. The Kingwood and Greysteel Texas Method variants are presented at the end of the chapter.

**"YOU MAY ALL GO TO HELL, AND I WILL GO TO TEXAS."** —Davey Crockett

## The Texas Method

The Texas Method is *the* classic intermediate program, with a long record of success and a rational structure firmly based on the Stress-Recovery-Adaptation cycle. It is flexible and easy to implement, and will drive progress for a long time if used carefully. With minor modifications, it is suitable for most Masters under 60 (and some above) committed to regular heavy training. The Texas Method is an excellent example of weekly progression and fluctuated loading – two hallmarks of intermediate level programming. The Texas Method usually runs on the same 3-day Monday/

Wednesday/Friday schedule as the standard novice program, although there are options for 2- and 4-day/week schedules, and variations that stretch the period out to 3 cycles per month instead of four. In all cases, the simple structure of this program allows for a smooth transition from novice to intermediate level programming.

There are three fundamental components of a Texas Method program, reflecting the Stress-Recovery-Adaptation formulation of Selye's syndrome.

The overload event begins with *volume day*, when the primary training stress is delivered. Classically, volume day falls on Monday, which makes Monday even more challenging for the intermediate Master than it is for everybody else in the world. Without question, this is the most difficult workout of the week. Training stress is produced by performing the exercises at moderately high intensity *and* high volume, to produce a very high stress or "dose." This level of training stress is now needed to force an adaptation. This level of stress will exceed the trainee's capacity to recover and adapt before the next training session.

This brings us to *recovery day*, which traditionally falls on Wednesday. This will be familiar to those trainees forced to take a lighter squat day during the late stages of their novice progression (Chapter 19). The idea now, however, is to actively *promote* recovery between difficult sessions while avoiding any level of stress that interferes with adaptation to the volume workout. The low-intensity, low-volume work of recovery day flushes tired muscles with blood and keeps motor pathways fresh between heavy sessions. It stimulates the ongoing biology of recovery triggered by volume day, without impeding it.

Adaptation over each cycle is manifested as *intensity day*, which typically falls on Friday. On intensity day, the targeted strength increase is displayed, but at low volume, so as to avoid excessive stress. Intensity day workouts usually call for just a single work set on each exercise. This is critical: Unlike the novice progression, where each workout both displayed a new level of strength and imposed a new training stress, in the Texas Method *a different aspect of the cycle is emphasized in each session.* Intensity day workouts are heavy and hard, to be sure, but not so much as volume day, and not so much as to prevent the delivery of a new, heavier volume training stress on the next Monday.

Program 5A presents the standard Texas Method template. We emphasize that *the structure represented in 5A is not fixed or universal,* but rather serves as a highly flexible model that can be modified and tailored to serve the needs of virtually any intermediate athlete under the age of 60.

Program 5A *as written* would be an excellent introduction to intermediate training for most trainees under 40. An athlete in the fifth decade will almost always require some adjustment to this model, and an athlete in his 50s will usually require quite radical modifications to train productively with the Texas Method. For an athlete over 60, the standard Texas Method will usually not be suitable, although we have worked with trainees over sixty enjoying excellent progress with *modified* Texas Method programming.

Before moving on to a detailed examination of how the Texas Method is employed and modified in practice, we wish to highlight some critical attributes of this program that coaches and athletes should consider carefully, before they decide to use it.

## The Texas Method Focuses on Intensity Day

The objective of every training period (1 week in the standard Texas Method) is to display a performance increase on intensity day. The other two days (volume and recovery) are to be modulated in a way that allows this to happen. Think of Monday and Wednesday workouts as manipulating volume and intensity dials on a machine, carefully calibrating stress and recovery so that a *performance increase* is consistently achieved on Friday. An important feature of post-novice programming is the emphasis on lower-volume work as the primary metric for measuring progress. Higher-volume work is reserved for the imposition of training stress (at relatively

**PROGRAM 5A: THE TEXAS METHOD**

| | VOLUME DAY | RECOVERY DAY | INTENSITY DAY |
|---|---|---|---|
| Week 1 | SQUAT 5x5 | SQUAT 2x5 | SQUAT 1x5 |
| | BENCH 5x5 | PRESS 3x5 | BENCH 1x5 |
| | DEADLIFT 1x5 | CHINS 3x8 | POWER CLEAN 5x3 |
| Week 2 | **VOLUME DAY** | **RECOVERY DAY** | **INTENSITY DAY** |
| | SQUAT 5x5 | SQUAT 2x5 | SQUAT 1x5 |
| | PRESS 5x5 | BENCH 3x5 | PRESS 1x5 |
| | DEADLIFT 1x5 | CHINS 3x8 | POWER CLEAN 5x3 |

**PRESCRIPTION**: Weeks 1 and 2 are alternated. Squats and pressing movements on volume day are at 85–90% of intensity day targets. Recovery day squats and pressing movements are at 80–90% of volume day targets, at decreased volume, as shown. Adaptation with increased performance is displayed on intensity day – weight increases from one intensity day to the next (week to week). Notation is sets x reps.

**INDICATIONS**: <40: Yes 40–49: Yes 50–59: Discretion >60: Discretion

**PARAMETERS**: Initiated at the termination of novice training. Most Masters will continue in some version of Texas method indefinitely or alternate between novice training (e.g., after layoffs) and Texas Method. A very few Masters may progress to advanced training.

high intensity) to create the conditions necessary for display of increased strength. *The entire week's work is focused on the realization of the intensity day goals.*

### The Texas Method Is Grueling

This is the most stressful of all the intermediate programs treated in this text. Although the nature of the workouts change, the Texas Method calls for two very difficult workouts each week. Volume day is more *stressful* than intensity day, and intensity day is *heavier* than volume day…but *both* sessions are *hard.* This is an important difference between the Texas Method and some of the other routines in this text: This program prescribes two very difficult sessions every week, one by virtue of high volume and one by virtue of high intensity. This structure is highly productive – for athletes who can tolerate and sustain it. For this reason, the Texas Method is considered an "athlete's program." That does *not* mean it is only meant for competitive athletes. But the Texas Method may be too grueling for intermediate Masters training for general health, or who are engaged in other physical activities that compete for limited recovery capacity. The Texas Method is most appropriate for Masters in their 40s or 50s (and some in their 60s) who have made serious strength training their primary mission. These trainees should be committed to their recovery with the same vigor as they approach their training. Diet, supplementation, active rest, and sleep are to be monitored with exceptional care, and the athlete shouldn't be too turned off by some persistent soreness.

### The Texas Method Is Versatile

This bears repeating: it is *not* a rigid, static program. The Texas Method is a general structure upon which a wide variety of different set-rep and progression schemes may operate. It can be modified to support training for virtually any sport, profession, or life situation. More to the point, the availability of multiple training variables and parameters for manipulation of these variables means the program is subject to exquisite adjustments to permit ongoing progress. Athletes must keep accurate records of their training and must pay attention to how they *feel* under the bar and during recovery. Coaches must review training logs frequently and learn to judge the way the athlete looks and performs under the bar. The best athletes and coaches learn to anticipate an oncoming stall or performance regression before it happens. This takes time, experience, and objectivity.

# Initiating the Texas Method

The Texas Method offers a smooth transition to intermediate training because of superficial similarities to the novice program, with the same exercises, a 3-day/week schedule, and an emphasis on sets of 5 (at least at first). But this program does not simply start up where the novice program left off. Initiating the Texas Method in this simplistic way is a form of training greed, and will sabotage the long-term potential of the program before it's even begun.

### Setting up the squat program

Coach and trainee begin by determining the weight used for the last completed sets of 5 across in the novice program. To illustrate, let's assume the last novice work sets were 275x5x3. This same weight for a *single set* of 5 will be the amount of weight used for the *intensity day* workout for the first week of the Texas Method – representing a moderate back-off in volume stress for the training period. A common and costly error is to use the weight on the bar for the last completed novice workout for the *volume day*. This is far too aggressive for any athlete, especially a Master. This approach will result in a stall within just a few weeks of beginning the program.

Volume day weight will instead be set at about 90% of the goal for the first intensity day weight, and performed for 5 sets of 5. For a target intensity day work set of 275x5, the volume day squat target will be 250x5x5. Recovery day squats will be about 90% *of volume day*, at about half the volume. 225x5x2 would be appropriate for recovery day.

### Pressing movements on the Texas Method

Programming the press and the bench on Texas Method may be more complex than the squat, due to the very natural desire to give the press and the bench equal levels of prioritization in the program. For many years the standard recommendation has been to alternate weeks of press-focus with a week of bench-focus, as illustrated in Example 23-1.

This approach works well for younger athletes, and even for some in their 50s and 60s. But we have found that many Masters will stall on this classic approach to Texas Method programming for the pressing movements. We believe the culprit here is the Master's intensity dependence. After the intensity day's 5RM on the press or bench, more than 10 days elapse before the next heavy workout is done for that exercise. For many Masters, this is simply too long to maintain strength, even with the light day squeezed in the middle.

One approach to this problem is covered in the Greysteel Texas variant discussed at the end of this chapter (Example 23-17). Another solution that seems to work well is to choose one pressing movement as the primary focus and train that exercise with priority. For most Masters, that priority should probably be the bench press. This is not because the bench is superior to or more useful

**Example 23-1: Standard Press-Bench Alternation in Texas Method**

| Week | Monday | Wednesday | Friday |
|---|---|---|---|
| 1 | Press 5x5 | Bench 2x5 | Press 1x5 |
| 2 | Bench 5x5 | Press 2x5 | Bench 1x5 |

than the press. In fact, for basic utility and carryover to everyday life, it certainly is not.

Our rationale for emphasis on the bench is threefold. First, heavy bench work will drive improvement on the press more than heavy pressing will drive improvement on the bench. The heavier loads trained on the bench have significant impact on the nervous system as well as the triceps. Both will promote a heavier press – and the reader should take note that this approach most explicitly does *not* abandon the press.

Second, the bench-press-bench setup allows for more effective utilization of the close-grip bench press. Normally, assistance exercises are not part of the big picture when designing a program. However, the positive effects of close-grip bench work carry over to both the standard bench and the press. The most effective implementation of the close-grip bench is when the exercise is used for back-off work after the intensity day bench workout. A limited volume of very heavy bench pressing sets the stage quite nicely for the close-grip bench. The elbows are warm (very important for an older athlete) the nervous system is primed, and local muscular fatigue is not too high. This work is not as effective when placed in the middle of the week on the light day.

Third, and most critically, *the press can still be done heavy on the recovery day*. Limit sets of 5 on the press are still much lighter than anything done on the bench press. We find that heavy press work on recovery day usually does not generate enough stress to interfere with a demonstration of increased bench performance on intensity day.

The astute reader will realize, however, that this approach creates an inherent problem in the program. The reason an athlete moves to intermediate programming is because novice programming is no longer working. A big part of the novice program is the 3x5 formula. One reason the Texas Method works is because it varies this set-rep scheme to manipulate both volume *and* intensity. If the overhead press is to be used as the recovery day pressing movement, it's a good idea to alter the set-rep scheme at first, or the press will get stuck. Adding volume is not a good idea. It is better to maintain a target of 15 *total* reps, but instead of 3x5, aim for 4 sets of 3–4. This will generate 12–16 total repetitions, but will allow the trainee to add a small amount of weight to the bar to keep progress moving in the right direction. After several weeks or months of this, he can likely move back to 3x5 without a problem.

*This approach does not commit the athlete to a permanent bench (or press) focus.* Athletes could decide to switch priority every couple of months. If the bench press is to be placed mid-week, 5x3 for work set weights is a reasonable place to start.

Either way, sets and reps on volume and intensity day for the pressing movements are set up as they were for the squat. The last completed 3x5 workout on the novice program will determine the starting weights for the first intensity day of the Texas Method. Target weights will also be reckoned as for the squat: volume day work sets are performed at about 90% of intensity day targets, and recovery day weights are 90% of volume day targets.

## Programming pulls on the Texas Method

At the start, most Masters do best when they begin with their last set of 5 deadlift on the novice program. However, the Texas Method pulling program can be challenging and often demands a high degree of individualization. For the Master, there are two factors that present potential difficulty. First, the Olympic lifts will do little to promote deadlift performance, because most Masters have a limited explosive capacity. This means that Masters usually train the Olympic lifts at a lower percentage of their maximum deadlift than their younger counterparts. Lower-intensity power cleans or snatches are poor drivers of increasing pulling strength. So a high volume of cleans or snatches may only serve to fatigue the Master and actually interfere with a display of improved deadlift performance.

On the other hand, some athletes do need more than one heavy set of pulls each week to spur new progress. If cleans and snatches do not provide an adequate stimulus, the athlete will need a different strategy for increasing pulling volume. With younger athletes, an excellent solution is the addition of

2–3 sets of stiff leg deadlifts (SLDLs) at the end of the volume day. This approach is sometimes used by strong deadlifters who aren't proficient in the Olympic lifts. They simply cannot generate enough stress with the low weights of a clean or snatch to do anything positive to a 500–600-pound deadlift. But adding SLDLs to a Master's routine will push them past their recovery capacity and sabotage the deadlift.

In most instances, however, the actual pulling volume is not the problem, it's the frequency with which it is performed. Older athletes generally do better by consolidating all their "slow pulls" on one day of the week. This means performing additional sets of deadlifts or a deadlift variant after the main work set of the deadlift is performed. Just 1–2 additional sets will provide the requisite volume. If conventional deadlifts are to be used as the back-off, then a 10–20% reduction is about right. For example, the athlete might perform his target deadlift set at 405x5, followed by back-off sets of 365x5x2. A less stressful variation would be to follow the 405 work set with back-offs at 365x5 and 335x5.

The exact volume of back-off work and the exact percentage offset should be calculated at an individual level. There is no hard and fast rule about *exactly* how to set this up. The general idea is to add a little more pulling work without throwing the athlete into a recovery deficit.

## Putting it All Together

Example 23-2 illustrates the transition from novice training to Texas Method for a strong female Master in her late 40s, ending her novice linear progression and transitioning into the Texas Method the following week.

Notwithstanding this example, upper back work such as assisted chins, pull-ups, and bodyweight rows need not be done on both recovery and intensity day. Trainees may decide to limit assistance work to just one day of their preference. The workload from squats and benches on volume day is often so draining and time consuming that the athlete doesn't have much left in the tank for chins or pull-ups. Athlete and coach are encouraged to experiment with multiple setups to find what works best.

The approach used in the preceding example works very well as a starting point for the Texas Method. But *progressing* on the Texas Method gets complicated sooner rather than later. The basic setup will not last forever. In fact, it likely won't last longer than just a few weeks – possibly a few months if the trainee is recovering well. One of the biggest mistakes trainees of all ages make is trying to stay with an unmodified Texas Method template for far too long. Trainees and coaches should remember that by this point in the training evolution, sets of 5 have been used almost exclusively for every major exercise. Most trainees stagnate quickly without significant changes to the program. And we emphasize that such changes will *not* come in the form of multiple ***resets*** – reducing the load and then working back up again – since this will result in stagnation at around the same point as before. To restore progress, modification of the program structure is required.

## Modifications of the Texas Method

Initial modifications to the Texas Method are focused on adjusting the set-rep targets for intensity day. Up to this point, the trainee has been using a single set of 5 reps to display adaptation on intensity day. As the weight gets heavier, displaying new strength with a 5-rep set every week becomes increasingly untenable.

Two alternate methods are presented for intensity day programming: *running it out*, and *rotating rep ranges.*

### Running it out

This is the simpler of the two methods. When the athlete can no longer achieve a single set of 5 reps, he will continue to add weight to the bar, but only aim for a set of 3–4 reps. He will continue to target

**Example 23-2: Transition from Novice to Texas Method**

**Last Week of Novice Linear Progression**

| **Monday** | **Wednesday** | **Friday** |
|---|---|---|
| Squat 175x5x3 | Light Squat 160x3x3 | Squat 180x5x3 |
| Bench 125x5x3 | Press 90x5x3 | Bench 127x5x3 |
| Lat Pulls 3x8–10 | Deadlift 230x5 | Bodyweight Rows 3x10 |

**First Week of Texas Method**

| **Volume Day** | **Recovery Day** | **Intensity Day** |
|---|---|---|
| Squat 165x5x5 | Squat 150x3x3 | Squat 180x5 |
| Bench 115x5x5 | Press 85x5x3 | Bench 127x5 |
| Deadlifts 230x5 | Assisted Chins 3x8–10 | Bodyweight Rows 3x10 |

**Second Week of Texas Method**

| **Volume Day** | **Recovery Day** | **Intensity Day** |
|---|---|---|
| Squat 170x5x5 | Squat 155x3x3 | Squat 185x5 |
| Press 86x5x5 | Bench 117x5x3 | Press 91x5 |
| Deadlift 235x5 | Assisted Chins 3x8–10 | Bodyweight Rows 3x10 |

3–4 reps for as long as possible while continuing to add weight to the bar each week. This pattern will progress to intensity day with 2 or 3 heavy doubles instead of triples, and after several weeks or months the athlete will display adaptation with multiple heavy singles across (5x1) on intensity day. If possible, the athlete should stop the progression before he has a missed any of these modified targets. In *Practical Programming for Strength Training,* it is recommended that the trainee attempt to keep a total volume of 5–6 reps, even though reps/set are dropping every 2–3 weeks. This means that triples are generally done for two sets, doubles for 3 sets, and singles for 5 to 6 sets across.

For a Master in his late 50s or early 60s, this is probably not the best course of action, especially if the trainee is still pushing volume hard for 5 sets on Monday. *Using a sets-across approach for intensity day will often overwhelm the Master's recovery capacity.* Our experience suggests that if sets across are to be used on intensity day, 3 to 5 total reps are adequate and well-tolerated. This means that triples are done for a single set (1x3), doubles for 2 sets (2x2), and singles for 3–5 sets across (3–5x1). Older Masters who continue to push the volume on volume day will usually make progress with an even more conservative approach using single sets (1x3, 2x2, 1x1).

In Example 23-3, a Master in her 50s runs out her progression on intensity day. This example illustrates not only how a Master can run out the Texas Method, but also how she might *cycle back up and run it out a second time.* For clarity, only the squat is used in this example, although this strategy can be used for any of the exercises.

Example 23-3 *is not prescriptive,* nor is it meant to be a reflection of "typical" performance for a female athlete in her late 50s. It does illustrate what is *possible* for a female Master, and how she *might* progress her training.

In week 1, she begins with 4 sets of 5 reps on volume day and a single set of 5 reps on intensity day – with an approximate 10% offset between the two days. The changes we see in her volume day will be discussed later. Suffice to say that for a trainee of this age and level of strength, it is likely that 3–4 sets will provide *plenty* of stress. Recovery day weights are set at just under a 10% offset and volume is reduced to just 2 sets of 3 reps. The athlete increases intensity targets from week to week in increments of about 2 pounds, an acceptable rate for a female Master of this age.

Note that for the first 12 weeks weight was added to the bar on every intensity day, even as reps began to fall from 5 to a top single of 165 in week 12.

As difficulty increases on intensity day, so does the difficulty of volume day, and often the subjective feedback of the athlete will indicate that volume reductions are needed. Staying with 4 total sets for the duration of the cycle, the athlete gradually reduces the target rep range from 5 reps to 3 reps over the course of this hypothetical 24-week progression.

The most critical elements of this example are seen in weeks 12–14 (in bold) as the athlete reaches relative limits on both intensity and volume days and undergoes a slight offload on both days. Week 12 culminates in a heavy single on intensity day. This is not an all-out 1RM, but rather a heavy-*ish* single indicating that a modification is likely in order.

The following volume day (beginning of week 13) decreases the load, but volume increases to 4 sets of 5 reps. Additionally, the intensity day is lowered by 20 pounds but the lifter resumes her 5-rep sets. On both of these days the trainee should perceive an easier workout even though volume has been increased and *she is starting anew with heavier 5s than she used at the beginning of the example.* In week 14, this allows her to make a larger-than-normal 5-pound jump on her intensity day.

Another important feature of Example 23-3 is the amount of work our female Master is able to perform on volume days relative to intensity day. A female athlete can productively absorb a higher volume of work, and at a higher weight relative to her intensity day targets, compared to her male counterparts. These matters are discussed in more detail in Chapter 27.

### Rotating rep ranges

This option is usually more effective than running it out. Rotating rep ranges, a type of rep progression approach, gives the athlete exposure to limit sets on all the rep ranges more frequently, making it a critically important strategy for preventing stagnation on the Texas Method. A common rotation is a 3-week cycle, as illustrated in Example 23-4. The athlete decreases intensity day targets from 5 to 3 to 1 over the course of three weeks. Beginning the rotation again in week

**Example 23-3: Running it Out**

| Volume Day | Recovery Day | Intensity Day |
|---|---|---|
| 125x5x4 | 115x3x2 | 140x5 |
| 127x5x4 | 117x3x2 | 142x5 |
| 130x5x4 | 120x3x2 | 144x5 |
| 132x5x4 | 122x3x2 | 146x5 |
| 134x5x4 | 124x3x2 | 148x4 |
| 136x4x4 | 126x3x2 | 150x4 |
| 138x4x4 | 128x3x2 | 152x4 |
| 140x4x4 | 130x3x2 | 154x3 |
| 142x3x4 | 132x2x2–3 | 156x3 |
| 144x3x4 | 134x2x2–3 | 158x2 |
| 146x3x4 | 136x2x2–3 | 160x2 |
| **148x3x4** | **138x2x2–3** | **165x1** |
| **130x5x4** | **120x3x2** | **145x5** |
| **132x5x4** | **122x3x2** | **150x5*** |
| 134x5x4 | 124x3x2 | 152x5 |
| 136x5x4 | 126x3x2 | 154x5 |
| 138x5x4 | 128x3x2 | 156x5 |
| 140x4x4 | 130x3x2 | 158x4* |
| 142x4x4 | 132x2x2–3 | 160x4 |
| 144x4x4 | 134x2x2–3 | 162x3* |
| 146x3x4 | 136x2x2–3 | 164x3 |
| 148x3x4 | 138x2x2–3 | 166x3 |
| 150x3x4 | 140x2x2–3 | 168x2* |
| 152x3x4 | 142x2x2–3 | 170–180 x 1* |

*rep PRs

4, the athlete repeats this cycle with slightly heavier weights. For clarity, we show only the squat.

The problem encountered by athletes who utilize this cycle is that the heavy single comes around too often, and the athlete stalls. If this pattern manifests, it indicates an adjustment to this basic rotation that puts the heavy single at a frequency of once every 6 weeks, with a slower progression through 5s and 3s. This approach is very powerful for younger athletes (including some younger Masters) using the Texas method.

For older Masters, however, we have found that a composite approach, applying a simple rep progression scheme to the intensity day rep rotation, works beautifully. This very simple approach has made Texas Method programming more accessible to older Masters by *slowing down the rate at which weight is added to the bar each week*, while still providing a means of displaying increased performance capacity.

Example 23-5 is a comprehensive illustration of this important technique, using just the squat as an example. Please study it carefully.

Using this protocol, the athlete sets up a very simple 3-week cycle of 5s, 3s, and 1s with an approximate 5% offset between each rep range. Once the athlete goes through the first 3-weeks, he cycles back through using the exact same weights, simply adding a single rep to the set each week. A set of 5 becomes set of 6 on the next intensity day. The triple becomes a set of 4, and the single becomes a double.

*But there is no increase in weight until the pattern is complete.* This is the critical factor making the approach sustainable in the long term for Masters, with their slower rates of recovery and adaptation. Only when the athlete has completed the 6s, 4s, and 2s will he then increase the weight on the bar and repeat the process for 5s, 3s, and 1s.

**Example 23-4:Rotating Rep Ranges on Intensity Day**

| Volume | Recovery | Intensity |
|---|---|---|
| 280x5x5 | 252x5x2 | **315x5** |
| 285x5x5 | 255x5x2 | 320x3 |
| 287.5x5x5 | 260x5x2 | 325x1 |
| 290x5x5 | 255x5x2 | **320x5** |
| 292.5x5x5 | 260x5x2 | 325x3 |
| 295x5x5 | 265x5x2 | 330x1 |
| 297.5x5x5 | 260x5x2 | **325x5** |
| 300x5x5 | 265x5x2 | 330x3 |
| 302.50x5x5 | 267.5x5x2 | 335x1 |

**Example 23-5: Intensity Day Rotation with Rep Progression**

| Volume Day | Recovery Day | Intensity Day |
|---|---|---|
| 275x5x5 | 245x5x2 | **305x5** |
| 277x5x5 | 247x5x2 | 320x3 |
| 279x5x5 | 249x5x2 | 335x1 |
| 281x5x5 | 251x5x2 | 305x6 |
| 283x5x5 | 253x5x2 | 320x4 |
| 285x5x5 | 255x5x2 | 335x2 |
| 287x5x5 | 257x5x2 | **310x5** |
| 289x5x5 | 259x5x2 | 325x3 |
| 291x5x5 | 261x5x2 | 340x1 |
| 293x5x5 | 263x5x2 | 310x6 |
| 295x5x5 | 265x5x2 | 325x4 |
| 297x5x5 | 267x5x2 | 340x2 |

## Volume day manipulations

Always bear in mind that the point of the Texas Method is to *consistently sustain progress on intensity day performance.* If progress is not occurring on intensity day (and a sound system of progression is in place), athlete and coach should examine what is happening (or *not* happening) on volume day. Remember that volume and intensity are control knobs on the programming machine, and it is the appropriate modulation of these training variables that ensures steady progress. When volume and recovery days are planned and executed correctly, the Texas Method is a very useful program and can be sustained for a long time. But the athlete must exercise patience and always be willing to fine-tune the program until the calibrations are correct for the present training situation. The volume day knob is like the temperature dial on an oven – a little too much heat and the food gets burned. Not enough, and the food never gets cooked at all. Calibrating volume day can be the biggest challenge to succeeding with the Texas Method, especially for Masters. Too much volume at too much weight, and the athlete can't recover by Friday. Not enough volume, with too little weight, and the athlete hasn't been adequately stimulated to adapt and display a new performance increase. The older the athlete, the more critical this balance becomes. Since older athletes are much more sensitive to volume than their younger counterparts, a push in the wrong direction can easily result in overtraining.

If there are problems on intensity day, the challenge is to determine whether volume day loads are appropriate. A principal clue in the diagnosis (assuming, as always, that recovery has been properly addressed) is whether the athlete is demonstrating stagnation or regression on intensity day.

*Stagnation* means the athlete is able to maintain gains from previous cycles, but is unable to advance, even on a rotating rep model. *Regression* is the more serious scenario, in which the athlete is actually losing performance from one intensity day to the next.

Stagnation on intensity day indicates that volume day is not imposing a sufficient training stress. The athlete should look to increase either volume or load, or both, on volume day.

*If the athlete is still training with 5x5 on volume day, there is no reason to add volume.* In this circumstance, it is far more likely that volume day loading is too light. An increase in load exceeding the normal 2–5-pound jump will likely get the athlete unstuck. In such cases, the increase in weight may actually necessitate a reduction in total volume. This could be as simple as switching from 5x5 to 4x5 in order to accommodate the increase in load.

On the other hand, sometimes load is correct, but total volume is simply not high enough. If the athlete is using a modified volume approach, then it may be that he needs to increase the number of work sets. Unfortunately there is no fixed formula that will work for every trainee. Coaches and athletes must make an educated guess about what variable needs to be adjusted, change only that variable, and then observe the results.

If the athlete starts to experience actual *regression* on intensity day, the culprit is usually excessive stress on volume day: too much volume, too much weight, or both. Volume day sets of 5 should maintain about a 10–15% offset from intensity day sets of 5. If work sets on volume day are closer to a 5% offset, then loading should be decreased, or the athlete will burn out rather quickly. As an example, consider an athlete in regression who fails 350x5 on intensity day after squatting 335x5x5 on volume day. This Master should reduce the load on the bar for his volume day work, as the offset is not wide enough. The athlete and coach must be wary of allowing a narrow offset to persist for too long. For the Texas Method, fluctuation in load between all three sessions in the week is critical.

In most cases, however, excessive volume is to blame for burnout. Remembering that *Masters Athletes are volume-sensitive and intensity-dependent*, most adjustments will come in the form of decreasing set/rep totals, rather than the percentage offset.

Many of the volume reduction strategies used for the Texas Method volume day mirror those that were used in the Novice Linear Progression.

**Reduction in set number.** The first strategy is to reduce the total number of sets the athlete performs on volume day. If the standard 5x5 scheme is producing too much stress, simply perform 3 or 4 sets of 5 at the same load. For most Masters (and many younger trainees) the standard 5x5 volume accumulation scheme will eventually become excessive. The older and stronger the athlete, the more this will be the case. When an athlete first enters into intermediate level training, 3 sets of 5 may not be enough volume to disrupt homeostasis and stimulate adaptation. But this will change, especially for the trainee who has made substantial progress over a prolonged period of time. In most cases, the athlete will have grown much stronger (pronounced increase in ability to create stress) and will also be older than when he started training (decreased ability to recover). At almost a year older and 100–300 pounds stronger, a heavy workout of 3x5 work sets is not the same stimulus it once was. It is now a much more stressful event.

Some athletes prefer to keep the 5 volume day work sets, but do better with a decrease in reps per set. Instead of 300x5x5, the athlete may perform 300x3x5 or 300x4x5. Staying between 3 and 5 reps per set is optimum for volume day training. This strategy works particularly well for Masters who are working on issues with technique or perhaps have an injury they are trying to train around. Reducing reps/set can prevent form deterioration, if athlete and coach note a consistent breakdown in form at the end of a set of 5.

**Work in a Range.** Working within a rep range applies the rep progression principle to the volume day. Most volume day strategies rely on the sets-across method, where the goal of the day is to lift a given amount of weight for the same number of repetitions across multiple sets. The sets-across structure is very taxing and requires long rest times between sets. Athletes of all ages can often benefit from working within a repetition range that allows them to shorten total training time by reducing rest time between sets. When rest between sets is reduced, it is likely that reps per set will fall by 1 or 2 each set because the athlete is operating in a state of incomplete recovery. An excellent option is using 4 sets of 4–6 reps each. *The athlete can add weight to the bar when at least one of his sets is performed for a set of 6, and none of his sets drops below 4 reps.* The progression on this type of system is somewhat fluid, and relies heavily on careful record-keeping and log analysis. Example 23-6 illustrates what 8 weeks of progress might look like. Each week the exact amount of work fluctuates.

**Back-Off Sets.** If the athlete wishes to maintain the strict 5x5 rep scheme, he can try using back-off sets at a slight reduction in load. The number of work sets and back-off sets may vary. Many prefer just one top work set followed by 4 back-off sets.

**Example 23-6: Working in a Range on Volume Day**

| Week | Volume Day |
|---|---|
| 1 | 250 x 5, 4, 4, 4 |
| 2 | 250 x 5, 5, 5, 5 |
| 3 | 250 x ***6***, 5, 5, 5 |
| 4 | ***255*** x 4, 4, 4, 4 |
| 5 | 255 x 5, 4, 4, 4 |
| 6 | 255 x ***6***, 4, 4, 4 |
| 7 | ***260*** x 5, 4, 4, 4 |
| 8 | 260 x ***6***, 5, 5, 5 |

An example might be 300x5; 285x5x4. Or there could be some other arrangement such as 2 top work sets, followed by 3 back-off sets, or perhaps 3 top work sets, followed by 2 back-off sets. There is no set protocol that must be followed. This strategy requires careful observation and fine-tuning by the trainee and coach. Back-off sets tend to invite the critical mistake of trying to keep volume high by sacrificing the intensity upon which the Master is so dependent. Back-off sets should be at not more than a 5% reduction from the top work sets. For example if the athlete were doing 2 heavy work sets and 3 back-off sets for volume, 280x5x2 followed by 225x5x3 would not be appropriate. The correct target would be 280x5x2 followed by 265x5x3.

**Descending sets** are a variation of the back-off set method. Descending sets allow weight to drop a little each set, usually over the course of 4–5 total sets. Example 23-7 illustrates.

**Example 23-7: Using Descending Sets on Volume Day**

**Warm-up Sets:** 45x5x2, 135x5, 185x3, 225x1, 275x1, 315x1, 365x1

**Top Set: 405x5**

**Descending Sets:** 395x5, 385x5, 375x5, 365x5

Descending sets used for volume day work will drop weight from set-to-set in small increments, usually as little as 5–10 pounds. Specific amounts will have to be titrated for each individual athlete. Only enough weight should be taken off of the bar to allow target reps to be performed without breakdown in technique.

**Ascending sets** can also be used as a volume day strategy – although they are the most difficult of volume day modifications to adjust and get right. The problem with ascending sets is that the first 2–3 "work sets" are usually not of sufficient intensity to disrupt homeostasis and produce an adaptation. Many of the early sets in an ascending sets protocol are just very fatiguing warm up sets. Example 23-8 illustrates. As in Example 23-7, the athlete is using 405 as his top set target, but in this case he uses ascending sets *up to* 405 to accumulate volume, rather than descending sets *down from* 405.

Note the difference in weight increments between these two approaches. Descending sets are far more stressful than ascending sets, but at the same time they are less likely to fatigue the athlete prematurely, before he can put up his top-end work set. Attempting ascending sets with narrow weight increments does not work well. If the athlete in Example 23-8 performed ascending sets at the same increments as the athlete in Example 23-7, he'd be utterly smoked by the time he made it to his top set. Even if he could put up 405x5, he would probably display atrocious form. More likely he would miss reps.

Even if the intervals are appropriate, the ascending-sets approach is difficult to work with, and is our least preferred volume day modification. The exception is in the individual circumstance that a given athlete just happens to be extremely volume sensitive, as may be the case with a athlete in his late 50s or 60s. Because ascending sets utilize less intensity, they create the least stress. If the athlete is routinely finding himself under-recovered and unable to make progress on his intensity day work, ascending sets may be an appropriate solution.

**Example 23-8: Using Ascending Sets on Volume Day**

**Warm-up Sets:** 45x5x2, 135x5, 185x5, 225x5

**Ascending Sets:** 275x5, 315x5, 365x5, 385x5

**Top Set:** 405x5

### Implementing the Dynamic Effort Method

After extended work in the Texas Method and other intermediate programs, most athletes will reach a point of physical and mental stagnation. Progress becomes difficult and nothing seems to work. Everything feels slow and heavy, and training weights are stagnant across the week. At this point, the program may be revitalized by the use of ***dynamic effort sets***, in which barbell movements are performed at lower intensity but higher speed. Developed by legendary powerlifting coach Louie Simmons as part of his Westside Barbell Method, the dynamic effort approach is easily integrated into the traditional Texas Method structure. The intermediate Master will use dynamic effort sets as a volume day replacement for sets of 5. The intensity day protocol will remain the same – focused on a single heavy set of 5, 3, 2, or 1 (see *Work in a Range*, above).

For Masters who have not been working with the Olympic variants, dynamic effort sets explicitly introduce a new factor, *power*, which is the product of force and velocity. *Power is strength displayed quickly.* Classically, barbell training focusing on power incorporates the clean, the snatch, and their derivative movements (Chapter 12). As we have been at pains to point out, however, these movements will be relatively contraindicated for many older trainees due to the problems associated with mobility, explosiveness, stress, and potential for injury. High volumes of heavy snatches can really aggravate a creaky old shoulder, just as a high volume of cleans can annoy the wrists and elbows. Both movements can be problematic for the knees due to the shock of receiving a heavy bar in a quarter-squat rack position.

Dynamic effort sets, however, allow movements focused on power production to be incorporated *by utilizing basic barbell movements the trainee has already mastered*, bypassing the special challenges of the Olympic lifts. It follows, therefore, that dynamic effort sets should *not* be used unless the athlete can demonstrate nearly flawless form on the exercise. If so, then squats, presses, deadlifts, and bench presses are all suitable exercises to use with the dynamic effort method.

Like the standard Texas Method volume day, dynamic effort sets are performed at high volume – but at lower intensity. The athlete will perform 8–12 sets of *submaximal* triples, doubles, and singles, usually with limited rest time between sets. About 20–30 total repetitions seems to be the right amount of volume for dynamic effort training. Squats will be trained for 10–12 sets of 2, and pressing movements will be trained for 8–10 sets of 3, each exercise using about 1 minute of rest between sets. Deadlifts respond best to singles for 10–15 total reps, with 30–60 seconds between sets.

*The primary concern of the dynamic effort set is bar speed.* This is why reps are capped at 3. More than 3 reps/set and the barbell is likely to slow down. During a dynamic effort set, trainees are focused on moving the barbell *as fast as possible* through the entire range of motion. This requires tremendous *focus* from the athlete – and also from the coach. If the athlete is not moving the barbell as fast as possible on each and every rep, the method is not effective. Moving a lighter weight slowly for multiple sets of 2 is not a stressful event. Moving a lighter weight *as fast as possible* for multiple sets of 2 on limited rest, however, imposes a powerful training stress.

Bar speed is influenced not just by the volitional effort of the athlete, but also by the critical factor of loading. The optimal weight will probably take several workouts to calibrate. For squats, the athlete should be able to *accelerate* the load enough that the plates rattle at the top of the movement, but it should not be so light that the weight is flying off his back. A load of 70–80% of the athlete's 1RM is usually about right if utilized for doubles. This is also a good starting point for deadlifts. Press and bench work well at about 60–70%.

As always, these percentages are a rough guideline. Bar speed is the most important variable to get right. Over the course of 8–12 total sets the athlete should not lose the ability to accelerate the load through the range of motion. If the athlete is losing bar speed during the workout, the load is too heavy. While the athlete should be able to maintain high bar speed over the course of 20–30 total reps, he should have to work and focus to do so. If the weight doesn't require significant effort and concentration to accelerate, it's probably too light. This assessment definitely has a strong subjective component, but it's valuable enough that trainee and coach should spend the time to get it right.

Limited rest time is an important component of the dynamic effort method. Trainees are attempting to create stress, not just through bar speed, but also through increased ***training density,*** a training variable that describes the ratio of training work performed to the time taken to perform it. Eight sets of 3 performed in 20 minutes is a higher training density than eight sets of 3 performed in 60 minutes. Because the number of reps is low, less fatigue is accumulated on each set. This means that instead of 5–10 minute rests between sets as on a standard volume day, trainees using dynamic effort for volume will reduce rest times to 1 or 2 minutes. Five heavy sets of 5 (25 total reps) might take a athlete over half an hour to complete if rest times are about 5 minutes. However, the same volume (12 sets of 2) moved with maximum velocity might take less than 15 minutes to complete. This can be a very powerful new stimulus to boost an athlete out of a training rut.

It should be obvious that, given the high volume and training density of the dynamic effort method, it brings along a significant conditioning component as a fringe benefit. Abbreviated rest times and the explosive, high-power nature of the training will produce elevated heart rates and a soaring metabolic demand. The longer the trainee does this sort of work, the better conditioned he will become.

The dynamic effort method tends to benefit from a cyclical approach, rather than attempting to add weight to the bar in a linear fashion from week to week. If we determine that the trainee is capable of maintaining adequate bar speed between 70% and 75% on the squat, then we might set up a 3-week cycle that looks like Example 23-9.

Starting in week 4, the athlete would cycle back to 70% with the idea that he will move the weight *faster* than the last time. After running through each cycle 2–3 times, the athlete may then add a *small* amount of weight to the bar for each week. The challenge of dynamic effort programming is to keep the weight progression in balance with the bar speed, all while monitoring the progress of Friday's intensity day workout – which, we wish to emphasize, *is still the main focus of the program.* Trainees who want to utilize the dynamic effort method should allow 3–6 months of experimentation before the right balance is found, and possibly up to a year of continuous tweaking before the system is truly mastered.

Once the trainee has mastered the method, then cycling dynamic effort sets with traditional volume sets of 5 can be a very effective mechanism for prolonging weekly intermediate progress before more complex programming is warranted.

Because the 5-rep set is such a powerful metric for measuring strength, it is useful to find a way to keep them in the intermediate training template for the majority of the year. The program in Example 23-10 does just that. The program operates in two phases that can be alternated over and over again to drive steady progress while allowing some diversity in the training plan.

Phase I, consisting of the standard Texas Method and modifications to draw out progress, is the more difficult of the two. This is due to the greater volume of slow, heavy, grinding reps, which challenge every trainee, but particularly the Master. After several weeks or months running through Phase I, most athletes will welcome the transition to Phase II. Volume is still high on Mondays, but the switch from volume 5s to the dynamic effort method is usually *perceived* as easier. After pushing for volume sets of 5 for several weeks or months,

**Example 23-9: Using Dynamic Effort Sets for Volume Day**

Week 1: 70% 1RM x2 x12

Week 2: 72.5% 1RM x2 x12

Week 3: 75% 1RM x2 x12

the trainee will now utilize that capacity to push for new 5RMs on intensity days. For the purposes of illustration, this program has the deadlift operating on a completely different schedule than the squats and the bench presses, but still adheres to the same principles. In Phase I, the deadlift is done on Friday. Because heavy 5x5 squats are so difficult, no pulling is scheduled for Mondays during Phase I. Instead the trainee attempts a new single set of 5 each week, and volume is accumulated via 1–2 back-off sets following the 5RM attempt. In Phase II, the trainee increases load on the deadlifts and cycles through some new triples, doubles, and singles. Dynamic effort deadlifts are done later in the week to maintain total volume.

It is difficult to precisely plan the transition between these two phases. With intermediate level programming, the trainee is attempting to display new performance increases on a weekly basis regardless of the rep range. Once each phase goes stagnant, the trainee can transition to the next phase and run it for as long as they are making weekly progress. This could be as little as a few weeks or as long as several months. Done correctly, this process can last as long as 2 years. Trainees are encouraged to exercise patience in fine-tuning the details of the program. Volume and intensity must all be carefully modulated over time.

## The Texas Method and Exercise Variation

Just as sets and reps on the Texas Method can get stagnant, so can the selection of exercises. Usually a stalled lift is best unstuck through modification of either volume or intensity. These changes can be applied to volume day, intensity day, or both. But sometimes an athlete is buried in such a rut

**Example 23-10: Alternating Standard Texas Method with Dynamic Effort Sets for Volume**

**Phase I**

| **Volume** | **Recovery** | **Intensity** |
|---|---|---|
| Squat 5x5 | Light Squat 2x5 | Squat – Standard or Rep Progression |
| Bench 5x5 | Press 3x5 | Bench – Standard or Rep Progression |
| | Chins 3x8 | Deadlift 1x5; 1–2x5 |

**Phase II**

| **Volume** | **Recovery** | **Intensity** |
|---|---|---|
| Squat (DE) 12x2 | Light Squat 2x5 | Squat 1x5 |
| Bench (DE) 10x3 | Press 3x5 | Bench 1x5 |
| Deadlift 1x5 ***or*** 1x3 ***or*** 1x1 | Chins 3x8 | Deadlift (DE) 10x1 |

on an exercise that nothing seems to work to get it going again. When this occurs, the substitution of a *supplemental exercise* may be indicated. A supplemental exercise will almost always be barbell-based and will resemble the parent movement both in performance and in load as closely as possible. Depending on the movement, and the degree of regression that may have set in on the primary exercise, the supplemental movement can be used as a replacement on either volume or intensity day. Sometimes the supplemental movement may be used for many weeks, or it may be utilized in a short rotation with variations that cycle every 2–3 weeks. In our experience, the bench and deadlift benefit most from supplemental exercises, while the press and squat do not respond nearly as well, if at all. Stagnation on the squat and the press are usually better resolved by manipulations in volume, intensity, and frequency.

**Supplemental exercises for the deadlift.** Rack pulls and SLDLs make the best supplemental movements for the deadlift. If the deadlift is experiencing significant regression, it can be supplanted altogether for 6–12 weeks with a simple weekly rotation of rack pulls and SLDLs performed on the intensity day. Rack pulls allow the trainee to handle heavier loads than the deadlift, and place significant amounts of stress on the spinal erectors. Rack pulls are trained for a single set of 3–8 reps, with perhaps one much lighter back-off set. Rack pulls are very stressful and cannot be effectively trained every week. They almost always have to be set up in a rotation with other pulling variants.

SLDLs involve much less weight than either rack pulls or deadlifts, but are effective at adding tremendous stress to the hamstrings. As such, they are a valuable supplemental exercise for the deadlift. But *Masters must take care with stiff-leg deadlifts.* They place a pronounced stretch on the hamstrings and challenge the ability of the athlete to keep his low back in extension. SLDLs should be done for 1–3 sets of 5–8 reps. The fluctuation from week to week in load between rack pulls and SLDLs is ideal for getting a trainee out of a rut. And the emphasis of each exercise on the erectors and hamstrings will prevent the trainee from losing ground on the deadlift. If the trainee has good success with these exercises he may wish to keep SLDLs in an intensity day weekly rotation with the deadlift, training each movement every third week.

**Supplementing the bench press.** As previously discussed, close-grip bench presses can be plugged in as an alternate movement on either intensity day or volume day. Either way, an excellent strategy is to utilize them as back-off sets, after a top set is performed with the standard bench press. So a volume

| **Example 23-11: Basic 4-Day Texas Method** | **Monday (Vol)** | **Tuesday (Vol)** | **Thursday (Int)** | **Friday (Int)** |
|---|---|---|---|---|
| | Bench 5x5 | Squat 5x5 | Bench 1x5 | Squat 1x5 |
| | | | | Deadlift 1x5 |

| **Example 23-12: 4-Day Texas Method – Bench Focus** | **Monday (Vol)** | **Tuesday (Vol)** | **Thursday (Int-Rec)** | **Friday (Int)** |
|---|---|---|---|---|
| | Bench 5x5 | Squat 5x5 | Bench 1x5 | Squat 1x5 |
| | | | Press 4x4 | Deadlift 1x5 |

| **Example 23-13: 4-Day Texas Method – Bench + Press** | **Monday (Vol)** | **Tuesday (Vol)** | **Thursday (Int-Rec)** | **Friday (Int)** |
|---|---|---|---|---|
| | Press 1x5 | Squat 5x5 | Bench 1x5 | Squat 1x5 |
| | Bench 5x5 | | Press 5x5 | Deadlift 1x5 |

day bench workout might be 275x5, followed by the close-grip bench at 245x5x4. On intensity day the athlete might bench 295x2 and then do a set of close-grips with 265 for a 3–5RM. Close-grip bench presses can also be part of a rotation with regular bench presses. An effective rotation is to train 1–3 reps sets across on the regular bench press one week, followed by 1–3 rep sets across on the close-grip bench the following week. This simple rotation can keep bench press progress going for many months.

### The four-day Texas method

Athletes and coaches may prefer to take the workload of the standard 3-day Texas Method and spread it across a 4-day training week. Usually this is done to reduce either the time or the stress of the volume day workout. Squats at 5x5 with 8–10 minute rest periods is both time-consuming and exhausting. Any other exercise performed in the same training session tends to suffer from the fatigue of the volume squat. Example 23-11 illustrates a 4-day entry-level Texas Method program for a athlete focused on the squat, bench press, and deadlift.

The primary benefit of this arrangement is that volume workouts are less fatiguing and *much* shorter, allowing them to fit more readily into a busy schedule.

The primary drawback is the absence of a true light day. This can be a problem, especially for the squat. A light squat day can be very helpful for those who struggle with recovery or are plagued by form or technique issues. If a trainee has grown accustomed to the rejuvenating effects of the mid-week light squat, he may not perform as well on intensity day if the light squat day is removed.

The pressing schedule for a 4-day program will usually boil down to trial and error. The program in Example 23-12 is organized with bench as the primary pressing exercise. The secondary pressing exercise usually fits most easily into the intensity day, because there is less accumulated fatigue than on volume day.

If a trainee can recover from the workload, he may be able to benefit from doing volume and intensity days on both the bench and the press. There is a high likelihood that volume may have to be moderated for each lift when using this approach.

### The two-day Texas method

Like the 3-day novice program, the standard 3-day Texas Method can be spread out over a 2-day training week or performed on a 1-on, 2-off schedule. The extra rest days may be essential for long-term progress, especially for older Masters. When a program reduces frequency, intensity must go up slightly on any light days if regression is to be prevented. If the recovery day offset in the 3-day program was 10%, it might now be a 5% offset.

**Example 23-14: 2-Day Texas Method – 1-On-2-Off Structure**

**Monday (Vol)**
Squat 5x5
Bench 5x5
Pull-ups 3x6–8

**Sunday (Int)**
Squat 3x2
Bench 3x2
Deadlift 1x5

**Saturday (Rec)**
Light Squat 4x3
Press 3x5
Chins 3x8–10

**Friday (Vol)**
Squat 5x5
Bench 5x5
Pull-ups 3x6–8

**Thursday (Int)**
Squat 1x5
Bench 1x5
Deadlift 1x5

**Thursday (Rec)**
Light Squat 4x3
Press 3x5
Chins 3x8–10

**Wednesday (Vol)**
Squat 5x5
Bench 5x5
Pull-ups 3x6–8

**Tuesday (Int)**
Squat 2x3
Bench 2x3
Deadlift 1x5

**Monday (Rec)**
Light Squat 4x3
Press 3x5
Chins 3x8–10

**Sunday (Vol)**
Restart Cycle

**Example: 23-15: 2-Day Texas Method – Fixed Schedule**

**Monday (Vol)**
Squat 5x5
Bench 5x5
Pull-ups 3x6–8

**Thursday (Rec)**
Light Squat 4x3
Press 3x5
Chins 3x8–10

**Monday (Int)**
Squat 3x2
Bench 3x2
Deadlift 1x5

**Thursday (Vol)**
Squat 5x5
Bench 5x5
Pull-ups 3x6–8

**Monday (Rec)**
Light Squat 4x3
Press 3x5
Chins 3x8–10

**Thursday (Int)**
Squat 2x3
Bench 2x3
Deadlift 1x5

**Monday (Vol)**
Squat 5x5
Bench 5x5
Pull-ups 3x6–8

**Thursday (Rec)**
Light Squat 4x3
Press 3x5
Chins 3x8–10

**Monday (Int)**
Squat 1x5
Bench 1x5
Deadlift 1x5

**Thursday (Vol)**
Restart Cycle

If necessary, the trainee can change up the set and rep scheme to accommodate this. For example, a recovery day with a 5% offset might use sets of 3 instead of 5. This keeps the weight on the bar, but reduces the subjective (and actual) difficulty of each set – preserving the easier nature of this training session. Four sets of 3 reps is a good recovery day scheme for a Master using this protocol.

Example 23-14 illustrates a 2-day Texas Method variant using a 1-on-2-off structure. This particular program will use an intensity day rotation for the squat and the bench.

The same approach could be utilized across 2 fixed days/week, such as Monday/Thursday, Tuesday/Friday, Monday/Friday, or Wednesday/Saturday (Example 23-15).

## The Kingwood Texas Method

Another 2-day Texas Method option has been used for many years with trainees over 55 at Kingwood Strength & Conditioning. This variation keeps a light day as the second workout every week. On the first day of the week, the trainee alternates between a high-volume workout and a high-intensity workout every other week. In this particular version, deadlifts can be done every Monday or alternated with another heavy pulling exercise such as the rack pull.

**Example 23-16: The Kingwood Texas Method**

| Monday (Vol) | Thursday (Rec) |
|---|---|
| Squat 5x5 | Light Squat 4x3 |
| Bench 5x5 | Press 5x5 |
| Deadlift 1x5 | Chins 3x8–10 |
| **Monday (Int)** | **Thursday (Rec)** |
| Squat 3x2 | Light Squat 4x3 |
| Bench 3x2 | Press 5x5 |
| Deadlift 3x1 | Chins 3x8–10 |
| **Monday (Vol)** | **Thursday (Rec)** |
| Squat 5x5 | Light Squat 4x3 |
| Bench 5x5 | Press 5x5 |
| Deadlift 1x5 | Chins 3x8–10 |
| **Monday (Int)** | **Thursday (Rec)** |
| Squat 2x3 | Light Squat 4x3 |
| Bench 2x3 | Press 5x5 |
| Deadlift 3x1 | Chins 3x8–10 |
| **Monday (Vol)** | **Thursday (Rec)** |
| Squat 5x5 | Light Squat 4x3 |
| Bench 5x5 | Press 5x5 |
| Deadlift 1x5 | Chins 3x8–10 |
| **Monday (Int)** | **Thursday (Rec)** |
| Squats 5x1 | Light Squat 4x3 |
| Bench 5x1 | Press 5x5 |
| Deadlift 3x1 | Chins 3x8–10 |

In Example 23-16, the deadlift rotates between a single set of 5 and a series of heavier singles. The bench is used as the primary pressing exercise, but this is doesn't have to be the case. The press could be the Monday exercise, with the bench on Thursdays, usually for a moderate volume of around 15 total repetitions.

## Michigan Lone Star: The Greysteel Texas Method

Finally, we present the Texas Method approach used at Greysteel Strength & Conditioning for carefully selected Masters Athletes. Readers will recognize many of the themes that we have discussed throughout this chapter in this variation, including the use of fewer sets (4x5) on volume day. The Greysteel Texas Method is a 2-day/week (Monday/Friday) approach that spreads the training period over a full 7 days (Monday/Friday/Monday, instead of the Monday/Wednesday/Friday pattern in the traditional program). It alternates the bench and press from one period to the next, as in the standard Texas Method, *but the off-period pressing movement is modified on recovery day to maintain high intensity* by "chasing singles." If the bench is the primary pressing movement for this cycle (trained on volume and intensity days), then the press is trained on recovery day. After warming up, the athlete performs a series of progressively heavier singles, attempting to approach, achieve, or surpass his previous 1RM on the exercise. Three or at most 4 singles are attempted, and the increment of added weight for each single is small – between 1 and 2.5 pounds. An unusual feature of the Greysteel Texas Method, therefore, is that the athlete will frequently achieve new PRs in the pressing movements *on recovery day.* The Greysteel variant can be utilized with any of the other modifications to the Texas Method discussed in this chapter, including manipulation of volume and intensity day targets, the implementation of dynamic effort sets, rotating rep ranges, and exercise supplementation.

The reader may be forgiven at this point for feeling overwhelmed by the vast number of variations and modifications to the Texas Method template presented here. And readers who picked up this book looking for a simple, one-size-fits-all, cookbook approach to training...well, they stopped reading a *long* time ago.

Our discussion of the Texas Method underscores that cookie-cutter programs *simply do not exist for the serious athlete,* particularly

**Example 23-17: The Greysteel Texas Method**

| Period | Volume | Recovery | Intensity |
|---|---|---|---|
| 1 | **Monday** | **Friday** | **Monday** |
| | Squat 4x5 | Light Squat 2x5 | Squat 1x5 |
| | Bench 4x5 | Press to heavy singles | Bench 1x5 |
| | Power Cleans or Chins | | Deadlift 1x5 |
| 2 | **Friday** | **Monday** | **Friday** |
| | Squat 4x5 | Light Squat 2x5 | Squat 1x5 |
| | Press 4x5 | Bench to heavy singles | Press 1x5 |
| | Power Cleans or Chins | | Deadlift 1x5 |
| 3 | **Monday** | **Friday** | **Monday** |
| | Squat 4x5 | Light Squat 2x5 | Squat 1x5 |
| | Bench 4x5 | Press to heavy singles | Bench 1x5 |
| | Power Cleans or Chins | | Deadlift 1x5 |

Masters training at the intermediate level. It is precisely because the underlying structure of the Texas Method is subject to so many useful variations and modifications that it is so powerful and versatile. Armed with this structure, a firm grasp of the Stress-Recovery-Adaptation cycle, and conservative increases in loading, selected and very dedicated intermediate athletes and their coaches can systematically fashion Texas Method-based programs exquisitely tailored to their needs. Such an approach will produce regular, steady progress for many months or even years.

Many Masters, however, will not be able to train this intensely or this diligently. For them, other intermediate options exist, as discussed in the next chapter.

# 24

# Heavy-Light-Medium and Split Programs

Heavy-Light-Medium programs spread the Stress-Recovery-Adaptation cycle over a one week training period to produce a versatile intermediate training approach that is less grueling than the Texas Method and therefore more suitable for the majority of Masters. Some athletes will make progress on 2-day, Heavy-Light variants. Like the Texas Method, Heavy-Light-Medium programs allow for individuation and emphasis on different training goals, and are amenable to multiple models of advancement, including rotating reps, rep progressions and "running it out." Dynamic effort sets make a useful addition to the HLM approach for some Masters. Split routines, which disperse workloads over several shorter workouts, may be indicated for many Masters based on practical considerations or recovery capacity.

## Heavy-Light-Medium for Athletes Over 40

The Heavy-Light-Medium (HLM) training system is an excellent approach for most intermediate Masters. Popularized by the late Bill Starr in his classic text *The Strongest Shall Survive,* the HLM system consists of 3 full-body training sessions each week, producing varied levels of training stress. Starr originally designed his training program for competitive collegiate athletes. These athletes were attempting to balance the demands of playing their sport with the process of getting stronger in the weight room. Starr had to design the strength program to accommodate athletes who were frequently training sore, beat-up, and under-recovered. This might sound familiar to a hard-training Master! Starr knew that athletes derived immense benefit from frequent exposure to the basic compound barbell exercises, but were not capable of training with maximum loads more than about once a week. Other training days required lighter loads to permit recovery, or both training and practice would suffer.

For most Masters, who have to contend with blunted adaptive and recovery processes, the HLM system will be a better alternative than the Texas Method. The two methods look remarkably similar, but key differences make HLM less stressful and easier on recovery.

The Texas Method has a *Heavy-Light-Heavy* structure. While Monday and Friday differ in intensity and volume, both training sessions are *hard.* In the Texas Method, volume day must be heavy enough to drive a performance increase on Friday. And Friday must realize that performance increase or program modification must occur for continued progress.

In the HLM system, only the heavy day is high-stress day. Other training days contribute low or medium levels of stress to the overload event. The light day allows active recovery, forcing blood into tired muscles and stimulating the remodeling process. Medium day disperses training volume across the week. Not everyone will need a medium day, and some will make progress on a Heavy-Light structure. For most, however, medium days are necessary to prevent detraining. The athlete is not yet ready to display a new performance increase on Friday, but enough time has elapsed since Monday's heavy day that if he does not train with at least a moderate weight, he could regress. The light day is not enough of a stress to preserve strength gains, but the medium day should be.

In this approach, the light and medium days may be thought of as "maintenance days": they promote active rest and allow practice of the movement pattern. The lifter is not looking to display new performance increases on these days, instead they support the overload event. *In the HLM system, the heavy day is the focal point of the program.* The construction and execution of the program and the arrangement of all training variables support continual progress on the heavy day.

## Defining heavy, light, and medium

There is an unavoidable taint of subjectivity in the terms *heavy, light,* and *medium.* In practice, this terminology will depend heavily on the perceptions of the coach and athlete, as well as on the athlete's actual performance. *Heavy* could be defined as a situation in which the lifter must struggle to complete the specified number of repetitions and hold his form together under load. This could occur with a single rep or a set of 5. *Medium* is a load under which the lifter feels he is working hard to achieve the prescribed volume, but is in no danger of missing a rep, and there's still gas in the tank at the end of each set. *Light* should always be perceived as fairly easy. Form should be perfect and reps should all move smoothly.

Percentage offsets give us a more quantitative handle on the program. The light and medium day offsets should be based on the athlete's most recent *heavy* set(s) of 5 reps. Even though other rep ranges will be utilized on the heavy day, this number will provide the most useful starting point. Experience shows that younger athletes do well when the light day is about 20% less than the heavy day load, and the medium day is about 10% less than the heavy day load. Most Masters, however, run the risk of detraining with offsets this large, due to their characteristic intensity-dependence. Accordingly, reductions in the percentage offset will often be appropriate in this population, as in Example 24-1.

With the above considerations in mind, we can construct a rational HLM program for the Masters Athlete. Like the Texas Method, this program spreads the Stress-Recovery-Adaptation cycle over multiple workouts, and like the Texas Method it is incredibly versatile and subject to modification. For reasons discussed in our examination of the Texas Method, our HLM template (Program 6A) uses the bench press on heavy and medium days, and relegates the press to light days. We emphasize, however, that *the press is still trained heavy.* With a little imagination and his growing understanding of programming, the reader can easily see how this program might be modified to increase the emphasis on the overhead press, or indeed to meet any number of other criteria specified by the particular athlete's situation.

**Example 24-1: Intensity Modulations for Heavy-Light-Medium Design**

| Heavy | Light | Medium |
|---|---|---|
| Squat | Squat | Squat |
| 250x5x5 | 220x5x2 | 235x5x3 |
| | (-12%) | (-6%) |

**PROGRAM 6A: HEAVY-LIGHT-MEDIUM**

| HEAVY DAY | LIGHT DAY | MEDIUM DAY |
|---|---|---|
| SQUAT 4x5 | SQUAT 2x5 (90%) | SQUAT 1–3x5 (95%) |
| BENCH 4x5 | PRESS 3x5 | BENCH 1–3x5 (95%) |
| DEADLIFT 1x5 | | CHINS 3x8–10 |

**PRESCRIPTION:** Execute program as indicated. Variations described in the text. Notation is sets x reps.

**INDICATIONS:** <40: Discretion 40–49: Yes 50–59: Yes >60: Discretion

**PARAMETERS:** Initiated at the termination of novice training or as indicated during intermediate training. Most Masters will continue in some variant of HLM indefinitely or alternate between novice training (after layoffs) and HLM. A very few Masters may progress to advanced training.

## Setting Up the HLM Program

As with the Texas Method or any other intermediate program, athletes should begin the HLM program with a small step back from where they left off the novice phase. Most athletes terminate the novice progression in a state of heightened fatigue, and a slight deload is now indicated. This allows the athlete to catch up on recovery while calibrating his new program.

An excellent way to enter the HLM program is to keep the heavy day weights achieved at the end of the of the novice program, but at a lower volume. So if the athlete ends his novice progression with 3 sets of 5 reps at 250, he may begin his HLM program with a heavy day target of 250 pounds for a single set of 5, or perhaps 2–3 sets of 3. Now he can calculate light and medium days at their respective 10% and 5% reductions, and make adjustments going forward. After starting out with just a single set of 5 or a pair of triples on his first heavy day, the athlete can build volume up to tolerance over the next couple of weeks. Once he has achieved his target volume he can start pursuing weekly increases in intensity.

In Example 24-2 the athlete drops volume from his last week of the novice program while maintaining intensity through the first week of intermediate programming. During weeks 2 and 3 of the new program he builds up his heavy day

**Example 24-2: Transitioning from Novice to HLM Intermediate**

**Last Week of Novice Phase**

| | Monday | Wednesday | Friday |
|---|---|---|---|
| | 245x5x3 | 225x3x2 (Light day) | 250x5x3 |

**Heavy-Light-Medium**

| Week | Heavy | Light | Medium |
|---|---|---|---|
| 1 | 250x5 | 215x5x2 | 235x5x3 |
| 2 | 250x5x3 | 215x5x2 | 235x5x3 |
| 3 | 250x5x4–5 | 215x5x2 | 235x5x3 |
| 4 | 255x5x4–5 | 220x5x2 | 240x5x2 |

volume to his target of 4–5 total work sets. In week 4 the athlete has entered the program proper, and can now make increases in intensity for heavy day work sets. Notice also that the athlete makes a corresponding adjustment to his medium day, dropping one set from the workout to accommodate the new levels of stress he is absorbing on heavy day.

### Sets and reps

The stress that drives adaptation must occur on the heavy day, meaning that intensity and volume need to be appropriate to this purpose. Reps never need to exceed 5–6 per set, but could go as low as multiple heavy singles. Total work sets on heavy days can be as high as 4 or 5. To keep things simple, these can be performed as sets across, but when needed volume modification schemes such as back-off sets or descending sets can be used to achieve total volume goals without burning out the trainee. For the light days, the trainee should perform either 2 sets of 5 reps or 3 sets of 3 reps. Both achieve about the same number of total reps and should use similar loads.

Medium days incorporate 1–3 sets of 5 reps. More volume than this on a medium day means that intensity probably isn't high enough to prevent detraining. Furthermore, excessive medium day volume can prevent the lifter from performing at peak strength on his heavy day 72 hours later. There are other ways to arrange sets and reps, but for purposes of simplicity and providing some structure for a starting point, these recommendations should work well for most Masters who have reached true intermediate status.

After experimenting with these recommendations for a couple of weeks, the athlete will likely decide to make adjustments to the arrangement of sets and reps performed on each day to tailor the program to his individual needs. Perhaps he starts with 5 sets across on his heavy day, but drops to just 3 sets across as weight on the bar increases. Or maybe he begins the program with 3 sets on his medium day at a 10% offset from his heavy day work, but after several weeks he might drop the medium day to just a single set while narrowing the offset to just 5%. Here again we see the importance of record-keeping and log review, with liberal doses of training experience and good judgment.

### Exercise selection

Starr's original program in *The Strongest Shall Survive* consisted of only 3 exercises – the squat, bench, and power clean. All 3 were performed each Monday, Wednesday, and Friday for 5 sets of 5 reps. The only difference between sessions was the load on the bar – it fluctuated across the week in accordance with the Heavy-Light-Medium concept. We prescribe a broader selection of exercises for the Masters Athlete.

**Squats.** Squats are the simplest exercise to program on the HLM system, and often benefit most from this type of programming. This is due in part to the technical nature of the squat. The squat is prone to "form creep" and benefits from frequent practice, like any other skill. Frequent squatting with light and moderate loads allows the older and less mobile athlete ample opportunity to practice the lift without placing too much strain on his recuperative capacity. Our HLM program has the athlete squatting 4–5 sets of 1–6 reps on heavy day, depending on the variant utilized. These could be performed as sets across, or a less stressful variation incorporating back-off sets, ascending sets, or descending sets.

Light squats will be performed for 2 sets of 5 or 3 sets of 3 at 10–20% less than the last heavy set of 5. Medium days will use 1–3 sets of 5 reps at 5–10% less than the last heavy set of 5.

**Pressing Movements**. A comprehensive 3-day pressing program will include the bench, the press, and either a third exercise or the press or bench repeated a second time during the week at a more moderate volume and intensity. Four variations on the HLM pressing program are presented in Examples 24-3:6.

In Examples 24-3 and 24-4, only one pressing movement is performed each week. This approach is indicated only if the athlete has an orthopedic barrier to one exercise or the other. If not, he should pick a pressing program that incorporates both the press and the bench. If an exercise is only

**Example 24-3: HLM Bench Only**

| Heavy | Light | Medium |
|---|---|---|
| Bench 4x5 | Bench 2x5 (-10%) | Bench 3x5 (-5%) |

**Example 24-4: HLM Press Only**

| Heavy | Light | Medium |
|---|---|---|
| Press 4x5 | Press 2x5 (-10%) | Press 3x5 (-5%) |

**Example 24-5: HLM Bench Priority**

| Heavy | Light | Medium |
|---|---|---|
| Bench 4x5 | Press 3–4x5 | Bench 3x5 (-5%) |

**Example 24-6: HLM Press Priority**

| Medium | Heavy | Light |
|---|---|---|
| Press 4x5 | Bench 3–4x5 | Press 3x5 (-5%) |

to be performed once a week, then volume might be increased slightly on that exercise. Notice also that the press priority variant (Example 24-6) does not conform to a strict heavy-light-medium sequence. It would be more accurate to say that it follows a medium-heavy-light order for the week. This minor deviation from the HLM structure allows for a more balanced training week that places the bench between the two press days.

In *Practical Programming for Strength Training,* three press variants are presented, all of which work well on medium days for younger athletes. The *push press* is an extremely useful variant for heavy overhead work, but it is relatively contraindicated for Masters due to a potential for knee injury. The other two exercises, the close-grip bench press and the incline press, are both useful for any Master capable of benching and pressing with acceptable form and technique. Long-paused bench or overhead presses are also acceptable medium day variations.

**Example 24-7: HLM High-Frequency Pulling Variant**

| Heavy | Light | Medium |
|---|---|---|
| Deadlift 1x5 | Power Snatch 3–5x2 | Power Clean 3–5x3 |

**Example 24-8: HLM Power Clean-Only Variant A**

| Heavy | Light | Medium |
|---|---|---|
| Deadlift 1x5 | Power Clean 2–3x3 (-5%) | Power Clean 6x2 |

**Example 24-9: HLM Power Clean-Only Variant B**

| Medium | Heavy | Light |
|---|---|---|
| Power Clean 6x2 | Deadlift 1x5 | Power Clean 2–3x3 (-5%) |

**Pulling Program.** In *Practical Programming for Strength Training* the standard 3-day pulling program was arranged such that the 3 primary pulls from the floor (deadlift, power clean, and power snatch) fell neatly into the Heavy-Light-Medium structure. The primary concern for the Master will be total training volume when pulling from the floor this frequently. *Again*: Many Masters cannot or should not engage in a program that puts a high level of focus on the Olympic lifts and their variants. However, the Master who enjoys *and tolerates* training the Olympic variants may do well with the modification presented in Example 24-7.

Some Masters will be able to train one Olympic variant, but not the other. Perhaps a bad shoulder prevents the trainee from racking a snatch, or anthropometry prohibits the power clean. In this instance, trainees can focus on one Olympic variant. In this case, the athlete will modify both volume and intensity in order to make performance of the lift fit into the structure of an HLM system. Percentage offsets between light and medium days for the Olympic lifts will be small. In most cases

5% is enough, at most 10%. Many athletes prefer to place the deadlift between the Olympic lifting days. Examples 24-8:11 illustrate.

Many competitive Masters-class powerlifters do well on a Heavy-Light-Medium program that allows them to deadlift up to 3 days per week. Not all trainees, certainly not all Masters, will respond well to such a program, but some have found that dispersing deadlifting volume throughout an entire week is both effective and well tolerated. The key variable is volume. It must be kept low or any trainee, young or old, will not be able to recover from 3 deadlift sessions/week. The percentage offset between heavy, light, and medium sessions will be much broader than between Olympic lifts. A 10–20% offset should be used on a high-frequency deadlifting routine, and just a single set per session should be sufficient. In Example 24-12, a single set of 5 is used, but some competitive Masters have found that high-frequency deadlifting routines do well when deadlifts are trained with singles only. Anywhere from 1–3 singles across would be appropriate.

An easier arrangement for most athletes is to pull from the floor twice a week, on the heavy and medium days, replacing the light day pull with an upper back exercise that does not place stress on the lower back. Example 24-13 illustrates a program for an athlete who wants to work on both the clean and snatch.

**Example 24-13: HLM Alternating Clean-Snatch**

| Week | Heavy | Light | Medium |
|---|---|---|---|
| 1 | Deadlift 1x5 | Chins 3x8 | Power Clean 3–5x3 |
| 2 | Deadlift 1x5 | Chins 3x8 | Power Snatch 3–5x2 |

**Example 24-14: HLM Low-Frequency Pulling Variant**

| Heavy | Light | Medium |
|---|---|---|
| Squat 4x5 | Squat 2x5 | Squat 3x5 |
| Bench 4x5 | Press 4x5 | Close-Grip Bench 3x5 |
| Pull-ups | Deadlift 1x5 | Chins |

**Example 24-10: HLM Power Snatch-Only Variant A**

| Heavy | Light | Medium |
|---|---|---|
| Deadlift 1x5 | Power Snatch 3x2 (-5%) | Power Snatch 6–8x1–2 |

**Example 24-11: HLM Power Snatch-Only Variant B**

| Medium | Heavy | Light |
|---|---|---|
| Power Snatch 6–8x1–2 | Deadlift 1x5 | Power Snatch 3x2 (-5%) |

**Example 24-12: HLM Increased Deadlift Frequency Variant**

| Heavy | Light | Medium |
|---|---|---|
| Deadlift 1x5 | Deadlift 1x5 (-20%) | Deadlift 1x5 (-10%) |

Many Masters will have already determined, perhaps during the novice phase, that pulling from the floor multiple times per week is not a good option. In this instance, athletes should forego trying to arrange the pulling program in terms of heavy, light, medium. Instead, they should deadlift once a week, and train the back with less stressful upper back-only movements such as chins or lat pull-downs on the other two sessions of the week. This can easily be integrated into a program with squats and presses trained on the HLM model, as in Example 24-14.

This type of arrangement works well because the heavy deadlifts are placed on the light squat day. This allows the deadlift to be thoroughly warmed up by a few sets of light squats without being pre-exhausted by multiple sets of heavy squats.

# Progression on the Heavy-Light-Medium System

Depending on the needs of the athlete and his response to initial training on HLM, multiple approaches are available for sustaining and monitoring progress. These approaches will be familiar from our exploration of the Texas Method.

### Running out the heavy day

Assume that the volume goal of the heavy day is 4 total sets. The athlete will aim to maintain 4 sets while reducing the target rep range every couple of weeks until he has attained four heavy singles across. At this point the athlete may decide to progress with another methodology or run it through once again. Example 24-15 illustrates such a progression, showing only the squat.

In this approach, the light and medium days have to be progressed by "feel" and on an individual basis, rather than by strict percentages. It is permissible to hold weights static for 2–3 weeks if necessary, with attendant alterations to the set-rep scheme. The athlete must keep in mind that light and medium days promote recovery and prevent detraining without creating excessive new fatigue and stress. In Example 24-15, the athlete switches his light day from 2x5 to 3x3 after 5 weeks, and after 8 weeks, the light day load is actually reduced by a small margin. As the heavy day intensity continues to climb, the athlete reduces medium day volumes to maintain moderately heavy sets of 5 in the program, without letting the medium day become too stressful. This approach can be applied to any trainee, but the loads and volumes in this example must not be regarded as prescriptive. This is strictly an illustration of how one *might* progress on these training days.

### Basic cycling routine

As in the Texas Method, after the athlete has attempted to run it out once or twice, a rotating progression becomes useful for the HLM structure.

**Example 24-15: Running Out the HLM Heavy Day**

| Heavy | Light | Medium |
|---|---|---|
| 275x5x4 | 245x5x2 | 260x5x3 |
| 280x5x4 | 250x5x2 | 265x5x3 |
| 285x5x4 | 255x5x2 | 270x5x3 |
| 290x5,5,4,4 | 260x5x2 | 275x5x3 |
| 295x4x4 | 260x5x2 | 275x5x3 |
| 300x4x4 | 265x3x3 | 280x5x3 |
| 305x4x4 | 265x3x3 | 280x5x3 |
| 310x4,3,3,3 | 265x3x3 | 280x5x3 |
| 315x3x4 | 255x3x3 | 285x5x3 |
| 320x3x4 | 255x3x3 | 285x5x3 |
| 325x3,2,2,2 | 255x3x3 | 285x5x3 |
| 330x2x4 | 260x3x3 | 290x5x2 |
| 335x2x4 | 260x3x3 | 290x5x2 |
| 340x2,1,1,1 | 260x3x3 | 290x5x2 |
| 345x1x4 | 265x3x3 | 295x5 |
| 350x1x4 | 265x3x3 | 295x5 |

The fluctuation in stress is useful to generate longer runs of progress and prevent stagnation. Typically, the rotation is only applied to the "heavy" exercises while light and medium movements are held fairly static in volume with a very conservative progression in load. A tried-and-true method is a 3-week cycle of 5s, 3s, and 1s. Each time the athlete repeats a cycle he does so with a little more weight on the bar than the last time. If one rep range (for instance the 3s) gets stuck, the lifter does not abort the cycle or reset, but rather *continues to attempt progress with his 5s and singles.* This is what gets him *un-stuck.* Cycling the rep range is a powerful tool for long-term progress.

**Example 24-16: HLM Basic Cycling Routine**

| Week | Heavy | Light | Medium |
|---|---|---|---|
| 1 | Squat 300x5x3 | Squat 270x5 | Squat 285x5x2 |
| | Bench 250x5x3 | Press 175x5x3 | Bench 235x5x2 |
| | Deadlift 375x5 | Power Snatch 120x2x3 | Power Clean 165x3x3 |
| 2 | Squat 315x3x3 | Squat 270x5 | Squat 285x5x2 |
| | Bench 262x3x3 | Press 185x3x3 | Bench 235x5x2 |
| | Deadlift 395x3 | Power Snatch 120x2x3 | Power Clean 165x3x3 |
| 3 | Squat 335x1x3 | Squat 270x5 | Squat 285x5x2 |
| | Bench 274x1x3 | Press 176x5x3 | Bench 235x5x2 |
| | Deadlift 420x1 | Power Snatch 120x2x3 | Power Clean 165x3x3 |
| 4 | Squat 305x5x3 | Squat 275x5 | Squat 290x5x2 |
| | Bench 252x5x3 | Press 186x3x3 | Bench 240x5x2 |
| | Deadlift 380x5 | Power Snatch 122x2x3 | Power Clean 168x3x3 |
| 5 | Squat 320x3x3 | Squat 275x5 | Squat 290x5x2 |
| | Bench 264x3x3 | Press 177x5x3 | Bench 240x5x2 |
| | Deadlift 400x3 | Power Snatch 122x2x3 | Power Clean 168x3x3 |
| 6 | Squat 340x1x3 | Squat 275x5 | Squat 290x5x2 |
| | Bench 276x1x3 | Press 187x3x3 | Bench 240x5x2 |
| | Deadlift 425x1 | Power Snatch 122x2x3 | Power Clean 168x3x3 |
| 7 | Squat 310x5x3 | Squat 280x5 | Squat 295x5x2 |
| | Bench 254x5x3 | Press 178x5x3 | Bench 245x5x2 |
| | Deadlift 385x5 | Power Snatch 125x2x3 | Power Clean170x3x3 |
| 8 | Squat 325x3x3 | Squat 280x5 | Squat 295x5x2 |
| | Bench 266x3x3 | Press 188x3x3 | Bench 245x5x2 |
| | Deadlift 405x3 | Power Snatch 125x2x3 | Power Clean 170x3x3 |
| 9 | Squat 345x1x3 | Squat 280x5 | Squat 295x5x2 |
| | Bench 278x1x3 | Press 179x5x3 | Bench 245x5x2 |
| | Deadlift 430x1 | Power Snatch 125x2x3 | Power Clean 170x3x3 |
| 10 | Squat 315x5x3 | Squat 285x5 | Squat 300x5x2 |
| | Bench 256x5x3 | Press 189x3x3 | Bench 250x5x2 |
| | Deadlift 390x5 | Power Snatch 128x2x3 | Power Clean 172x3x3 |

| Week | Heavy | Light | Medium |
|---|---|---|---|
| 11 | ***Squat 330x2x3*** | Squat 285x5 | Squat 300x5x2 |
| | Bench 268x3x3 | Press 180x5x3 | Bench 250x5x2 |
| | Deadlift 410x3 | Power Snatch 128x2x3 | Power Clean 172x3x3 |
| 12 | Squat 350x1x3 | Squat 285x5 | Squat 300x5x2 |
| | Bench 280x1x3 | Press 190x3x3 | Bench 250x5x2 |
| | Deadlift 435x1 | Power Snatch 128x2x3 | Power Clean 172x3x3 |
| 13 | Squat 320x5x3 | Squat 290x5 | Squat 305x5x2 |
| | Bench 258x5x3 | Press 181x5x3 | Bench 250x5x2 |
| | Deadlift 395x5 | Power Snatch 130x2x3 | Power Clean 175x3x3 |
| 14 | ***Squat 330x3x3*** | Squat 290x5 | Squat 305x5x2 |
| | Bench 270x3x3 | Press 191x3x3 | Bench 255x5x2 |
| | Deadlift 415x3 | Power Snatch 130x2x3 | Power Clean 175x3x3 |
| 15 | Squat 355x1x3 | Squat 290x5 | Squat 305x5x2 |
| | Bench 282x1x3 | Press 182x5x3 | Bench 255x5x2 |
| | Deadlift 440x1 | Power Snatch130x2x3 | Power Clean 175x3x3 |

Example 24-16 presents a basic cycling protocol for an HLM routine using the Olympic lifts. This structure would be appropriate for a trainee in his 40s or 50s.

Note that in week 11 the athlete's attempt to squat 330x3x3 fails, resulting in 330x2x3. This does not change his attempts in the following week. He still attempts his prescribed weights for his singles and sets of 5 in week 12 and week 13. In week 14 he *repeats* 330 and attains his prescribed volume of triples.

Note also that in this example the press is cycled through only 2 rep ranges – 5s and 3s. Even though the press is lighter, heavy singles across are not an appropriate light day prescription for HLM.

### Using a rep progression

A more conservative approach to progress in the HLM system is by applying a basic rep progression to all heavy exercises. Again, adding reps comes in lieu of adding weight to the barbell each week. Rep progressions maintain load from week to week, but allow an older athlete who struggles with recovery to adapt to each new increment of added weight for several weeks before more weight is added. Each time more weight is added to the bar, the trainee will counter that stress with a drop in volume. This allows a slight offload in training volume about every 4th week *without ever decreasing load.*

**Example 24-17: HLM Rep Progression**

| Week | Heavy | Light | Medium |
|---|---|---|---|
| 1 | Squat 250x5x3 | Squat 220x5 | Squat 235x5x2 |
| | Bench 220x5x4 | Press 155x5x4 | Bench 205x5x3 |
| | Pull-ups max reps x3 | Deadlift 375x5 | Chins max reps x3 |
| 2 | Squat 255x3x3 | Squat 225x5 | Squat 240x5x2 |
| | Bench 223x3x4 | Press 157x3x4 | Bench 205x5x3 |
| | Pull-ups max reps x3 | Deadlift 380x3 | Chins max reps x3 |
| 3 | Squat 255x4x3 | Squat 225x5 | Squat 240x5x2 |
| | Bench 223x4x4 | Press 157x4x4 | Bench 205x5x3 |
| | Pull-ups max reps x3 | Deadlift 380x4 | Chins max reps x3 |
| 4 | Squat 255x5x3 | Squat 225x5 | Squat 240x5x2 |
| | Bench 223x5x4 | Press 157x5x4 | Bench 208x5x3 |
| | Pull-ups max reps x3 | Deadlift 380x5 | Chins max reps x3 |
| 5 | Squat 260x3x3 | Squat 230x5 | Squat 245x5x2 |
| | Bench 226x3x4 | Press 160x3x4 | Bench 208x5x3 |
| | Pull-ups max reps x3 | Deadlift 385x3 | Chins max reps x3 |
| 6 | Squat 260x4x3 | Squat 230x5 | Squat 245x5x2 |
| | Bench 226x4x4 | Press 160x4x4 | Bench 208x5x3 |
| | Pull-ups max reps x3 | Deadlift 385x4 | Chins max reps x3 |
| 7 | Squat 260x5x3 | Squat 230x5 | Squat 245x5x2 |
| | Bench 226x5x4 | Press 160x5x4 | Bench 210x5x3 |
| | Pull-ups max reps x3 | Deadlift 385x5 | Chins max reps x3 |
| 8 | Squat 265x2x3 | Squat 235x5 | Squat 250x5x2 |
| | Bench 230x2x4 | Press 162x3x4 | Bench 210x5x3 |
| | Pull-ups max reps x3 | Deadlift 390x3 | Chins max reps x3 |
| 9 | Squat 265x3x3 | Squat 235x5 | Squat 250x5x2 |
| | Bench 230x3x4 | Press 162x4x4 | Bench 210x5x3 |
| | Pull-ups max reps x3 | Deadlift 390x4 | Chins max reps x3 |
| 10 | Squat 265x4x3 | Squat 235x5 | Squat 250x5x2 |
| | Bench 230x4x4 | Press 162x5x4 | Bench 212x5x3 |
| | Pull-ups max reps x3 | Deadlift 390x5 | Chins max reps x3 |

| Week | Heavy | Light | Medium |
|---|---|---|---|
| **11** | Squat 265x5x3 | Squat 235x5 | Squat 250x5x2 |
| | Bench 230x5x4 | Press 164x3x4 | Bench 212x5x3 |
| | Pull-ups max reps x3 | Deadlift 395x3 | Chins max reps x3 |
| **12** | Squat 270x3x3 | Squat 240x5 | Squat 255x5x2 |
| | Bench 232x3x4 | Press 164x4x4 | Bench 212x5x3 |
| | Pull-ups max reps x3 | Deadlift 395x4 | Chins max reps x3 |
| **13** | Squat 270x4x3 | Squat 240x5 | Squat 255x5x2 |
| | Bench 232x4x4 | Press 164x5x4 | Bench 215x5x3 |
| | Pull-ups max reps x3 | Deadlift 395x5 | Chins max reps x3 |
| **14** | Squat 270x5x3 | Squat 240x5 | Squat 255x5x2 |
| | Bench 232x5x4 | Press 166x3x4 | Bench 215x5x3 |
| | Pull-ups max reps x3 | Deadlift 400x3 | Chins max reps x3 |
| **15** | Squat 275x3x3 | Squat 245x5 | Squat 260x5x2 |
| | Bench 235x3x4 | Press 166x4x4 | Bench 217x5x3 |
| | Pull-ups max reps x3 | Deadlift 400x4 | Chins max reps x3 |

Typically, rep progression programs will be used by older Masters who need very conservative progression. Example 24-17 illustrates how this approach is applied to a Master who is pulling from the floor once per week.

**Cycling with a Rep Progression.** While this approach may seem confusing and overly complex at first, it is one of the more effective and reliable ways to program for an older lifter whose progression is slow. For clarity, Example 24-18 illustrates this approach using only the heavy day squat.

In Example 24-18, the first 3-week cycle consists of sets of 5, 3, or 1. In the second 3-week cycle, all those weights are repeated, but one rep is added to each week. Sets of 5 become sets of 6, sets of 3 become sets of 4, and singles become doubles. Only after this entire process is repeated does the athlete add weight to the bar, and a new cycle of 5s, 3s, and 1s begins in week 7. The alternation between 5/3/1 and 6/4/2 works extremely well, albeit slowly. The exact number of sets will vary with the individual. Four sets were used in this example, which may be too much volume for some Masters. Modify the program by reducing the number of work sets when necessary.

**Example 24-18: HLM with a Cycling Rep Progression**

| Week | | Week | |
|---|---|---|---|
| **1** | 250x5x3 | **12** | 275x2x3 |
| **2** | 260x3x3 | **13** | 260x5x3 |
| **3** | 270x1x3 | **14** | 270x3x3 |
| **4** | 250x6x3 | **15** | 280x1x3 |
| **5** | 260x4x3 | **16** | 260x6x3 |
| **6** | 270x2x3 | **17** | 270x4x3 |
| **7** | 255x5x3 | **18** | 280x2x3 |
| **8** | 265x3x3 | **19** | 265x5x3 |
| **9** | 274x1x3 | **20** | 275x3x3 |
| **10** | 255x6x3 | **21** | 285x1x3 |
| **11** | 265x4x3 | | |

## Heavy-Light-Medium and the Dynamic Effort Method

Dynamic effort (DE) sets are an excellent approach to tailoring the HLM system for a Master. In contrast with the Texas Method, athletes using HLM have had the most success with DE sets when they are used on medium day, at moderate volume. Using DE sets on the heavy day at high volume does not work as well in the HLM program because the lighter DE sets are not offset by a heavier day on Friday as they are in the Texas Method. Most Masters will need to push a heavy weight at least once a week to avoid detraining. Although DE training can certainly impose a powerful training stress, the weights used for DE sets are too low to keep a Master from detraining if not used in conjunction with another heavy day later in the week. For this reason, DE sets fit best on medium day.

When we used DE sets as a volume day stressor for the Texas Method, we recommended that total volume be as high as 24 to 30 total repetitions – or 10 to 12 sets of 2–3 repetitions. When used with the HLM system on medium day, we don't need the volume to be this high. Six to eight sets of 2 to 3 reps will be sufficient. As always, athlete and coach retain the prerogative to adjust the volume up or down based on results of the programming. Example 24-19 illustrates.

**Example 24-19: HLM with Dynamic Effort Sets**

| Heavy | Light | Medium |
|---|---|---|
| Squat<br>5x3 | Squat<br>5x2 (-10%) | DE Squat<br>2x8 @ 70% |
| Bench<br>5x3 | Press<br>5x3 | DE Bench<br>3x8 @ 65% |
| Pull-ups | Deadlift<br>5x1 | Chins |

## The Two Day Variant: Heavy-Light

For some Masters, progress is sustainable using a 2-day variant that eliminates the medium day. This is useful for older intermediate athletes with less avid recovery, or those who engage in other heavy physical pursuits that would interfere with a 3-day program. The Heavy-Light approach keeps the deadlift on heavy day, uses a 10% offset for the squat on light day, and alternates bench (heavy day) and press (light day).

The Heavy-Light variant is subject to all of the modifications discussed for sustaining progress with HLM, including rotating reps, running it out, and rep progressions. Dynamic effort sets are rather more tricky to use with this approach, because they are best used with HLM on medium day, which we have eliminated. DE sets *might* be productive in the Heavy-Light model if used on light day, but the greater percentage offset required by DE sets exposes the athlete to the risk of detraining.

### PROGRAM 6B: HEAVY-LIGHT

| HEAVY DAY | LIGHT DAY |
|---|---|
| SQUAT 4x5 | SQUAT 2x5 (90%) |
| BENCH 4x5 | PRESS 3x5 |
| DEADLIFT 1x5 | CHINS 3x8–10 |

**PRESCRIPTION:** Execute as indicated. Variations described in the text. Notation is sets x reps.

**INDICATIONS:** <40: Discretion 40–49: Discretion 50–59: Yes >60: Yes

**PARAMETERS:** Initiated at the termination of novice training or as indicated during intermediate training. Most Masters will continue in some variant of HL indefinitely or alternate between novice training (after layoffs) and HL. A very few Masters may progress to advanced training.

# Split Routines

Two- or 3-day/week whole-body routines are the simplest way to organize a training program. Full-body programs force the athlete to focus only on the most effective multi-joint barbell exercises and create the systemic stress that most effectively drives favorable adaptations.

However, as noted in our discussion of 4-day Texas Method variants (Chapter 23), there are reasons to disperse the organization of training into more discrete components. These reasons usually revolve around balancing training with the rest of life. Many working adults will find that around 60–90 minutes per day is all they can allot for a strength training program. For others, the prospect of a 2-hour full body volume day workout will seem intractable.

Conditioning work will now be an important part of training for many late-stage intermediates – an additional challenge to time management. Most trainees will prefer to combine their strength training and conditioning into the same training session. This means that barbell work needs to be completed in 45–75 minutes, to allow for a 10–20 minute conditioning session afterwards. The intermediate stage of training is also the time in which trainees will experiment the most with various types of assistance exercises and variations of the primary lifts.

For all of these reasons, many intermediates will find split routines, in which standard programming is dispersed across the week, essential.

One of the more effective split routine programs used by early intermediate trainees was presented in Chapter 23. The 4-Day Texas Method variants are in fact split routines. A typical Texas Method split incorporates a volume bench or press workout on Monday, a volume squat workout on Tuesday, an intensity workout for the bench or press on Thursday, and intensity day for the squat and deadlift on Friday.

Here we present two other split routine models: The Heavy-Light Split, and the One Lift a Day Split. Both are effective approaches to program organization for the intermediate Master. Both models impose a stress workout for each lift once per week.

## The heavy-light split

Not to be confused with the Heavy-Light variant of HLM (6B) presented earlier, the Heavy-Light Split is a 4-day program incorporating two main exercises each day – one at heavy weights, one light. A typical setup would have the athlete perform a heavy bench and light press on Monday, a heavy squat and light pull on Tuesday, a heavy press and light bench on Thursday, and a light squat and heavy deadlift set on Friday.

The purpose of the light exercise is to facilitate recovery and keep motor pathways stimulated so that a detraining affect does not creep in. *The light exercise is not intended to create a primary stress.* It should be moderate in both volume and intensity, and the athlete should never approach technical breakdown or failure with a light set.

Example 24-20 is a 3-week snapshot illustrating the Heavy-Light split.

Where 4 total sets are indicated, the Master is not necessarily required to do 4 sets across at the same weight, although in some cases that may be appropriate, as in the first few weeks of the program. Usually, however, the trainee will perform just one work set at the prescribed rep range of either 5 or 3 repetitions, followed by 3 back-off sets at about a 5% reduction from the work set – or whatever percentage offset allows them to get 3 additional sets across at the required rep range. Light exercises are performed for 3 sets across at a 5–10% reduction from the last completed heavy set of 5. In some instances this may be very near the same amount of weight used for the back-off sets on that lift's heavy day. Where two deadlift sets are indicated, this calls for one work set and one back-off set with a 5–10% offset. The back-off set should achieve the same amount of reps as the work set or perhaps one or two additional reps if the trainee wants to push hard. Where 5 singles are indicated, the same weight will usually be used on each set (sets across). Some trainees may do better with a top single followed by 4 back-off singles at a slight reduction.

**Example 24-20: The Heavy-Light Split**

| Week | Monday | Tuesday | Thursday | Friday |
|---|---|---|---|---|
| 1 | Press 3x5 | Squat 4x5 | Bench 4x5 | Light Squat 3x5 |
| | Light Bench 3x5 | | Light Press 3x5 | Deadlift 2x5 |
| 2 | Press 4x3 | Squat 4x3 | Bench 4x3 | Light Squat 3x5 |
| | Light Bench 3x5 | | Light Press 3x5 | Deadlift 2x3 |
| 3 | Press 5x1 | Squat 5x1 | Bench 5x1 | Light Squat 3x5 |
| | Light Bench 3x5 | | Light Press 3x5 | Deadlift 2x1 |

This is a 3-week training cycle that repeats itself over and over again. Starting in week 4, the trainee would rotate back to doing sets of 5 at a higher weight, but with a little more weight than he used on the previous cycle.

Clearly, this structure allows for all manner of variations to sustain progress, far too many to be explored here. Most of the heavy day programming options presented earlier in the text for the Heavy-Light-Medium system can be applied to the Heavy-Light Split. The goal of the program is the same – structure all variables of the training week so that progress can occur on the heavy day workout. This means two things: First, the heavy loads and volume for each lift must be stressful enough to drive adaptation over about a week, but not so stressful as to overwhelm recovery during this interval. Second, light loads and volume must be stressful enough so as to prevent a detraining effect from occurring within a 1-week window, but not so stressful as to actually prevent recovery from the heavy day stress.

Keeping that in mind, there are some very rough guidelines that can be established for this type of low-frequency programming. First, heavy day loads will generally require at least 1 limit set between 1 and 6 reps. This is the range in which strength is developed and therefore, new levels of strength performance must be consistently produced on a weekly basis for the intermediate trainee to make maximum progress. Additional volume may be required for complete homeostatic disruption to take place. This additional volume can be imposed in a variety of ways: sets across, back-off sets, and descending sets are all useful approaches for the accumulation of volume. Most trainees will require at least 2, but never more than 5 total sets in the 1–6 rep range on the heavy day to build an effective program (this includes PR work sets as well as back-off sets, descending sets, and so on).

Light day work will consist of 2–5 sets of about 3–5 reps at a reduction of anywhere from 5–20% from the heavy day loads for that lift. It is worth repeating that percent offsets for light work vary with the lift and the athlete. Bigger, stronger Masters and heavier lifts require larger offsets than smaller athletes and lighter lifts. And always remember that older Masters will require lower volume but higher intensity for effective light day work.

## One lift a day split

The One Lift a Day Split is similar to the Heavy-Light Split. A typical schedule is illustrated in Example 24-21.

Frequency can be modulated, if desired, by deviating from a standard weekly structure. One Lift a Day works exceptionally well on a 2-days-on, 1-day-off schedule that puts the trainee in the gym 5 days per week instead of just 4. Scheduling could also be less frequent, at just 3 days per week. A powerlifting specialist might reduce the schedule to Monday (squat), Wednesday (bench) and Friday (deadlift), with the press relegated to the role of an assistance exercise. Again, this structure lends itself to a wide range of variations and progression options.

A programming approach uniquely suited to the One Lift a Day structure is the *rotating linear progression,* very similar to running out the intensity day in the Texas Method. This approach is simple and straightforward on paper but requires objectivity and experience from the athlete and coach. Load is increased for each of the exercises independently of all the others in the program. This is a radical departure from the usual approach, in which all of the primary exercises are progressed in parallel. With the rotating linear progression the athlete will begin at the upper end of the strength training repetition range. Six reps is a good choice at the beginning of the program. The process begins in week 1, with some trial and error to determine the weight that allows for 6 difficult reps, followed by 1 or 2 back-off sets at a very slight offload. In week 2 the athlete adds weight to the bar and again attempts a set of 6. In the following weeks, intensity will increase and volume will decrease, until the trainee tops out at a heavy double or single. At this point he will cycle back to 6 reps and begin the process again, but with more weight.

In this approach, each exercise will usually operate on its own individual time line. Certain exercises will make very long runs of 12–16 weeks from 6 to 1 reps, some will repeat every 4–6 weeks. What matters is that the athlete is setting new PRs along the way and ending at a higher weight than the previous rotation did. Using this method in the context of One Lift a Day can allow these cycles to repeat over and over with little or no change in the complexity of the program. This only works if the trainee has reached a level of training experience that allows him to impose a very high level of training stress with just a single set of a given exercise. If he cannot, he will require a higher frequency, higher volume model of intermediate level programming such as the Texas Method or the HLM system.

Example 24-22 is a 16-week snapshot of the One Lift a Day program for the squat, bench, and deadlift, and illustrates how the 3 exercises progress on different schedules. This example is by no means prescriptive.

This type of programming works very well after extended training in the Texas Method, which can result in accumulated systemic fatigue. A switch to lower-volume programming allows some of that fatigue to dissipate. Here we see a hint of advanced programming.

**Example 24-21: One Lift a Day Split**

**Monday** – Bench

**Tuesday** – Squat

**Thursday** – Press

**Friday** – Deadlift

**Example 24-22: Staggered Progress on One Lift a Day**

| Mon<br>Squat | Wed<br>Bench | Fri<br>Deadlift |
|---|---|---|
| **315x6** | **275x6** | **405x6** |
| 320x6 | 277x6 | 410x5 |
| 325x5 | 280x6 | 415x5 |
| 330x5 | 282x5 | 420x4 |
| 335x5 | 284x5 | 425x3 |
| 340x4 | 286x5 | 430x3 |
| 345x4 | 288x5 | 435x3 |
| 350x3 | 290x5 | 440x2 |
| 355x3 | 292x4 | **410x6*** |
| 360x3 | 294x4 | 415x6 |
| 365x2 | 296x4 | 420x5 |
| **325x6*** | 298x3 | 425x5 |
| 330x6 | 300x3 | 430x4 |
| 335x6 | 302x2 | 435x4 |
| 340x6 | 305x2 | 440x3 |
| 345x5 | **282x6*** | 445x3 |

*** Start of a new cycle**

## Other Intermediate Programs

The vast majority of Masters will make excellent, long-term progress on Split Routines, the HLM structure, the Texas Method, or one of their variants. Other intermediate programs are available, of course, including those described in detail in *Practical Programming for Strength Training*. They are almost never indicated for the athlete over 50. This is doubly true of the huge selection of programs yielded by a cursory Internet search. A tiny fraction of such programs *might* be suitable for the intermediate Master. Most are not, and a few may lead directly to derailment, detraining, or disaster.

Before even considering alternatives to a Split, an HLM, or Texas variant, athlete and coach should ask themselves several critical questions. Is another program *really* required for the intermediate Master, or does the search for "something new" represent an early symptom of the CPH syndrome? Will the program allow for individualization and tailoring to the blunted recovery, intensity-dependence, and volume-sensitivity of the Master? Most importantly, *does the program reflect the Stress-Recovery-Adaptation structure*, and does it modulate volume and intensity over an appropriate interval (1 week or so) to achieve specific training objectives? Without these attributes, it is no program at all. It's just another random thrashabout.

The intermediate Master who cannot make long-term progress on a *properly* designed and modulated Texas, HLM program, or split routine is a rare creature indeed. The Master who *truly* transcends the intermediate category and requires more protracted and complex programming is rarer still – almost a unicorn. *This unusual person trains primarily for competitive performance, not for health and function*. Such an athlete is an advanced Master.

# 25
# The Advanced Master

The vast majority of Masters will never require advanced programming. Training at this level is not conducted for health or fitness, but rather to optimize performance for competition. Those few Masters who train for competition cannot expect to use programs employed by younger athletes without modification, because they ignore the principle that older trainees are volume-sensitive and intensity-dependent. After examining a classic advanced training model of accumulation and intensification, this chapter briefly presents a more suitable option for the Master: the Two Steps Forward, One Step Back model. An illustration of how this approach is used for competition is provided. We emphasize that no advanced training model can ever be prescriptive. Programming at this level must be exquisitely tailored to the individual athlete and his performance goals.

## You Are *Not* an Advanced Athlete

Sorry, but you are (almost certainly) not an advanced Master. *And you probably never will be.* This does not mean you are not going to get strong. If you train with the exercises and programs we have put forward to this point, you *will* get strong – possibly very strong – and you will do wonders for your health and physical performance. But it is rare for an athlete of *any* age to string together enough uninterrupted training time to exhaust intermediate programming options.

For example, the process of completing the novice progression, exhausting the Texas Method, moving through several variations of the Heavy-Light-Medium model, and continuing from there to variations on a split routine, could consume *years* of training, with weekly progress. But the vast majority of trainees will never realize this ideal. We train to live, and Life Happens. A family vacation, illness, injury, wedding, divorce, or a special project at work – living your life *will* derail your training sooner or later. So the training career of virtually any Master is a stop-and-start process that repeats over and over.

*This does not mean that the intermediate Master cannot make progress over the long term* – he can, and will. And it most emphatically does *not* mean that Masters should be complacent about interruptions in training. They should fight to string together as much consistent training time as possible. But for all save the most stubborn, dedicated, and *lonely* Masters, there will be discontinuities. So the need for programming beyond the intermediate level will likely never present itself, because the trainee never truly develops an adaptation to the stress significant enough to warrant complex advanced programming.

We follow Rippetoe in asserting that the advanced Master is not only exceptional, *he is a competitor in a strength sport.* This means participation in powerlifting, Olympic weightlifting, or Strongman competition. Only an individual committed to such competition will have cause and sufficient motivation to make the sacrifices that ensure his training is *not* interrupted by external life events. This has serious implications, not just for programming, but also for healthy aging – for the Game of Life. Competitive strength athletes plan their lives around their training. Families, friends, careers, and *even personal health* take a back seat to the competitive calendar. Family vacations are only scheduled where good barbells and racks are easily accessible. And while the rest of the family is on the beach, Dad is in the gym…again. Baker once coached a competitor who went about 3 months with a horrible toothache because the trainee refused to submit to oral surgery for fear of losing a week or more of valuable meet preparation.

This is not training for health. This is not training for life. *This is training to win a trophy.*

So let's be clear: the authors would *never* recommend that a Masters Athlete sacrifice health, safety, prosperity, adventure, or time with loved ones just to avoid missing a squat workout. If you are fortunate and dedicated enough to ever get to the point where you would even consider advanced programming, you will be healthy, strong, and fit. You will have made great headway against the atrophic effects of aging. Pursuit of advanced progress under the barbell is done because *you want to* – you are already doing what you *need to.*

## Organization of Advanced Programming

The term "advanced" can be misleading, because it seems to imply *better*. Trainees erroneously believe that undertaking an "advanced" program is how they can pursue "advanced" strength – a fundamental misapprehension of what the program-athlete categories mean.

Remember the important lesson from Chapter 18: athlete-program categories are not based on absolute strength. *Novice, intermediate* and *advanced* refer to the rate at which we can apply stress, recover from stress, and demonstrate new performance increases (Table 25-1). For a novice this cycle usually takes about 48–72 hours and programming is maximally simple. For intermediate trainees, the cycle takes about a week and programming is more complex. Advanced programming stretches the Stress-Recovery-Adaptation cycle out over a month or even longer. This means that both the overload event – with multiple stresses and longer recovery – will take more than a week's worth of training to complete. This is not "better." This is slower, more complicated, and a much bigger pain in the ass. The truly advanced athlete looks back on his novice and intermediate days much as he looks back on his lost youth – rather wistfully.

Advanced programming is a highly individualized endeavor. It is impossible to draw up cookie-cutter templates of advanced programs that work in all situations. Advanced trainees must be very precise in their application of all of the training variables – volume, intensity, recovery time, nutrition, sleep, supplementation, and so on. Advanced athletes use programs designed on the basis of years of training data from their logs. They have truly *evolved* into their advanced routine, built up from a long history of consistent and well-documented work, cherry-picking what has worked and discarding what has not.

| | STRESS | RECOVERY | ADAPTATION |
|---|---|---|---|
| NOVICE | A single workout. | 2–3 days of active rest. | Displays performance increase at each workout, which also imposes a training stress for the next cycle. |
| INTERMEDIATE | One or more workouts over a longer period of time. | Takes place throughout the overload event. | Displays performance increase across the components of the overload event. |
| ADVANCED | Accumulated in multiple training sessions over longer time periods. | Program-dependent. | Displays performance increase across the components of the overload event. |

***Table 25-1.*** Programming categories as expressions of the Stress-Recovery-Adaptation cycle.

That all being said, it is possible to draw up very general approaches to programming in this range. In *Practical Programming for Strength Training,* Rippetoe and Baker present several advanced program models. All are uniquely variable, but can be usefully considered as falling into two broad types. These approaches exploit the Stress-Recovery-Adaptation cycle (of course), over extended phases of ***accumulation*** and ***intensification***. In a more standard approach, stress is imposed during the accumulation phase with heavy volume over an extended period, usually about 4–6 weeks. After 1–3 weeks of deloading for recovery, ever-increasing weights are pursued at low volume during the intensification phase, which lasts about 3–5 weeks.

A useful variation on this structure is the Two Steps Forward, One Step Back Model. TSFOSB also relies on accumulation and intensification, but the training period is drastically shortened. In TSFOSB programming, all phases of accumulation, deloading, and intensification (or peaking) are executed within a 1-month time frame. This is in stark contrast to the more standard approach, which may take 2 or 3 months from beginning to end just to complete 1 cycle.

For Masters, we strongly prefer the condensed TSFOSB model. To understand why, we must first examine both models in some detail.

The pyramid model is a classic example of accumulation and intensification, and is an excellent way to illustrate this approach to advanced programming. Example 25-1 shows only the squat for simplicity.

The goal of the accumulation phase is to bring the trainee to the brink of overtraining – what we call *overreaching*. At this point, performance begins to stall or even decline due to the build-up of fatigue over weeks of heavy work. The deload week that follows the accumulation phase allows the trainee to shed much of the built-up fatigue and then continue that process through the intensification phase at greatly reduced frequency and volume. As the fatigue dissipates, adaptation manifests and performance rises sharply.

For the Masters Athlete there are two major drawbacks to this type of programming. Both occur during the accumulation phase, and both represent violations of a critical principle of Masters programming.

First, this model does not allow for the *volume-sensitivity* of the Master. The accumulation phase imposes very high volume at high frequency over a protracted training interval. Such a prescription will crush most Masters, especially in the later weeks where workloads are approaching maximal at each training session. Under this regimen, virtually any athlete over fifty will cross from overreaching to overtraining, which can wreak havoc on his entire training career. *Overtraining must be avoided at all costs, especially in the Master.*

The obvious solution would seem to be simply cutting down the volume at each training session, or perhaps reduce the frequency of the sessions to just twice per week. But this will not do, because the success of the program hinges on the accumulation of volume-induced stress. Low-volume, low-frequency programs will not impose an adequate training stress on any advanced athlete (not even a Master) – and will fail to produce the desired adaptive response.

Second, this model fails to address the *intensity-dependence* of the Master. Without frequent high-intensity loading, he quickly loses his ability to produce high levels of force, even in the presence of stressful, high-volume work. In a younger trainee, 4–6 weeks of sets of 5 at moderately high intensity would preserve, if not increase, his ability to demonstrate performance increases at even higher intensities – a contest 1RM, for example. For a Master, this same regimen will result in a decrease in maximal force production.

The solution to both problems is to simply shorten the duration of both the accumulation and intensification phases, which brings us finally to the Two Steps Forward, One Step Back model.

**Example 25-1: An 8-Week Advanced Program**

**Accumulation Phase (4 weeks)**

| Week | Monday | Wednesday | Friday |
|---|---|---|---|
| 1 | 275x5x5 | 255x5x5 | 285x5x5 |
| 2 | 295x5x5 | 275x5x5 | 305x5x5 |
| 3 | 315x5x5 | 295x5x5 | 320x5x5 |
| 4 | 325x5x5 | 305x5x5 | 330x5x5 |

**Deload Phase (1 week)**

| Week | Monday | Thursday |
|---|---|---|
| 5 | 295x3x3 | 315x3x3 |

**Intensification Phase (3 weeks)**

| Week | Monday | Thursday |
|---|---|---|
| 6 | 335x3x3 | 345x3x3 |
| 7 | 355x3x3 | 360x3 |
| 8 | 365x3 | 375x2–3 |

## The Two Steps Forward, One Step Back Model

In the TSFOSB model, the trainee is never exposed to prolonged bouts of elevated volume, and he handles loads at or above 90% of 1RM at least once a month, condensing the entire process of loading, deloading, and peaking into a period of 4 weeks – a tidy monthly training pattern. Each cycle is complete unto itself, but a series of carefully planned 4-week cycles can be neatly "stacked" to form a composite program to prepare for an approaching competition.

The "two steps" part of the model denotes a 2-week period of loading, in contrast to the 4–6 weeks needed for the first model. "One step back" refers to a 1-week deload period in week 3, with week 4 as the performance week.

Notice the highly generalized structure of the model we have presented below. We do not and cannot prescribe specific sets, reps, or exercise selection for this approach, because at this level of training the program must be tailored to the individual athlete and the specific demands of the competitive event. The 2-week loading period carries a lower risk of overtraining, and the shorter 1-week deload carries a lower risk of detraining. On the other hand, performance improvements with this structure are small. Incremental monthly increases, as little as 5–10 pounds or even less, are to be expected for a Master training on this model.

## PROGRAM 7A: TWO STEPS FORWARD, ONE STEP BACK

WEEK 1: PREPARATORY LOADING – Moderate-to-high volume, moderate intensity.

WEEK 2: PRIMARY LOADING – Highest volume; highest intensity possible at that volume.

WEEK 3: DELOADING – Low volume, low intensity.

WEEK 4: PERFORMANCE – Very low volume, very high intensity.

**PRESCRIPTION:** Highly variable, depending upon the competitive focus and capacities of the trainee. Programming at this level mandates individualization. See text for application examples.

**INDICATIONS:** <40: Discretion 40–49: Yes 50–59: Discretion >60: Caution

**PARAMETERS:** For use in Masters who have made significant progress in intermediate training and wish to engage in strength competition. May be terminated at the end of the competitive career and supplanted with long-term intermediate programming.

### The TSFOSB training cycle: week by week

Weeks 2 and 4 (primary loading and performance) of the TSFOSB program are the "money weeks" for the lifter. The program is built around these 2 weeks, and weeks 1 and 3 (preparatory loading and deloading) are designed around what happens in weeks 2 and 4.

**Week 1 is Preparatory Loading**, often called the "base week." If multiple cycles are to be linked together, then week 1 will usually fall between two very demanding weeks. This requires the athlete to moderate the stress by manipulation of both volume and intensity. In this sense, week 1 serves a recovery function, while laying the groundwork for the rest of the cycle.

**Week 2 is Primary Loading**. This is by far the most stressful component of the cycle. The intensity is reduced, but the volume is turned up from week 1, with extra sets or reps. During primary loading the athlete is aiming to push the limits of volume accumulation with multiple strength-building sets across, all in the 3–5 rep range, sometimes augmented by back-off sets at slightly less intensity. If possible, the athlete should attempt new personal bests for volume-based work. If not, he can lower the weight to what is manageable. *The primary goal here is to achieve the prescribed volume (sets x reps) for each day during this week at the highest intensity the athlete can manage.*

**Week 3 is Deloading.** Volume and intensity are both reduced, but intensity is not dropped so far that detraining can occur. Deloading for an advanced Master requires that intensity be kept higher than for younger trainees.

**Week 4 is Performance.** During Performance week, the athlete will focus on setting new personal records in the competitive lifts, or at least hitting the target volume for intensities at or above 90% of 1RM. It is critically important that the advanced athlete work at or above 90% at least every 4th week. A less frequent exposure to weights at this intensity will likely detrain his ability to push maximum loads. Performance weeks usually incorporate 1–3 work sets of 1–3 reps each.

### A TSFOSB POWERLIFTING PROGRAM FOR MASTERS

The following program, built on the TSFOSB model, has been utilized extensively to prepare Masters for powerlifting competition. Three consecutive 4-week TSFOSB cycles are linked to form a complete 12-week program. Cycle 1 (i.e., the first month) loads with sets of 5 and peaks with heavy triples. Cycle 2 loads with sets of 4 and peaks with heavy doubles. Cycle 3 (or the pre-competition cycle) loads with triples and peaks with singles across or testing for new 1RMs.

This is an excellent way for the Master to arrange his programming at the advanced level. This approach keeps both volume and intensity at appropriate levels, but creates enough fluctuation that the trainee does not go stale over the course of a long series of repeated cycles.

Let us assume that this advanced athlete is capable of a 500-pound squat, a 350-pound bench, a 545-pound deadlift, and a 225-pound press. The first cycle begins with set percentages, and all other cycles to follow will be derived from these numbers. Always remember that percentages are just rough guidelines. Under actual circumstances the numbers would always be adjusted for each trainee at the start of every training week. Rather than focus on the percentages used in this example, *the reader should study how volume and intensity are manipulated throughout the training cycle.*

In this program performs each lift or one of its variations is performed twice per week. This includes the 3 competitive power lifts (squat, bench, deadlift) as well as the press which has been included for balance. The squat, bench, and deadlift are trained as early as possible in the week while the athlete is relatively fresh. Later in the week, he will perform the lifts again at a slightly lower weight, or he can perform a variation of the lift that works for his body type and perceived weaknesses. All lifts during the week are done for the prescribed set and rep range unless otherwise noted. Deadlifts may use back-off sets to achieve the prescribed volume at each session. For example, if 5x5 is prescribed, a lifter may do 1 heavy set of 5, followed by 4x5 at the minimum reduction in load that the athlete can manage.

**Example 25-2: A 4-Month Competitive Training Program**

Starting point based on current 1RMs: Week 1: 75%, Week 2: 80%, Week 3: 70%, Week 4: 90%

**Cycle 1**

| Week | Monday | Tuesday | Thursday | Friday |
|---|---|---|---|---|
| **1: Preparatory Loading (4x5)** | Squat 375x5x4<br>Deadlift variant ***or*** Olympic lifts | Bench 265x5x4<br>Press or Variant | Deadlift 405x5x2<br>Squat or Variant | Press 170x5x5<br>Close-Grip Bench |
| **2: Primary Loading (5x5)** | Squat 400x5x5<br>Deadlift variant ***or*** Olympic lifts | Bench 280x5x5<br>Press or Variant | Deadlift 445x5x3<br>Squat or Variant | Press 180x5x5<br>Close-Grip Bench |
| **3: Deloading (2x5)** | Squat 350x5x2<br>Deadlift variant ***or*** Olympic lifts | Bench 245x5x2<br>Press or Variant | Deadlift 385x5<br>Squat or Variant | Press 160x5x2<br>Close-Grip Bench |
| **4: Performance (3x3)** | Squat 455x3x3<br>Deadlift variant ***or*** Olympic lifts | Bench 315x3x3<br>Press or Variant | Deadlift 495x3<br>Squat or Variant | Press 205x3x3<br>Close-Grip Bench |

If not performing a meet on the final week, the athlete might use the opportunity to test himself under simulated meet conditions and let his body rest with the prolonged deload shown here.

The foregoing example is extremely rigid, specific, detailed, and streamlined for ease of illustration. It cannot be overemphasized that *true advanced programming is highly individualized.* Any athlete who undertakes such a program must have the flexibility to make changes within the general and nonspecific TSFOSB structure. Blind adherence to a set and rep prescription or rigid percentages is not to be expected of an advanced trainee of *any* age.

If you make it to this level, you'll *know* what adjustments to make.

**Cycle 2**

| Week | Monday | Tuesday | Thursday | Friday |
|---|---|---|---|---|
| **1: Preparatory Loading (4x4)** | Squat 415x4x4<br>Deadlift variant ***or*** Olympic lifts | Bench 285x4x4<br>Press or Variant | Deadlift 435x4x2<br>Squat or Variant | Press 185x4x4<br>Close-Grip Bench |
| **2: Primary Loading (5x4)** | Squat 435x4x5<br>Deadlift variant ***or*** Olympic lifts | Bench 300x4x5<br>Press or Variant | Deadlift 465x4x3<br>Squat or Variant | Press 195x4x5<br>Close-Grip Bench |
| **3: Deloading (2x4)** | Squat 385x4x2<br>Deadlift variant ***or*** Olympic lifts | Bench 275x4x2<br>Press or Variant | Deadlift 415x4<br>Squat or Variant | Press 175x4x2<br>Close-Grip Bench |
| **4: Performance (3x2)** | Squat 475x2x3<br>Deadlift variant ***or*** Olympic lifts | Bench 340x2x3<br>Press or Variant | Deadlift 525x2<br>Squat or Variant | Press 220x2x3<br>Close-Grip Bench |

**Cycle 3**

| Week | Monday | Tuesday | Thursday | Friday |
|---|---|---|---|---|
| **1: Preparatory Loading (4x3)** | Squat 425x3x4<br>Deadlift variant ***or*** Olympic lifts | Bench 305x3x4<br>Press or Variant | Deadlift 475x3x2<br>Squat or Variant | Press 190x3x4<br>Close-Grip Bench |
| **2: Primary Loading (5x3)** | Squat 465x3x5<br>Deadlift variant ***or*** Olympic lifts | Bench 325x3x5<br>Press or Variant | Deadlift 505x3x3<br>Squat or Variant | Press 210x3x5<br>Close-Grip Bench |
| **3: Deloading (2x3)** | Squat 405x3x2<br>Deadlift variant ***or*** Olympic lifts | Bench 295x3x2<br>Press or Variant | Deadlift 425x3<br>Squat or Variant | Press 180x3x2<br>Close-Grip Bench |
| **4: Performance – MEET WEEK** | **Tuesday**<br>Squat 385 x 3 x 2<br>Bench 285 x 3 x 2 | **Saturday – MEET** | | |

# 26
# Conditioning

Conditioning, also known as endurance training or "cardio," is an essential component of the complete exercise prescription, magnifying the metabolic, cardiovascular, and performance benefits of strength training. Conditioning is far more sport- and vocation-specific than strength training, and for many athletes the best training recommendation is to "lift weights and play your sport." For Masters who practice low-intensity sports or who train solely for health, however, this prescription does not suffice. Evaluation of the various modalities available through the prism of our exercise prescription criteria indicates that high-intensity interval training (HIIT) alternatives are superior to low-intensity, long slow distance (LSD) exercises. Conditioning at high intensity confers the health benefits of low-intensity training in less time, while producing less interference with strength training and promoting more comprehensive bioenergetic and performance adaptations. Multiple modalities for HIIT conditioning are available. The authors prefer sled work for its simplicity and lack of eccentric component. Intervals with Concept2 rowers, Airdyne bikes, and standard stationary bikes are also recommended. Sprints, high-impact aerobics, group classes, rowing machines, and Crossfit are not appropriate for the General Exercise Prescription. Program suggestions are provided. The chapter concludes with an examination of walking-based conditioning programs for particularly deconditioned Masters.

## The Importance of Conditioning

You will recall that our *complete* prescription for the Masters athlete incorporated both strength and conditioning components. The best data available suggests that this combination improves the general health and performance benefits of either modality alone.[1] Of the two, strength is the more critical, because the ability to produce force is the foundation of *all* physical performance – the foundation of *movement*, itself. All physical performance attributes depend on strength. And as we saw in Part I, strength training is the exercise medicine best suited to address the Sick Aging Phenotype.

But strength training is a means to an end, not an end in itself. The objective is strength for *life*: membership in a recreational sports league, skiing in the Rockies, or hiking along a nature trail with your beloved. Strength is *always* necessary, but it isn't always enough to ensure such activities are accessible and enjoyable. Once the foundation of strength is built, it must be complemented by appropriate conditioning, so the athlete can use that strength to engage in meaningful physical activities outside of the gym.

Conditioning work goes by many names: "aerobics," "cardio," "energy-system training" (for the nerds), "endurance training," and so on. The modalities available for conditioning work are even more numerous – jogging, running, cycling, kickboxing classes, step aerobics, a fast-paced Zumba class at the local Y. With so many choices, where does the Master begin to design an appropriate conditioning plan?

As usual, it depends on what you're trying to accomplish. The general public tends to view exercise (and certainly anything resembling aerobic or "cardio" exercise) as a weight-loss intervention. The idea that conditioning work will allow them to "burn off" bodyfat or atone for the calorie-dense, nutrient-poor garbage they load into their bodies has driven millions to the hamster wheel of endless cardio. Certainly, an appropriate exercise prescription will produce improvements in body composition, including the loss of truncal and visceral fat. But when it comes to obesity, diet is 90% of the problem. It is far more effective to *not eat* an additional 1000 calories than to try to *burn off* an additional 1000 calories.

Significant fat loss doesn't happen in the gym. *It happens at the dinner table.*

This is true for everybody, but particularly the Master. Not only is cardio alone ineffective for long-term body composition improvement, but it also entails high volume and high frequency, which will crush a Master. Attempts to "run off" a beer belly will sacrifice knees, ankles, and low backs in the process. Even worse, such high-volume conditioning will be detrimental to building and maintaining strength and muscle mass. That is a fool's trade-off.

## Criteria for the Design of a Conditioning Program

Appropriate conditioning must be approached from the standpoints of *health and performance*. Its purpose is to optimize cardiovascular and metabolic health and hone fitness: the ability to meet the physical demands of one's life and environment.

In other words, *conditioning is a component of our exercise prescription*. Our approach will therefore be consistent with the one we have taken throughout this text. The conditioning component of the exercise prescription must meet our familiar criteria:

### Criteria for the General Exercise Prescription

1. Our conditioning component must be ***safe***.
2. Our conditioning component must have a ***broad therapeutic window***.
3. Our conditioning component must be as ***comprehensive as possible***.
4. Our conditioning component must ***specifically and effectively combat the Sick Aging Phenotype.*** It should also be as specific as possible to the physical demands confronted by the individual athlete.
5. Our conditioning component should be as ***simple and efficient*** as possible.

#### Conditioning Safely

Safety is always the prime criterion for the formulation of our exercise prescription. Conditioning work must not expose the Master to undue risk of injury, and it must not degrade other physical attributes, but rather enhance them. This includes protecting one's hard-earned physical strength and muscle mass. Such protection extends to the trainee's ability to effectively train for strength *without interference* from the conditioning work. A protocol or modality that introduces significant interference with the development of strength should be excluded.

*Indeed, a properly constructed conditioning program will not only minimize interference, but will actually promote the athlete's ability to productively engage in strength training.* As the Master gets stronger, harder workouts are required to impose training stress and produce adaptation (Chapter 18). Conditioning prepares the athlete to absorb harder workouts without getting "gassed."

Conditioning work is not just about training to get into shape. It's also about *getting in shape to train.*

Bone and joint health must also be considered. Many wonderful activities are excellent for developing cardiovascular fitness and endurance, but are unnecessarily hard on the joints, tendons, and ligaments. The ideal conditioning modality will force positive adaptations in cardiovascular function and work capacity while interfering minimally with recovery and causing as little injury and inflammation as possible. This criterion puts jogging, running, martial-arts-based aerobics, and other high-impact activities in an unfavorable light. Some may choose to pursue them out of personal preference and passion, and that's fine. But they are not suitable candidates for the conditioning component of a *General* Exercise Prescription.

To meet the criterion of safety, our general conditioning prescription must meet certain parameters. It should be low in volume, to reduce interference effects, minimize residual fatigue, and avoid overtraining. It should incorporate low-impact, repeated motor activities requiring minimal technical proficiency. For example, pedaling on a stationary bike is a simple movement pattern that does not require practice, does not expose the athlete to unpredictable or impulsive forces, and does not excessively stress the involved joints. Our conditioning exercise will ideally avoid eccentric movement patterns, which produce soreness and interfere with recovery from strength training. Here, again, pedaling a stationary bike is a good example, as is pushing or pulling a sled. Jogging, running and sprinting do not fit the bill. A simple, stable, repetitive, low-impact exercise that produces the least soreness will be the safest.

### Therapeutic window of conditioning

Our conditioning modality must incorporate a broad therapeutic window, or range of available doses. Here we encounter some difficulty. Many popular conditioning modalities do not possess a broad range of intensities or favorable volume-dosing profiles.

Conditioning options may be broadly divided into *low-intensity* (walking, jogging, running) and *high-intensity* (interval training with sprints, bikes, rowers, sleds and kettlebells). Obviously, this classification lacks granularity, and there can be extensive overlap, but it will do for our purposes. As we saw in Chapter 3, walking, running, and other low-intensity approaches do not fit the bill for our General Exercise Prescription, in part because they lack a broad range of intensities, and are highly dependent on volume for dosing manipulation. High-volume, low-intensity work is poorly suited to the needs of the Master, does not train the entire bioenergetic spectrum (Chapter 4), and interferes with strength training. These are strong arguments in favor of high-intensity modalities for conditioning.

However, some high-intensity modalities suffer from a similar problem. Sprints, for example, are by definition all-out efforts – a sprint is always done at or near maximal intensity, or it's not really a sprint. Fortunately, there are several low-volume, high-intensity conditioning modalities, discussed below, that permit excellent modulation of intensity. This expands their therapeutic window, allowing for careful dosing and programming.

### Comprehensive conditioning

The protocol should have as broad an effect as possible and maximize the trainee's ability to perform tasks up and down the power spectrum, as well as improve their capacity to handle ever increasing loads in the weight room. Here again, high-intensity modalities are favored, for reasons that are best examined below, in our consideration of specificity and effectiveness.

## Specificity and Effectiveness

**Health-Specific Conditioning.** Conditioning does not produce significant progressive improvements in strength, power, muscle mass, bone density, or mobility. But the addition of a conditioning component to our barbell prescription enhances the ability of strength training to fight the Sick Aging Phenotype, and our conditioning modality must fulfill this criterion. This is not a problem, because *almost any type of exercise will improve cardiovascular and metabolic health.* Decades of research have established that virtually all forms of conditioning have *some* activity against the Sick Aging Phenotype, reducing visceral fat, improving insulin sensitivity, and resisting the development and progression of cardiovascular disease.

However, conditioning work also has implications for sport- and profession-specific performance, and for our ability to function in the Arena of Life. In this regard, specificity becomes an issue, and selection of the appropriate conditioning modality becomes more crucial.

**Performance-Specific Conditioning.** Hall of Fame NFL running back Earl Campbell was famous not only for battering opposing defenses into submission with a brutal combination of speed and power, but also for routinely missing his mandatory 2-mile conditioning test at the start of every NFL season. Recognizing that the test had no relevance to the demands of game play, his legendary coach Bum Phillips responded to a concerned sports writer's question with the classic response: "Well, I'll be sure to take him out of the game if it's 4th and 2 miles."

Bum Phillips understood the proper role of sports conditioning, and the need for conditioning specificity. Unlike strength, the most general of all physical adaptations, conditioning work may be very specific to the demands of the sport or environment. "Sport-specific strength" is largely nonsense, while the concept of "sport-specific conditioning" is quite valid. Building foundational strength in the core group of barbell exercises has tremendous *transfer* to activities in and out of the weight room. Adding 100 pound to the squat will make your deadlift stronger. It will also improve your ability to run, jump, lunge, lift, and love, as the need arises.

Conditioning transfer is less robust, especially as one becomes more advanced in their level of conditioning. For the rank novice, *any* physical activity causes broad general improvements in performance across a range of physical attributes, including endurance – for a short while. After this brief honeymoon, conditioning improvements become more performance-specific. Swimming does not improve running, cycling does not improve skiing, and of course none of these will help your squat.

So we have an interesting paradox. On the one hand, the addition of virtually any form of conditioning work – high- or low-intensity – would seem to complete our barbell prescription and work against the Sick Aging Phenotype. Specificity is not an issue here. On the other hand, the physical performance requirements of a particular sport or vocation may demand a very high degree of conditioning specificity. And this most explicitly includes the Game of Life.

Consider, for example, the training of a martial artist. His sport involves brief (2–3 min) rounds of *very* intense effort and high power output. A very common and *very silly* approach to training such an athlete is to have him train for strength by punching with dumbbells or kicking with ankle weights, with a few push-ups and crunches thrown in for good measure. His conditioning program is focused on 3–5 mile runs. Under this misinformed approach, his strength training is specific, emulating the peculiar movements of his sport with added resistance. His conditioning work is very generalized, looking nothing like his sport. It doesn't get much more nonspecific than running.

This approach is exactly back-asswards. As for any athlete, our fighter's strength training should be quite nonspecific – squats, presses, deadlifts, and cleans will improve his strength, power, body composition, balance, endurance, and mobility

– the *General* Fitness Attributes required by *all* athletes. *But his conditioning work must prepare him for the cardiometabolic demands of the ring*, which loping around the track a few times can *never* do. Running doesn't even approach the intensity of a 3-minute kickboxing bout. In fact, most sports demand power outputs that exceed those of running: tennis, volleyball, swimming, gymnastics, soccer, basketball, track and field, and so on. Our fighter would be better served by a conditioning modality that more closely resembles the power-capacity demands of his sport. He could incorporate sprints, sled pulls, high-intensity calisthenics, and the like. *But his most productive conditioning time will come from high-intensity interval work in his sport* – sparring, shadowboxing, heavy bag drills.

So it seems that strength training should be generalized while conditioning should be specific, reflecting the power-capacity demands of the sport or profession. And we maintain that this is true for sport- and profession-specific performance.

For most athletes, therefore, the prescription of a strength and conditioning program is simple: *lift weights and practice your sport.*

From the standpoint of *overall fitness for life*, however, it's just a little more complicated than that.

**Trading Places.** Consider a second example, that of a golfer. It's ridiculous for his strength training program to specifically emulate the movements of his sport. We're not going to have this poor bastard start swinging a 5-pound club for his rank novice program and try to work our way up to a 150-pound club…*because that would be stupid.* As for any athlete, nonspecific strength training with barbells will fit the bill for strength and power development.

On the other hand, the cardiometabolic demands of golf are relatively minimal, even if, unlike most North American golfers, this guy actually totes his own clubs, instead of tootling around the golf course in the Adipocart. Low-intensity modalities like jogging and hiking mimic, more or less, the movement patterns and power-capacity demands of his "sport,"[2] and will adequately condition him for golf. More to the point, *just playing golf* will condition him for golf.

But none of this will condition him for activities with a *higher* power output than golf.

This is critical to understand. Let us assume our martial artist does low-volume, high-intensity conditioning (appropriately sport-specific), while our golfer does high-volume, low-intensity conditioning (appropriately golf-specific). Both are well-conditioned for their respective activities.

Now, let's go all Mark Twain on these guys, and drop each of them into the other's arena. The results will be instructive, catastrophic, and entertaining.

The martial artist will play a truly execrable game of golf, culminating in a permanent ban from the grounds and, quite possibly, legal action. But he will have little difficulty lugging clubs around the golf course. True, he won't enjoy it. He might get tired, his feet might get sore, and the *overwhelming excitement of golf* might be too much for him. But he will easily meet the power-capacity demands of the situation.

Our golfer in the fighting ring, however, is immediately cooked. *He has no hope* of meeting the energy demands of MMA or kickboxing. Early in the first round, even before his opponent transplants his mandible to his eye sockets, he will be in a state of utter metabolic depletion and profound cardiorespiratory distress.

We submit that this has implications for the Arena of Life. The athlete who engages in a high-intensity sport and conditions in a high-intensity modality is prepared to take on a broad range of physical challenges, across a wide spectrum of power-capacity demands. The athlete who engages in low-intensity conditioning, however, will *not* be prepared to confront physical challenges demanding high power outputs. This is not a problem for him, as long as he stays on the golf course.

The problem for the Athlete of Aging is that *the physical challenges encountered in the Arena of Life are not limited to those on the low-power end of the spectrum.* The Arena of Life is free of rules and expectations. Here, the demands on performance, and the intensity, duration, and frequency are always changing. Moving day, an escaped grandchild, running for your life, a serious illness, or an unexpected invitation to a volleyball game at a nude beach party all exceed the cardiometabolic and power demands of golf.

The everyday activities that make up the fabric of our lives tend not to be at the metabolic extremes, and they are not readily subject to precise dosing and training progression. This means they cannot stand in as conditioning in the same way that sport-specific work serves the dual function of conditioning and practice.

So when it comes to the Arena of Life, the advice to "just lift weights and play your sport" breaks down, *unless* that sport involves regular, high-intensity work. But most Masters are not rugby players, fighters, or gymnasts. They're accountants, doctors, teachers, and grandparents.

Thus, our General Exercise Prescription mandates a low-volume, high-intensity conditioning program, sometimes called a *GPP (general physical preparedness program)*. Such a program ***specifically and effectively*** addresses the Sick Aging Phenotype while also fulfilling the requirement of a ***comprehensive*** preparation for a broad range of power-capacity demands.

## Conditioning simplicity

Coaches and trainees often get too clever by half in the design of conditioning programs. We reiterate that if you are engaged in regular sports practice, the best conditioning strategy is to simply practice and play your sport as much as possible, provided that sport is at the high-intensity end of the spectrum.

If conditioning work is indicated, it should be as simple and time-efficient as possible. Here again, low-volume, high-intensity modalities win the day. These fall under the rubric of HIIT (high-intensity interval training), as discussed in Part I. In HIIT, the trainee engages in short bouts of very intense effort alternated with short periods of rest. Bike intervals are a classic example. On the stationary bike, set at moderate-high resistance, the athlete pedals as hard and as fast as possible for, say, 60 seconds. This will suck a bit. The athlete then rests, or pedals lightly, for 60 seconds. Then he goes all-out for another 60 seconds. Then he rests again. The pattern is repeated about 4–8 times.

This approach has been studied extensively and compared to more traditional LSD (long slow distance) aerobic training.[3] The cardiovascular and performance adaptations produced by high-intensity training are similar, and in many cases superior, to those produced by continuous endurance training. For example, in a 2009 study Wisløff et al. found that 4 rounds of 4-minute runs at 90–95% of maximum heart rate followed by 3 minutes of active recovery at 70% of maximum heart rate resulted in 10% greater improvement in stroke volume (the amount of blood pumped with each contraction of the heart) than did long distance running.[4] Total oxygen consumption was similar in both protocols. Each protocol was performed 3 days per week for 8 weeks. Similarly, Gibala et al. found that sprint interval training (a form of HIIT) yielded performance improvements similar to those of traditional endurance training in a fraction of the time, with similar increases in muscle oxidative capacity, buffering capacity, and glycogen content.[5]

Another metabolic benefit of HIIT, especially for those concerned with fat loss, is known as ***excess post-exercise oxygen consumption*** (EPOC). HIIT training results in an elevated rate of oxygen consumption, and associated energy utilization, well after the training bout is over. This increased oxygen consumption and caloric expenditure is associated with the energy demands of restoring homeostasis in the muscle – repletion of energy stores, elimination of reaction products, repair of microtrauma, and adaptive responses. This "extended burn" draws on the favored fuel for oxidative metabolism – triglyceride – and promotes fat loss.[6]

At the date of this writing, therefore, it appears that high-intensity interval training confers all the benefits of LSD while being simpler, more time-efficient, safer, and more titratable. For the Masters Athlete who requires conditioning work, HIIT satisfies our exercise prescription criteria beautifully. It remains only to select the appropriate form of HIIT.

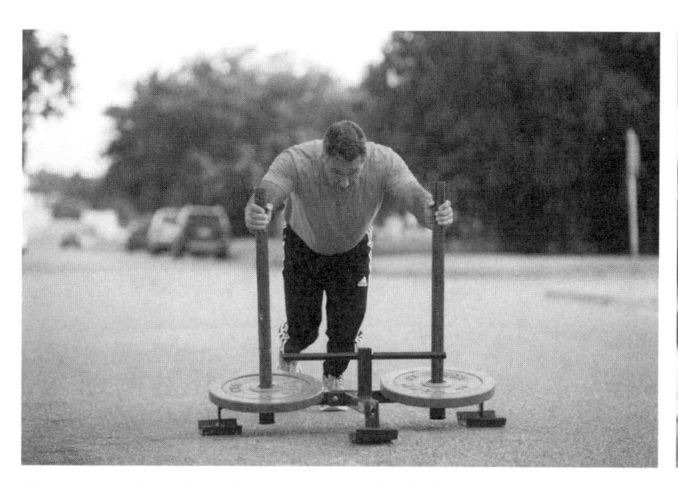
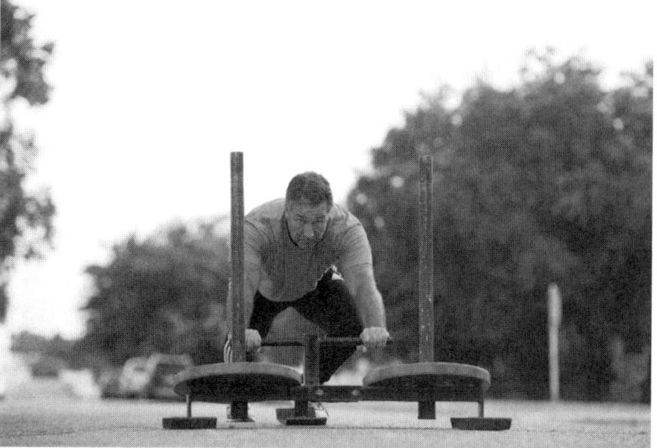

***Figure 26-1.*** Conditioning with sled pushes. (*Left*) Pushing the Prowler using the vertical handles. (*Right*) Pushing the Prowler using the horizontal handles. This position requires the athlete to keep his hips low, and is far more taxing than pushing against the uprights.

# Exercise Selection

### First choice: the Prowler & other sleds

For conditioning work, we strongly prefer the Prowler and other training sleds. Originally designed for football players, sleds have recently gone mainstream, and are increasingly popular in black-iron gyms and Crossfit boxes. The sled is simply a heavy platform with skids that the trainee must push a certain distance (Figure 26-1).

The challenge, of course, is that the sled does not *like* to be pushed.

Sleds are the ideal implement for HIIT, fulfilling all of our exercise prescription criteria. Prowlers and other sleds are ***safe***. Sled-pushing is a low-impact, repetitive motor activity performed on a stable surface, and it has no eccentric component, meaning there's no delayed soreness. In fact, many report that the concentric-only activity of sled pushes actually helps to dissipate soreness and improve the rate of recovery after heavy lower body work.

Most often, trainees run or sprint while pushing the sled, although older adults (especially older men) may want to avoid sprinting with heavily loaded sleds. There are anecdotal reports of strained calves and Achilles tendons from sprint work with loaded sleds. If this is a concern, the athlete can simply walk the sled. While not as hard as a sprint, this is no easy task in itself.

Sleds, especially those constructed like the Prowler (which can accommodate standard barbell plates), have a ***wide therapeutic window***, and are subject to dosing manipulations via several variables: load, speed, distance, rest intervals, total volume, and frequency, allowing the construction of a rational conditioning program tailored to individual needs and abilities. Athletes can begin pushing an unloaded sled a short distance at a slow pace once a week, and work their way up to multiple sprints over longer distances with heavy loads and short rest intervals. Dosing can be further modulated by the incorporation of heart-rate-guided protocols, such as those described by Reynolds and Bradford.[7]

Sled pushing imposes a ***comprehensive*** conditioning stress, because it is a form of HIIT, and works the trainee at the high-power, "anaerobic" end of the bioenergetic spectrum. Like any other form of HIIT, it therefore produces adaptations all across that spectrum, with improvements in both "aerobic" and "anaerobic" capacity. While the lower body is of course the primary engine in this exercise, the entire kinetic chain from the toes to the fingers is involved in a sled push – ideal for athletes and lifters.

Sled pushing is ***specific and effective against the Sick Aging Phenotype***. As a form of HIIT, it will improve insulin sensitivity and cardiovascular health, while decreasing frailty and improving the ability to train productively after the rank- and early-novice phases.

Finally, pushing the sled is ***simple and efficient***. All forms of HIIT are more time-efficient than LSD conditioning, and all of them tend to be perceived as more enjoyable, promising to improve program compliance. But for sheer simplicity, you just can't beat five or ten intervals of pushing a heavy sled back and forth over a short distance once or twice a week.

Sled work can be done either "heavy and short" or "light and long." Optimal conditioning levels are likely best attained by a combination of both, perhaps alternated by session.

Short sprints with heavy weight can be effective in as little as 10 yard increments. Longer sprints are typically done between 40–60 yards with lighter weights. If walking rather than sprinting with the sled, trainees will often go for time rather than distance, e.g., 1–3 minutes of work followed by 1–3 minutes of rest.

Rest intervals for sled sprints are dependent on the individual fitness of each trainee. Those just starting out will need longer rest between efforts. Rest time should be monitored as this is a variable that can be effectively manipulated to improve the quality of the workout and measure progression. Trainees can also progress by adding weight, increasing distance, or increasing volume (number of sprints).

Example 26-1 illustrates a simple progression for sled training. In this approach, the sled is pushed twice a week, for one short heavy session and one long light session.

**Example 26-1: Pushing the Sled for Conditioning**

| Session 1 (short, heavy) | Session 2 (light, long) |
|---|---|
| 90 lbs x 10 yds x 4 | 50 lbs x 50 yds x 2 |
| 100 lbs x 10 yds x 4 | 50 lbs x 50 yds x 3 |
| 110 lbs x 10 yds x 6 | 50 lbs x 50 yds x 4 |
| 120 lbs x 10 yds x 6 | 50 lbs x 50 yds x 5 |
| 120 lbs x 10 yds x 8 | 50 lbs x 60 yds x 5 |
| 140 lbs x 10 yds x 8 | 50 lbs x 50 yds x 7 |
| 140 lbs x 10 yds x 10 | 50 lbs x 40 yds x 10 |
| 160 lbs x 10 yds x 10 | 50 lbs x 50 yds x 9 |
| 160 lbs x 15 yds x 10 | 50 lbs x 50 yds x 10 |
| 180 lbs x 15 yds x 10 | 60 lbs x 50 yds x 10 |

## Second choice: sled drags

Dragging the sled is another terrific option, and it fits our exercise prescription for exactly the same reasons cited above for sled pushes. This approach has long been a cornerstone of conditioning, and is almost synonymous with Westside Barbell, a powerlifting gym home to many of the strongest lifters in the world. Westside Barbell owner Louie Simmons pushes his lifters with high-volume, fast-paced training routines using heavy weights. A Friday workout at Westside might see 12 sets of very explosive dynamic effort doubles at 70–80% of 1RM. Rest time is limited to just a minute or two. This pace, volume, and weight would not be sustainable if these lifters were not well conditioned – a classic example of *being in shape to train*. To achieve this level of conditioning, Simmons has for many years used high-volume, high-frequency sled work, and this approach has spread to gyms all across the world.

The sled is usually dragged by a rope or chain attached to a belt around the trainee's waist or a shoulder harness (Figure 26-2). Like the sled push, the drag is a concentric-only exercise that does not produce soreness. Light sled drags are an excellent way to speed recovery after heavy lower body work.

Drags are not quite as intense as pushes. Sled drags are typically done for total time (e.g., drag a moderate weight for 15–20 minutes without stopping) or done for longer intervals (50–100 yd interspersed with brief rest periods). But like pushes, weight, distance, rest intervals, and total volume can all be manipulated to increase or decrease the dose and specificity of the exercise.

Sled drags do have some advantages over pushes. With light weights, drags allow for a very upright posture and *long* strides, extremely beneficial

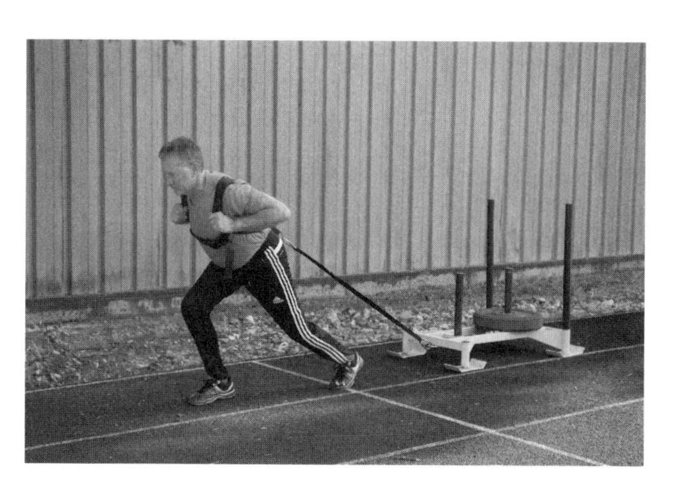

***Figure 26-2.*** Sled drags.

to the development of the hamstrings. This can be a useful variation for a lifter who struggles with squat depth, due to a weak posterior chain. It allows for extra work to the area without producing heavy soreness in the way that extra squatting and deadlifting might cause.

Second, sled drags are not as hard as pushes. That's fine. As we'll see in the programs below, moderately-paced conditioning has a role, and this will promote adherence to the program. Not every conditioning session needs to be at maximal intensity. Depending on the athlete and his training goals, sled drags may actually be preferable to pushes when done between workouts as active recovery.

Due to the excellent properties of sled conditioning, the Master training for general health and function has no need for high-volume, high-repetition lower body assistance work. Athletes can focus on heavy squats, heavy deadlifts, and any need for high-rep lower body work can be satisfied by sled pushes or drags, without the soreness, inflammation, interference and blunted recovery that accompany jogging, running, and the manifold unprogrammed thrashabout routines to be found in fitness magazines, exercise DVDs, internet videos, and "boot camps."

### Third choice: rowers and bikes

We consider these two distinct modalities together because of their similar performance, metabolic demands, and effects. Both are performed seated and both involve an upper and lower body component. Most athletes find rowers more difficult than bikes. Both exercises are tremendously challenging at higher intensities. We prefer Concept2 Rowers and Airdyne bikes, but many options are available. Airdyne bikes incorporate an upper body component, the advantages of which would seem to be obvious. Stationary bikes probably put less demand on the cardiovascular system due to the lack of an upper body component, but they are completely suitable for conditioning.

Rowers and bikes are both ***safe***, being low-impact, predominantly concentric exercises on stable surfaces. The lack of a foot-strike makes them excellent choices for trainees recovering from certain types of lower body injuries.

Both have fairly ***wide therapeutic windows***. Opportunities for manipulation of intensity, volume and other training variables are similar to those for sleds. Work intervals can be increased while rest stays at one minute. Or 1-minute intervals can be kept for work, while rest is reduced to just 30 seconds. Obviously, the model of bike or rower selected must allow for some adjustment of intensity.

As forms of HIIT, both modalities impose ***comprehensive*** conditioning stresses, and both are specific to and effective against the Sick Aging Phenotype, for reasons we have already treated at length.

Finally, both modalities are ***simple and efficient***. An easy way to begin is with simple 1 minute-on/1 minute-off protocols for 10–15 total minutes. As the trainee advances he may also benefit from much shorter workouts with much higher intensity. The classic Tabata interval program consists of 20-second work intervals followed by 10-second rest intervals. This process is repeated just 8 times. Protocols like this are highly effective, although they are best suited to trainees who have already achieved a more advanced level of conditioning. For the older, overweight, or very uncoordinated trainee, bikes have a much lower learning curve and are easier to mount and dismount than rowers. If both are available, novice Masters may prefer to begin with the bike rather than the rower.

## Also ran: traditional cardio machines

This category includes the ubiquitous treadmills, ellipticals, Stairmasters, and related species. They inhabit most commercial fitness facilities, workplace gyms, rec centers, and the invariably pathetic hotel "fitness clubs" we've all seen on the road. They also populate many home gyms. They are available in a range of sizes, shapes, quality, and price points. They are unlikely to be as effective as pushing a Prowler, dragging a sled, or intervals on an Airdyne or Concept2, but the authors understand that preferred modalities are not always available. Most of these machines can be adapted to fill in as a HIIT workout.

Treadmills are everywhere. Many of you have one somewhere in your home right now… gathering dust. The most useful feature of a treadmill is the ability to place the machine at an incline. High incline treadmill walking is an excellent exercise for a Master. In many ways, it is very close to the effects of dragging a sled. Like a sled, inclined walking can be done for a set period of time (15–20 minutes) without stopping, or used for intervals of varying lengths. It is most useful to utilize the degree of incline and not the speed of the machine to manipulate the difficulty of the exercise. The major drawback to this incline-based approach is that it can be tough on older knees, and some experimentation and monitoring is mandated when initiating a treadmill-based program. Speed should be kept moderate on a treadmill and trainees should avoid supporting their bodyweight on the handrails, which reduces the difficulty (and training stress) of the exercise. Use only the minimal support needed for balance, should it become an issue.

Stairmasters and Step-Mills are not as heavily utilized as treadmills, but are among the most misused items of cardio equipment in the gym. This is because Stairmasters and Step-Mills done with a full range of motion and minimal support from the arms are *extremely difficult.* Such effort can usually be sustained for seconds, especially at the start. At The Circus, gym members typically use the tiniest range of motion, perhaps just 2–3 inches, on the Stairmaster, while supporting most of their bodyweight on the handrails. If these machines are used, they must be used correctly, which means very short work intervals (perhaps only 20–30 seconds) followed by at least 30–60 seconds of rest. This can be repeated for as many times as the trainee's work capacity will allow. In other words, these machines are best used as a type of HIIT.

Ellipticals are useful when resistance and not speed is used as the primary training variable. Elliptical trainers at low resistance and high speed use momentum to the trainees' advantage and make the workout much easier. This means lower intensity, greater volume, and longer workouts – everything we're trying to avoid. Ellipticals work well for bouts of 30–60 seconds of high-resistance work, followed by 30–120 seconds of complete rest or slow-paced pedaling at a lower resistance for active rest. Again, this can be completed as many times as the trainee's work capacity will allow.

Most modern cardio machines have an automated setting to set up an "interval" workout for you. Some automated settings are better than others. All machines will also have a manual setting, which will allow for the construction of an individualized interval protocol.

Most traditional cardio equipment can be used for short periods of time after any training session (10–20 minutes) or utilized as its own workout on an off day from lifting.

## Not recommended: running and jogging

Running and jogging do not meet the criteria of our exercise prescription and are not recommended. Although running and jogging are certainly not particularly dangerous, they are high-impact exercises with prominent eccentric components, frequently performed outside on variable grades, and therefore are not as ***safe*** as other alternatives. These activities promote muscle soreness and fatigue, which will blunt the Master's recovery capacity. The negative orthopedic effects on the ankles, knees, and low back of the Master are unavoidable with these modalities.

Because they are not subject to the same degree of training variable manipulation as other conditioning modalities, running and jogging have a much narrower ***therapeutic window***.

As low-intensity modalities, running and jogging lack the ability to produce ***comprehensive*** metabolic and performance adaptations.

Like most forms of conditioning work, running and jogging clearly confer cardiovascular benefits and physical performance improvements, and so they are partially ***effective*** against the Sick Aging Phenotype. However, their tendency to interfere with the far more comprehensive and important activity of strength training against unhealthy aging limits their fulfillment of this criteria. The catabolic and interference effects of distance running will ultimately derail strength training progress (Chapter 4).[8]

Running and jogging are certainly ***simple*** activities, but they are hardly ***efficient***. As we have seen, the health and performance adaptations produced by running and jogging are also conferred by HIIT protocols, and in a fraction of the time.[9]

If you are a Master and you are passionate about running or some other LSD activity, we say to you: *that's your sport*, and that's great. *Lift weights and play your sport.* You won't get as strong as you could be, but you'll be strong*er*, and you'll be doing what you like to do, and you'll do it better when you're stronger. But we cannot recommend these activities as conditioning components of our General Exercise Prescription for the Masters Athlete.

### NOT RECOMMENDED: FITNESS CLASSES, BOOT CAMPS, AND OTHER GROUP THRASHABOUTS

Group thrashabouts like Zumba, BodyPump, Jazzercise, kickboxing aerobics and the like are still popular exercise options, especially for women. There is nothing magical about any of them – they are simply movement for the sake of movement. If your goal is raise your heart rate and get sweaty, group thrashabouts *will* do the job. But they are not titratable, have a poor therapeutic index, incorporate high volume, and often emphasize high-repetition eccentric movements such as squats and lunges. Even worse, some of these workouts use added weight (dumbbells or padded "barbells") for high-volume work with poor form. High volumes of eccentric work (even if light and used with partial ranges of motion) will interfere with heavy strength training. Additionally, many of these types of classes are a solid 60–90 minutes. If group class exercise is to be performed, look for options that are 30 minutes or less and done *without* a high volume of eccentric movements. This will eliminate most of them.

The criteria of our General Exercise Prescription will eliminate the rest. If you really love Zumba or kickboxing class, *go for it*. But be prepared for soreness and interference with your strength training. Group thrashabouts are not recommended for the Master.

### THE 800-POUND GORILLA: CROSSFIT

As a system, Crossfit has become too broad for neat definition, which makes it difficult to recommend as a component of the General Exercise Prescription. Crossfit programs vary based on the individual skill, expertise, and training philosophy of individual facility owners and coaches. Some Crossfit boxes are run by excellent coaches who understand how to modify and adapt the protocols for Masters Athletes. In general, however, Crossfit does not meet our exercise prescription criteria, and is not a wise conditioning option for Masters, who have no business doing high-repetition deadlifting in a state of fatigue, high-repetition box jumps, or heavy snatches for time. Masters shouldn't be using rings for dips or kipping their pull-ups. A highly individualized Crossfit program run by an experienced, well-informed, and careful coach *might* be appropriate for a few trainees in their 40s. But even the best Crossfit program won't be ideal for the 65-year old trainee.

## Conditioning Programs

It is common to see certain types of exercise programs divide strength and conditioning work into separate and distinct phases or blocks of training. For example, some trainers might recommend that preparation for a skiing trip include a 4–6 week block of training focused primarily on development of strength, with very little conditioning. This strength block would be followed by a 4–6 week conditioning block that curtails strength work in favor of running, cardio machines, or even HIIT. The problem with this approach is that both strength and conditioning will regress sharply when not trained, especially in Masters. "Peaking" strength during a 4–6 week strength block is of little value if that strength will not be available for the actual event 4–6 weeks later.

We prefer a concurrent system of training for Masters. ***Concurrent training*** works multiple physical performance attributes simultaneously. In concurrent training there is no need to drastically increase or decrease the relative volume or frequency of strength or conditioning work throughout the year. Instead, the frequency of both types of training will remain *relatively* fixed. The frequency, volume, and type of each activity are arranged so that both strength and conditioning training are complimentary. Increased strength feeds the athletes' ability to condition at high intensities, and improved conditioning enhances the effects of getting stronger and increases work capacity in the weight room.

Example 26-2 illustrates how conditioning might be integrated with various strength programs throughout the training career. *It is not prescriptive.* Coach and trainee must be guided by practical constraints, training goals, and other individual considerations. For each of the programs in the example, we have suggested how either sled work (drags or pulls) or HIIT (with a bike or rower) could be incorporated. But the particular conditioning modality in any individual case will be determined by the needs of the athlete, the judgment of the coach, and the facilities available.

During the rank and early novice phases, conditioning work is not indicated, and will only interfere with the recovery processes essential for strength acquisition. For the novice, improvement in conditioning comes from getting stronger. Conditioning work during the main novice phase is usually not indicated either, but if it is incorporated, the goal should be enhancement of exercise capacity. One day a week at most will do, ideally during the weekend, when the athlete has the longest recovery interval.

Intermediate and advanced programs allow more frequent conditioning work, but the inclusion of this work must be *to address the specific needs of the individual athlete, not to fill up available space in the program.* Athletes and coaches must assign the proper importance to active rest and recovery. Any imposition of conditioning work that interferes with progress in the program or performance in the Arena of Life is contraindicated. Example 26-2 represents the *maximum* amount of conditioning work a trainee at the specified levels should perform. For many Masters, the appropriate amount of conditioning will be less – usually *much* less.

## Conditioning for the Very Aged and Detrained: The Magic of Walking

For older and more deconditioned athletes, walking may constitute a significant and very valuable training stress. A brisk walk may be difficult even for some trainees in their 40s and 50s, depending on their individual strength and conditioning decline. Remember, a training stress is *any* activity that disrupts homeostasis and produces a meaningful physical adaptation. For the extremely feeble and/or deconditioned, the simple act of walking could even serve as a short-term stimulus for strength development (the novice effect). But for most it is simply the very beginning of a basic conditioning plan. Many older adults look to activities that include lots of walking (shopping, outdoor excursions, etc) with apprehension and dread. Strength training combined with a brisk daily walk can make these events more tractable and enjoyable. Eventually, walking will no longer disrupt homeostasis and will become a daily life activity, rather than a training stimulus. That's a good thing.

Walking is a great place to begin a conditioning plan because logistically it presents

**Example 26-2: Integrating Conditioning with Strength Training**

**2- and 3-Day Rank and Early Novice**

*No specific conditioning work.*

**3-Day Novice**

| | |
|---|---|
| Mon | Strength training |
| Tue | Rest |
| Wed | Strength training |
| Thu | Rest |
| Fri | Strength training |
| Sat | **Conditioning** (high-volume sled) |
| Sun | Rest |

**3-Day Advanced Novice**

| | |
|---|---|
| Mon | Strength training |
| Tue | Rest |
| Wed | Strength training w/ light squat day, **Conditioning** (moderate-volume sled) |
| Thu | Rest |
| Fri | Strength training |
| Sat | **Conditioning** (high-volume sled) |
| Sun | Rest |

**2-Day Novice or Intermediate Programs**

| | |
|---|---|
| Mon | Strength training |
| Tue | Active Recovery, **Conditioning** (HIIT) |
| Wed | Rest |
| Thu | Strength training |
| Fri | **Conditioning** (HIIT) |
| Sat | **Conditioning** (HIIT) |
| Sun | Rest |

**3-Day Intermediate Programs**

| | |
|---|---|
| Mon | Strength training: Volume day (TM) or Heavy day (HLM) |
| Tue | Light active recovery, **Conditioning** (low-volume, low-intensity sled) |
| Wed | Light full-body strength, **Conditioning** (low-volume, moderate-intensity sled) |
| Thu | Rest |
| Fri | Intensity day or medium full-body strength, **Conditioning** (bike or rower HIIT) |
| Sat | **Conditioning** (high-volume sled) |
| Sun | Rest |

**4-Day Intermediate Programs**

| | |
|---|---|
| Mon | Volume bench/press |
| Tue | Volume squat, **Conditioning** (low-volume HIIT) |
| Wed | Active recovery |
| Thu | Intensity bench/press |
| Fri | Intensity squat/ deadlift, **Conditioning** (low-volume HIIT) |
| Sat | Active recovery, **Conditioning** (high-volume HIIT) |
| Sun | Rest |

virtually no limitations. It doesn't require the acquisition of a new movement pattern. It requires no special equipment. Weather is no obstacle: most local malls and even some hospitals are crowded with "mall walkers" who gather at a prearranged time to trek several loops around the facility. A controlled climate and plenty of seating for brief respites takes away most of the excuses one might have for not going on a simple walk.

The benefit of walking is that it isn't very stressful. The downside is that it isn't very stressful. This means that, very quickly, simply walking *more* isn't going to produce progressive improvements in conditioning. Walking is not particularly subject to volume manipulation for progression, and just walking more often will be of limited value.

Instead, the trainee should look to make walks more challenging within a set period of time. Certainly, one can walk *faster.* And this is not a bad idea, but also runs its course very quickly as speed can only be built up to a certain level before a walk becomes a jog. Finding a course that incorporates hills, an inclined ramp or street, or even a long stair case into the route is an excellent idea for increasing the intensity of the walk. Ideally, long gradual slopes are best when beginning this type of activity, but most trainees will be limited by what is available to them in their local communities. The potential downside to incorporating hills, ramps, and stairs into the walking routine is the requirement to *go back down* the hill or ramp. Going downhill is often more uncomfortable than going uphill, especially for trainees with older, more sensitive knees. The forces absorbed by the knee to decelerate the body on a downhill slope can promote joint pain and inflammation. If the trainee is to introduce hills, ramps, and slopes into the routine, he should do so gradually and pay attention to the effects of the activity on the knees, ankles, hips, and lower back.

For those without access to hills or slopes, light loading of the torso is acceptable. The best equipment for this is a weighted vest. The ideal vest is one that evenly spreads the load from front to back, fits snugly with adjustable straps, and can allow for load to be scaled. Weighted vests are available as light as 10 pounds and in excess of 80 pounds. For the sake of the feet, ankles, and knees, trainees should start with the lightest weight available and very gradually increase weight based on overall tolerance. While walking with a weighted vest, trainees should pay careful attention to their posture. Stand up tall, keep the chest up, and maintain a slight arch in the lower back. The tendency will be to slouch forward once fatigue sets in. This puts undue pressure on the lower back. The day after the first weighted vest walking session, trainees can expect to feel some soreness in their abdominals, obliques, and spinal erectors. Soreness may be most pronounced in the trapezius. Soreness should be moderate and likely won't recur after a few sessions with the vest.

Another variation of weighted walking is the *farmer's walk*, consisting of walking for time or for distance while carrying a heavy load in each hand (*heavy* being relative to the individual). For professional strongmen, farmer's walks are done with as much as 250 pounds per hand. For the deconditioned older adult, loads starting at 10–20 pounds per hand or less may be appropriate. Farmer's walks can be a very simple indoor introduction to HIIT style training for the older, deconditioned adult, building endurance and work capacity and also grip strength, an often-overlooked victim of aging. Farmer's walks are done as intervals, usually for distance. The trainee will walk a chosen distance, say 20–50 yards, and then set the weight down and rest for a minute or so. He will repeat this process as many times as possible with a weight that challenges his ability to complete the distance without dropping it.

Most other types of loaded walking are not recommended. For instance, carrying weight in a backpack is not necessarily a good way to train – although backpacking may be an event to train for. It is preferable to distribute the load as evenly as possible around the torso as a good weighted vest will do.

Ankle weights are a quick recipe for patellar and hip flexor tendonitis when added to a long distance walk. We do not recommended adding weight to the legs while walking.

## Setting up the Walking Program

If the trainee is very deconditioned, walking routines should begin with *short but frequent* sessions. Trainees may start with as little as 5–10 minutes per day, but should aim for 5–6 days/week. Short, frequent walks are preferred over trying to go for a very long distance or time just 1–2 days/week. Shorter sessions allow time for the feet and lower body joints to adapt to the activity. High frequency speeds up the adaptation, but is also important for establishing the habit of walking. For a Master struggling psychologically and emotionally with beginning an exercise program, frequency is critical. Every day that training occurs (even a simple

10 minute walk) is a minor victory that builds confidence and momentum for the more difficult, more complex training to come.

Anyone for whom the simple act of walking serves as a training stimulus will be a novice strength trainee. By the time the trainee moves onto more complex programming, walking as a form of actual conditioning training will be a thing of the past. Even for most novices, after several weeks of consistent daily walks, it will no longer serve as an effective conditioning stimulus, *but rather as active rest.* Increased levels of conditioning will only be achieved through more intense modalities.

Example 26-3 illustrates a training week for a very deconditioned trainee layering a walking routine on top of a novice strength training plan. As the trainee builds strength and conditioning, walking duration can increase and eventually be replaced with more intense protocols. Walking sled drags or pushes at light weight are an excellent transitions from unloaded walking.

**Example 26-3: A Sample Walking Program for the Novice Master**

| | |
|---|---|
| Mon | (AM) Barbell training;<br>(PM) 10–15-minute walk |
| Tue | 10–15-minute walk |
| Wed | (AM) Barbell training;<br>(PM) 10–15-minute walk |
| Thu | Complete Rest |
| Fri | (AM) Barbell training;<br>(PM) 10–15-minute walk |
| Sat | 20–30-minute walk |
| Sun | Complete rest |

# 27

# The Female Master

The female Master will benefit from barbell training using the same exercises and programs as her male counterparts. A small number of minor modifications are often indicated. Female athletes have less strength, neuromuscular efficiency, power production, and muscle mass than men, and have less upper body strength relative to lower body strength. On the other hand, they are able to perform multiple repetitions at a higher percentage of their 1RM, tend to recover faster, and can tolerate higher training frequency and volume overall. Many female Masters can use the programs presented in this book as written. When indicated, the most common modifications for the female Master will be to switch from a 3 sets of 5 to 5 sets of 3 set design for high-volume training stress, switch from sets of 5 to sets of 1–3 for high-intensity/low-volume training stress, and increase the volume or frequency of deadlifts. Frequently voiced concerns that barbell training will endow the female Master with a "bulky," masculine phenotype and grotesque muscular hypertrophy are so completely unfounded as to be ridiculous. In this chapter, therefore, we ridicule them.

## Last But Not Least

We conclude this work with a short chapter dedicated to the female Master. We are at pains to make it clear that the position and brevity of this chapter should *not* indicate to the reader that the female Master is an afterthought in our deliberations. Rather, they should indicate to the reader that, with a few minor exceptions, the female Master should train in almost *exactly* the same way, and for *exactly* the same reasons, as her male counterpart.

Indeed, we would argue that barbell training, while beneficial to all aging adults, is *particularly* indicated for the female Master. Life is not fair, and the aging female loses muscle, bone, and strength at a greater rate than her male counterparts. Because the beneficial effects of resistance training are so acutely needed and easy to observe in this population, strength training is fortunately growing in popularity with female Masters…and sometimes even their doctors.

In this chapter we highlight some of the physiological differences between male and female athletes, and their implications for the female Master. But our broader objective is to emphasize to the reader that, notwithstanding a few minor modifications that may be indicated for some women, strength training for the female Master is almost identical to that for the male, proceeds in the same manner, is directed at the same goals, and has the same underlying structure.

First, however, it is incumbent upon us to disabuse the reader of a widespread and pernicious misconception about the effects of barbell training on female athletes.

## On the Chimerical Horrors of *Bulking Up*

Despite the growing body of data on the benefits of strength training for women and the increased popularity of barbell training for female Masters, we must concede that barriers to widespread application remain. Physicians, the commercial fitness industry, conventional wisdom, and that great purveyor of misinformation, the Internet, have quite thoroughly indoctrinated most women in the unfounded belief that their exercise prescription must be radically different from the male's. The answer is usually cardio, and lots of it, with little or no strength component. If resistance training is included at all, it inevitably involves low intensity and endless reps, usually with tiny pink neoprene dumbbells or some equally silly modality.

The exponents of this form of exercise medicine, which is *contraindicated* for the female Master and belied by the huge volume of data reviewed in Part I, rely on all manner of discredited arguments: an inflated risk of injury, groundless assertions that weight training is "bad for the knees" or "bad for the back," the disproven myth that weight training will "increase your blood pressure," or "give you a stroke," and so on. And if those arguments against strength training fail to keep the women-folk in their place, then YouTube fitness gurus, magazines, and misguided doctors have an ace-in-the-hole. They need only invoke the terror that lurks in the heart of every Decent Lady: the ghastly specter of ***Bulking-Up***.

Life, particularly for the aging adult, holds no shortage of horrors, but *Bulking-Up* surely ranks in the top tier of nightmares. After a few weeks or months of barbell training in the novice phase, the female Master awakens one morning to find herself confronted in the bathroom mirror by an appalling apparition: Schwarzenegger in a nightie. She is now a mass of grotesque muscular hypertrophy. Her once-willowy and tender frame is now distorted by rock-hard mounds of striated flesh that would embarrass a Marvel superhero. An unsightly arabesque of purple veins criss-crosses her once-smooth skin. Her breasts have been completely resorbed, replaced by the rippling pectoral muscles of a powerlifting Neanderthal. Her shoulders are as broad as a semi-truck, her hips as narrow as a teenage boy's. Her clothes don't fit. Her dog is scared of her. Her husband has run off with his anorectic secretary, revolted and terrified by the misshapen creature who now shares his bed.

Of course, *she had this coming*: Everybody warned her. "Weight training? You're going to *Bulk-Up*, Ellen! Come to Pilates class with me, dear."

But *no*, she wouldn't listen. Ellen just *had* to lift heavy weights and get strong, and now she has reaped the bitter harvest of her poor lifestyle choices: *Bulking-Up*. She'll have to live with that – but of course her husband, children, friends, employers, and pets won't have to. *Bulking-Up* is a lonely way of life. Who wants to be around Schwarzenegger in a nightie?

Nobody, of course, but then, he's just a bogeyman.[1] We can all wake up from this nightmare now, because it's just that – a silly fantasy with no basis in reality. Virtually any female Master can and should add muscle to her frame with strength training. When she does, she'll feel better, perform better, live better, and yes, she'll *look* better. But in the absence of very specific, long-term, extreme training combined with anabolic supplements (none of which are recommended or discussed anywhere in this text), the exaggerated hypertrophy of the *Bulking-Up* nightmare is a practical impossibility for the female Master.

## Physiological Differences

Women are not as strong as men. We quite deliberately skirt any discussion of the cultural, political, teleological, or social implications of this announcement, and simply report the fact of the matter.[2] Of course, *some* women are stronger than *some* men, but that is simply an instance of phenotypic variation. On the whole, women are smaller, have less muscle mass, and are not able to produce as much force, or as high a rate of force development, as their male counterparts. This is due to multiple factors, including much lower resting and post-exercise levels of testosterone,[3] lower muscle and muscle fiber cross-sectional area,[4] smaller Type II fibers relative to Type I fibers, and less acute angles (*pennation*) of muscle fiber attachment. Women appear to have somewhat lower power output and rate of force development than men, although the differences narrow when corrected for fat-free mass, and are probably due at least in part to differences in motor unit recruitment and the frequency of motor unit firing (*rate coding*), in addition to the hormonal and structural differences already mentioned.

The ability, or lack thereof, to recruit the maximum number of motor units into a movement pattern has programming implications for both sexes. The rank novice (regardless of age or sex) does not yet possess the neuromuscular efficiency to produce a significant amount of training stress in a single training session. So a novice can perform a "heavy" squat workout with 3 sets of 5 reps. The athlete can recover and return in 48–72 hours to repeat the 3 sets of 5 reps with even more weight. The ability to do this does not come from a superhuman capacity to recover and adapt, but rather the inability to produce a level of training stress that would prevent it.

As the novice (again, regardless of age or sex) grows in strength and experience, his ability to produce stress increases. At first, this is primarily (but *not* entirely) due to an increase in neuromuscular efficiency – the ability to recruit more muscle fibers into a loaded movement pattern. Later gains are dominated by the addition of muscle. So by the late novice phase, improved neuromuscular efficiency and the addition of more contractile tissue allow the athlete to impose a training stress that challenges the capacity to recover. All of these factors – improvement in neuromuscular efficiency, addition of muscle, and the capacity to recover and adapt – are governed by multiple innate factors, including genetic endowment, age, pre-existing medical conditions, and, not inconsequentially, sex.

The female athlete, and in particular the female Master, will find that long-term improvements in neuromuscular efficiency and muscle accretion will be more difficult and come more slowly. As a consequence, female Masters will retain many characteristics of the novice longer than will their male counterparts. This doesn't necessarily mean that female Masters will remain in the novice phase longer. But the *relatively* smaller training stresses that a female Master is capable of absorbing has implications for her programming. For the female athlete, an understanding of this concept is important when evaluating the potential effectiveness of a programming change. *The more a particular program relies on a single high-stress event, the less likely it is to be effective for a female athlete.* Instead, many female Masters will require multiple high-stress events per workout (i.e. more sets) performed multiple times per week, even as intermediate or advanced trainees. This is in contrast to many intermediate male Masters who *may* require decreases in both volume in frequency.

## Programming Implications

Although physiological differences discussed in the previous section limit the strength and power performance of women relative to men, it is critical to observe that the physiology of muscle tissue is far more similar between the sexes than it is different, and the Stress-Recovery-Adaptation cycle can be fully exploited by the female Master. While sex differences certainly have an impact on the *absolute* strength available to a Master, they have only minimal impact on *how* that strength can be attained. The female Master will pursue training in almost exactly the same way as her male counterpart. She will proceed through the same programs, use the same exercises, make the same indicated adjustments in the advanced novice and intermediate phases, and observe the same fastidious attention to recovery factors. Indeed, our experience shows that a large proportion of female Masters make excellent progress with the programs we have presented in this book *without modification.* That said, there are minor modifications that appear to optimize training for many in this population.

We have observed that a 5-rep max (5RM) for a male athlete is roughly 85–88% of his 1RM strength depending on the exercise and the trainee. For females, 5RM strength appears to be about 10% higher. This means that a female athlete might be able to perform 5-reps with roughly 95% of her 1RM. Again, depending on the individual and the exercise, the average male *might* manage a double at 95% of 1RM.

If we assume that females have lower neuromuscular efficiency (less complete motor unit recruitment and slower rate coding) we may reasonably attribute the difference in 1RM/5RM ratios to the fact that the trained male athlete is recruiting nearly all of his available motor units into a true 1RM attempt, while the female is not. Accordingly, she can perform more reps with a higher percentage of her 1RM strength than he can. This has several implications for programming.

### Women can train productively with fewer reps/set

During the intermediate or even the late novice phase, the female athlete and her coach *may* find that sets of 5 are not adequate to impose a training stress. Remember the novice effect – any reasonable training stimulus is sufficient to force a strength adaption at first, and for a short time. Eventually, however, the stimulus must be fine-tuned to fully exploit the Stress-Recovery-Adaptation cycle. In this regard, the 5-rep set for a female may be analogous to the 10-rep set for a male. It's just not heavy enough relative to her maximum to force a strength adaptation.

Accordingly, switching to sets of 3 across may be warranted when progress begins to slow on the 5-rep set. When working 3s across, most male athletes would be working in excess of 90% of 1RM – unsustainable for men for more than a few weeks before regression occurs. Females using 3s across at about 95% 1RM can often maintain progress for weeks or even months, provided progression is conservative from workout to workout.

For the female intermediate trainee, 4–6 sets of 3 can replace the 5-rep model for the accumulation of volume and training stress. If 3s are to be used to accumulate volume, then high-intensity work should be all singles and doubles across.

It is critical to keep in mind, however, that 3-rep sets across for a female might be 95% of 1RM strength. In practical terms this might mean a difference of just 5–10 pounds, or less. When first selecting weights for high-intensity work (think Texas Method intensity day) athlete and coach should be careful not to overload the barbell. The female Master might be able to squat 135x3x5, yet fail a single at 155 pound. Load conservatively when attempting high-intensity sets for the first time.

### Women recover faster – between sets and between sessions

Because women are producing less stress during a given set, they can and usually should train at proportionally higher volumes than men during each individual workout. When performing 3-rep sets across as novices, women will do well to perform 4–6 work sets. Fortunately, many female trainees can move through these higher-set volumes relatively quickly, perhaps more quickly than a male can get through 3 sets of 5. Less stress during the set means that shorter interset rest intervals are feasible.

In our experience, women also have considerably less trouble with delayed onset muscle soreness (DOMS). DOMS is primarily a result of the eccentric component of a movement, in which women appear to have a physiological and performance advantage. Less soreness means that women can often tolerate a higher frequency of training, particularly heavy sessions. The female novice Master is more likely to be able to stay with a 3-day training model much longer than her male counterparts, who often do better on lower frequency training. She won't need a mid-week light squat day as early, and she can deadlift more often, later into her program. She may do better with aggressive Texas Method-style programming than men of the same age. Training heavy twice a week (once for volume, once for intensity) will be too much for some male Masters, who often do better with Heavy-Light and Heavy-Light-Medium systems. Many female Masters will do much better with 2 heavy days/week. In fact, they may even detrain on programs that only ask them to lift heavy once a week.

### The pulling program

We have observed the most pronounced differences in programming between the sexes with the deadlift. For men, especially Masters, extraordinary care has to be taken in programming heavy deadlifts beyond the novice level in order to avoid overtraining the exercise – and the athlete.

Women, on the other hand, seem to do better with slightly higher deadlift volume during a particular session, and can also tolerate deadlifting at a higher frequency. Like the early novice, many female Masters can tolerate deadlifts multiple times per week and may need multiple sets per workout in order to progress, even as late-stage novices and early intermediates. In intermediate training, deadlifts can even be used for volume accumulation for sets of 3 across, and performed later in the week for singles or doubles.

Lower neuromuscular efficiency has important implications for power production. Power production is certainly a trainable quality for any athlete, to the extent that strength is a component of power. However, power is also highly dependent on the ability of the athlete to rapidly, *almost instantaneously* recruit a large amount of muscle mass. *That* particular ability is almost entirely genetic. This means that athletically gifted males have an innate genetic advantage over less gifted males in their ability to recruit muscle mass into explosive movement patterns. This also means that younger males will express power more efficiently than older males, and men will express power more efficiently than women – even women who become very strong.

So what are the implications for barbell training? As we have pointed out repeatedly, explosive exercises such as power cleans and power snatches have inherent limitations in their overall contribution to the Masters strength program. For many Masters, they will be relatively contraindicated, and will actually do little to promote the ability to move explosively. They are also not the best choice for volume accumulation in the pulling program. The athlete will simply not be able to move enough weight on a clean or a snatch to have any meaningful transfer to the deadlift. If the female Master can safely perform power cleans and power snatches, she will include them in her training program only because she *wants* to, not because she needs to.

The genetic limitations on power also have some implications for dynamic effort training. While dynamic effort sets have proven useful for many male Masters, they may not prove useful for a particular female Master. If dynamic effort sets are to be used, they will likely have to be done with heavier loads relative to males. On average, loads of around 85% of 1RM will be appropriate for a female Master using dynamic effort – certainly no less than 80%.

### Women have less upper body strength

This is a common observation, although some who work with younger female athletes have begun to question it. The difference in relative strength between the lower body and upper body appears to be less marked in highly trained females. It is certainly true that a female Master will have less absolute strength on all exercises compared to her male counterparts. But the *rate of increase* in her squat and deadlift strength will usually parallel that of the male Master – female and male strength curves for these exercises will have similar slopes. In our experience, however, the strength curves for the press and bench will diverge relatively early for the female Master. Women can train to put up impressive presses and bench presses, but their programming will usually have to accommodate the relatively lower upper body strength of the female and anticipate less rapid gains in these movements.

Example 27-1 shows some of the above principles at work in the setting of the novice-to-intermediate progression for a female Master.

### Example 27-1: Novice-to-Intermediate Progression for the Female Master

#### Phase I: Standard Novice Progression, Sets of 5 across

| | Monday | Wednesday | Friday |
|---|---|---|---|
| **Week 1** | Squat 45x5x3 | Squat 50x5x3 | Squat 55x5x3 |
| | Bench 45x5x3 | Press 33x5x3 | Bench 47x5x3 |
| | Deadlift 75x5 | Deadlift 85x5 | Deadlift 95x5 |
| **Week 2** | Squat 60x5x3 | Squat 65x5x3 | Squat 70x5x3 |
| | Bench 49x5x3 | Press 35x5x3 | Bench 51x5x3 |
| | Deadlift 105x5 | Deadlift 115x5 | Deadlift 120x5 |

#### Phase II: Novice Progression, Switch to multiple sets of triples

| | Monday | Wednesday | Friday |
|---|---|---|---|
| **Week 3** | Squat 75x3x4 | Squat 80x3x4 | Squat 85x3x4 |
| | Bench 53x3x4 | Press 37xx3x4 | Bench 55x3x4 |
| | Deadlift 125x3x2 | Deadlift 135x3x2 | Deadlift 140x3x2 |
| **Week 4** | Squat 90x3x4 | Squat 95x3x4 | Squat 100x3x4 |
| | Bench 57x3x4 | Press 40x3x4 | Bench 60x3x4 |
| | Deadlift 145x3x2 | Deadlift 150x3x2 | Deadlift 155x3x2 |

#### Phase III: Switch to Intermediate, Texas Method Style Program

| | Monday | Wednesday | Friday |
|---|---|---|---|
| **Week 5** | Squat 105x3x5 | Light Squat 95x3x2 | Squat 115x2x2 |
| | Bench 62x3x5 | Press 42x3x4 | Bench 68x2x2 |
| | Deadlift 160x3x2 | Lat Pulls 4x8 | Deadlift 170x2 |
| **Week 6** | Squat 107x3x5 | Light Squat 97x3x2 | Squat 117x2x2 |
| | Bench 64x3x5 | Press 44x3x4 | Bench 70x2x2 |
| | Deadlift 163x3x2 | | Deadlift 173x2 |

*Phases are shown as 2-week blocks *for the purposes of illustration only.*

### THE BOTTOM LINE: FEMALE MASTERS ARE A *LITTLE* DIFFERENT

We conclude this final chapter by emphasizing, again, that the female Master is *just not that different* from her male counterpart. She will pursue the same training goals, using the same exercises and programs. She will enter the novice program (Program 2A, Chapter 19) *as written* and proceed like any male Master, unless and until a modification is *indicated* to initiate training or maintain progress. Such modification will almost always take the form of a slight relative decrease in the rate of progression in the pressing movements, a switch from 3 sets of 5 to 5 sets of 3, and/or an increase in pulling volume or frequency. Many female Masters will continue to make progress without *any* of these modifications, or will require one or more of them only later in the training career.

In all cases, the fundamentals will remain the same: regular training, with a view to long-term progressive improvements in the General Fitness Attributes, proper performance of a small set of big multi-joint barbell exercises, assiduous attention to recovery factors, and proper record-keeping and analysis. Above all, athlete and coach must always bear in mind the underlying structure of *any* rational exercise prescription: the Stress-Recovery-Adaptation cycle.

# Acknowledgements

The production of this book benefited enormously from the contribution of many of our friends, family members, colleagues, and clients.

Above all, the authors thank their friend and mentor, Mark Rippetoe, for his support and guidance in all things barbell training. More than 35 years of experience on the platform have made him an incredible resource, and we continue to learn from him, year after year. Rip's many contributions to the literature on fitness are changing the way the world thinks about exercise, and this book simply would not exist without him.

We are indebted to stef bradford PhD for her guidance in preparing the manuscript for submission and editing, and for the beautiful layout and design of the book – not to mention all the other things she does to keep the world of Starting Strength going.

Mary Conover RN not only prepared the index but also made suggestions that improved the manuscript considerably. And her constant encouragement and support were invaluable at those times when the project seemed interminable and intractable. Can't thank you enough, Mary.

Simma Park transformed Sullivan's original sketches into beautiful illustrations. Jordan Feigenbaum MD made invaluable comments and suggestions for the recovery chapter and the section on nutrition. Our discussions with Joshua Lowndes contributed to our refinement of the sections on bioenergetics.

We must also thank our first readers and others whose advice, critical review, and support contributed to the completion of this project: Margaret Moran, Chris and Dan Lauffer, Val and John Rosengren, Nicholas Racculia, Janet Spangler, M.S. Patterson, Bob Grant, Lt Col Christian "Mac" Ward, Paul Horn, Tom Campitelli, Chris Kurisko, Lesia McQuade, Jeff Taylor, Scott Freeman MD, Anthony Lagina MD, Blaine White MD, Will Morris DPT, John Petrizzo DPT, Steve Hill, and Nick Delgadillo. We've probably left somebody out, for which we apologize in advance.

Finally, we express our gratitude to the clients, friends, and family members who have been so patient with us (and without us) during the long grind of hard work and self-mortification that produced this book.

Sorry, all. But *somebody* had to write it.

# Notes

## Chapter 1 – The Sick Aging Phenotype


1. Fauci and Morens, "Perpetual Challenge of Infectious Diseases," 454-461.
2. Fulginiti, "The Millennium in Infectious Diseases"
3. Jones, Podolsky, and Greene, "The Burden of Disease" 2333-2338; Armstrong, Conn, Pinner, "Trends in Infectious Diseases," 61-66.
4. Kata, "Anti-vaccine Activists," 3778-3789; Gross, "A Broken Trust," e1000114; Eggerston, "Lancet Retracts 12-year-old Article."
5. Rana et al., "Cardiovascular Metabolic Syndrome," 218-232.
6. National Vital Statistics Report 2002.
7. National Vital Statistics Report 2002; Ogden et al., "Prevalence of Obesity"; Park et al., "The Metabolic Syndrome," 427-436.
8. Omran, "The Epidemiological Transition," 509-538; Mackenbach, "The Epidemiologic Transition Theory," 329-331.
9. Park et al., "The Metabolic Syndrome," 427-436; Johannson and Sundquist, "Change in Lifestyle Factors," 1073-1080; van Dam et al., "Combined Impact of Lifestyle Factors."
10. Gary Taubes, *Good Calories, Bad Calories.*
11. Penninx et al., "Metabolic Syndrome and Physical Decline," 96-102.
12. Rana et al., "Cardiovascular Metabolic Syndrome," 218-232; International Diabetes Federation, "IDF Consensus Worldwide Definition."
13. Ford, Giles, and Dietz, "Prevalence of Metabolic Syndrome," 356–359.
14. Rana et al., "Cardiovascular Metabolic Syndrome," 218-232.
15. Monteiro and Azevedo, "Chronic Inflammation in Obesity," 228-32.
16. Barzilay et al., "Insulin Resistance and Inflammation," 635-641; Ottenbacher et al., "Diabetes Mellitus as a Risk Factor," M658-M653.
17. Roger et al., "Heart Disease and Stroke Statistics," e18-e209.
18. Horwich and Fonarow, "Glucose, Obesity, Metabolic Syndrome," 283-293.
19. Kurella, Lo, and Chertow, "Metabolic Syndrome and Chronic Kidney Disease," 2134-2140.
20. Esposito et al., "High Proportions of Erectile Dysfunction," 1201-1203; Amidu et al., "Metabolic Syndrome and Sexual Dysfunction," 42-50; Riedner et al., "Central Obesity is an Independent Predictor," 1519-1523.
21. Rasgon and Jarvik L, "Insulin Resistance, Affective Disorders,"178-183.
22. Rana et al., "Cardiovascular Metabolic Syndrome," 218-232.
23. Grundy, "Obesity, Metabolic Syndrome, and Cardiovascular Disease," 2595-2600.
24. Rana et al., "Cardiovascular Metabolic Syndrome," 218-232; Horwich and Fonarow, "Glucose, Obesity, Metabolic Syndrome," 283-293; Grundy, "Obesity, Metabolic Syndrome, and Cardiovascular Disease," 2595-2600; Inelman et al., "Can Obesity be a Risk Factor," 147-55; Despres and Lemieux, "Abdominal Obesity and Metabolic Syndrome," 881-887; Campos, "The Obesity Myth"; Campos et al., "Epidemiology of Overweight and Obesity," 55-60; Kim and Popkin, "Understanding the Epidemiology of Overweight," 60-67; Rigby, "Commentary: Counterpoint to Campos et al.," 79-80; Stevens, McClain, and Truesdale, "Obesity Claims and Controversies," 77-78.

25. Rana et al., "Cardiovascular Metabolic Syndrome," 218-232; Mokdad et al., "Type 2 Diabetes Trends," 1278-1283.
26. Ferreira et al., "Development of Fitness, Fatness and Lifestyle," 42-48; Cho, Park H, and Seo, "Lifestyle and Metabolic Syndrome," 150-159; Lakka et al., "Sedentary Lifestyle, Poor Cardiorespiratory Fitness," 1279-1286; Panagiotakos et al., "Impact of Lifestyle Habits,"106-112.
27. The insulin-receptor-downregulation model is a simple one, and does not capture the complexity of what is going on. But it will do for our purposes.
28. Menon, Ram, and Sperling. "Insulin as a Growth Factor," 633-647; Pollak, "Insulin and Insulin-like Growth Factor Signaling," 915-928; Hill and Milner, "Insulin as a Growth Factor," 879-886.
29. Berg, Tymoczko, and Stryer. "Food Intake and Starvation Induce Metabolic Changes."
30. Endothelial cells.
31. Eghbalzadeh et al., "Skeletal Muscle Nitric Oxide Synthases."
32. Esposito et al., "High Proportions of Erectile Dysfunction," 1201-1203; Amidu et al., "Metabolic Syndrome and Sexual Dysfunction," 42-50.
33. Rana et al., "Cardiovascular Metabolic Syndrome," 218-232; Strasser, Arvandi, and Siebert, "Resistance Training, Visceral Obesity," 578-591.
34. Grundy, "Obesity, Metabolic Syndrome, and Cardiovascular Disease," 2595-2600.
35. Maury and Brichard,. "Adipokine Dysregulation," 1-16; Bozaoglu et al., "Chemerin is a Novel Adipokine," 4687-4694; Whitehead et al., "Adiponectin: A Key Adipokine," 264-280.
36. NNT, "Statin Drugs Given for 5 Years"; Mahdavi et al., "Dyslipidemia and Cardiovascular Disease," 157-158; Ray et al., "Statins and All-cause Mortality," 1024-1031.
37. Hooper et al. "Reduced or Modified Dietary Fat"; Siri-Tarino et al., "Saturated Fat, Carbohydrate, and Cardiovascular Disease," 502-509; Chowdury et al., "Dietary, Circulating and Supplemental Fatty Acids" 398-406.
38. Taylor et al. "Statins for Primary Prevention"; Abramson and Wright, "Lipid-lowering Agents Evidence-based?" 168-169; Teicholz, "Questionable Link between Saturated Fat and Heart Disease."
39. Grundy, "Obesity, Metabolic Syndrome, and Cardiovascular Disease," 2595-2600.; Strasser, Arvandi, and Siebert, "Resistance Training, Visceral Obesity," 578-591.
40. Dominguez and Barbagello, "Cardiometabolic Syndrome and Sarcopenic Obesity," 183-189.
41. den Heijer et al., "Type 2 Diabetes and Atrophy," 1604-1610; Convit, "Cognitive Impairment in Insulin Resistance," 31-35; Willette et al., "Insulin Resistance, Brain Atrophy," 443-449.
42. Blaum et al., "Obesity and the Frailty Syndrome," 927-934; Fried et al., "Frailty in Older Adults," M146-M157.
43. NNT, "Statin Drugs Given for 5 Years"; Abramson and Wright, "Lipid-lowering Agents evidence-based?" 168-9.
44. Thompson, Clarkson, and Karas, "Statin-associated Myopathy," 1681-1690.
45. Culver et al., "Statin Use and Risk of Eiabetes Mellitus," 144-152; Sattar et al., "Statins and Risk of Diabetes," 735-742.
46. Hajjar, Cafiero , and Hanlon, "Polypharmacy in Elderly Patients," 345-351.
47. O'Gara et al., "Management of ST-elevation Myocardial Infarction," e362-345.
48. Johannson and Sundquist, "Lifestyle Factors and Health," 1073-1080; van Dam et al., "Combined Impact of Lifestyle Factors."; Malik et al., "Impact of the Metabolic Syndrome," 1245-1250.
49. Batsis et al, "Normal Weight Obesity and Mortality," 1592-1598.

## Chapter 2 – Exercise Medicine

1 Berryman, "Exercise is Medicine," 195-201.

2. Sallis, "Exercise is Medicine and Physicians," 3-4.
3. Dornerman et al., "Effects of High-intensity Resistance Exercise," 246-251; Engelke et al., "Exercise Maintains Bone Density," 133-142; Kemmler et al., "Benefits of 2 Years of Intense Exercise," 1084-1091.
4. Hoffman, "Arthritis and Exercise," 895-810.
5. Kubo et al., "Effect of Low-load Resistance Training," 25-32; Bucchanna and Marsh, "Effects of Exercise on Properties of Tendons," 1101-1107.
6. Morrisey, Harman, and Johnson, "Resistance Training Modes," 648-660.
7. Brach et al., "Physical Function and Lifestyle Activity," 502-509.
8. Borghouts and Keizer, "Exercise and Insulin Sensitivity," 1-12.
9. Pedersen, "Muscles and their Myokines," 337-346; Pedersen, "Exercise-induced Myokines," 811-816.
10. Kavanagh, "Exercise in Cardiac Rehabilitation," 3-6; Myers, "Exercise and Cardiovascular Health," e2-e5; Shephard and Balady, "Exercise as Cardiovascular Therapy," 963-972; Morriss et al., "Vigorous Exercise in Leisure-time," 333-339; Bonanno and Lies, "Effects of Physical Training on Coronary Risk," 760-764.
11. Pollack et al., "Resistance Exercise in Individuals," 828-833.
12. Nied and Franklin, "Promoting and Prescribing Exercise," 419-426; Li and Siegrist, "Physical Activity and Risk of Cardiovascular Disease," 391-407; Sattelmair et al., "Dose-response Physical Activity," 789-795; Ahmed et al., "Effects of Physical Activity," 288-295.
13. Borghouts and Keizer, "Exercise and Insulin Sensitivity," 1-12; Albright et al., "Exercise and Type 2 Diabetes," 1345-1360; Stensvold et al., "Strength Training v Aerobic Training," 804-810; Strasser, Siebert, and Schobersberger, "Resistance Training in the Treatment of Metabolic Syndrome," 397-415.
14. Vega et al., "Effect of Resistance Exercise on Growth Factors," 982-986; Kraemer and Ratamess, "Hormonal Responses and Adaptations," 339-361.
15. Cotman, Berchtold, and Christie, "Exercise Builds Brain Health," 464-472.
16. Petrides et al., "Exercise-induced Activation of the HPA-axis," 377-383; Ciloglu et al., "Exercise Intensity and Thyroid Hormones," 830-834.
17. Loeser et al., "Aging and Oxidative stress," 2201-2209; Navarro-Yepes et al., "Oxidative Stress, Redox Signaling," 66-85; Wohlgemuth, Calvani, and Marzetti, "Autophagy and Mitochondrial Dysfunction," 62-70; Dai et al., "Mitochondrial Oxidative Stress in Aging," 6.
18. Beltran et al., "Explosive-type of Moderate Resistance Training," 759-772.
19. Radak et al., "Adaptation to Exercise-induced Oxidative Stress," 90-107; Fischer-Wellman and Bloomer, "Oxidative Stress and Exercise," 3805-3830; Radak et al., "Exercise Results in Systemic Adaptation," 3855-3869.
20. Ferris,Williams, and Shen, "Effect of Acute Exercise on serum BDNF," 728-734.
21. Qiang, "Beneficial Effects of Physical Exercise," 265-270.
22. Stener et al., "Exercise Increases Mitochondrial \Biogenesis," 1066-1071.
23. Aarsland et al., "Is Physical Activity a Preventive Factor" 386-395.
24. Cotman, Berchtold, Christie, "Exercise Builds Brain Health," 464-472; Lange-Aschenfeldt and Kojda, "Alzheimer's Disease, Cerebrovascular Dysfunction," 499-504; Ahlskog et al., "Physical Exercise as a Preventative," 876-884; Graff-Radford, "Can Aerobic Exercise Protect Against Dementia?" 2-6.
25. Hillman, Erickson, Kramer, Be Smart, Exercise Your Heart," 58-65; Cotman and Berchtold, "Exercise: A Behavioral Intervention," 295-301; Colcombe et al., "Aerobic Exercise Increases Brain Volume," 1166-1170.
26. Duncan et al., "Home-based Exercise Program," 2055-2060.
27. Ahlskog, "Does Vigorous Exercise have a Neuroprotective Effect," 288-294.
28. Voss et al. "Exercise, Brain and Cognition," 1505-1513.
29. ten Have, de Graaf, Monshouwer, "Physical Exercise and Mental Health Status," 342-348.

30. Hirano et al., "Influence of Regular Exercise," e158-e163; Potter et al., "Review of the Effects of Physical Activity," 1000-1011; Cooney et al., "Exercise for Depression"; Carek et al., "Exercise for Treatment of Depression," 15-28; Bridle et al., "Effect of Exercise on Depression Severity," 180-185; Danielson et al., "Exercise Treatment of Major Depression," 573-585; Kalitesi, "Exercise and Quality of Life," 54-56; Chrysohoou et al., "High Intensity, Interval Exercise Improves Quality of Life," 1303-1306.
31. Cornelissen et al., "Impact of Resistance Training on Blood Pressure," 950-958.
32. Oka et al., "Impact of a Home-based Walking and Resistance Training," 365-369.
33. Headley et al., "Resistance Training Improves Strength and Functional Measures," 355-364.
34. Cheema et al., "Progressive Resistance Training in Breast Cancer," 9-26.
35. Dunstan et al., "High-intensity Resistance Training Improves Glycemic Control," 1729-1736.
36. Singh, Clements, and Fiatarone, "Randomized Controlled Trial of Progressive Resistance Training," M27-M25.
37. Kelley, Kelley, and Tran, "Resistance Training and Bone Mineral Density," 65-77.
38. Lemmey et al., "High-intensity Resistance Training," 1726-1734.
39. Heyn, Abreu, and Ottenbacher, "Effects of Exercise on Elderly Persons," 1694-1704.

## Chapter 3 – From Prescription to Program: Safety and Dosing

1. Smith, Schroeder, and Fahey, "Over-the-counter Medications for Acute Cough."
2. Guasch and Mont, "Exercise and the Heart"; Carter, Potter, and Brooks, "Overtraining Syndrome."
3. Jahnke et al., "Health Benefits of Qigong and Tai Chi," e1-e25.
4. Wayne et al., "Safety of Tai Chi?"
5. Pollock et al. "Resistance Exercise in Individuals," 828-833; Hamill, "Relative Safety of Weightlifting," 53-57; McCartney, "Responses to Resistance Training and Safety," 31-37.
6. Yongming, Cao, and Chen, "Similar Electromyographic Activities of Lower Limbs," 1349-1353; Saeterbakken and Fimland, "Muscle Force output and Electromyographic Activity," 130-136; Saeterbakken and Fimland, "Electromyographic activity and 6RM strength," 1101-1107.
7. These (SI) units are not used in the exercise science literature to express Intensity-Volume products (when they're expressed at all). I use this weird combination of units here for clarity and to simplify the discussion.
8. Paracelsus, *Die Dosis macht das Gift*. "The dose makes the poison."
9. Farinatti, Neto, and da Silva, "Influence of Resistance Training Variables."
10. Rippetoe and Baker, "*Practical Programming for Strength Training.*"
11. Kilgore and Rippetoe, "Redefining Fitness for Health and Fitness Professionals," 34-39.
12. Rippetoe and Baker, "*Practical Programming for Strength Training*"; Soleyn, "Training and Performance for the Novice."
13. Pleket, "On the Sociology of Ancient Sport," 29; Tilk, "Educational Narratives as a Pedagogical Paradigm."
14. Fries, Bruce, and Chakravarty, "Compression of Morbidity."

## Chapter 4 – Enduring Resistance, Resisting Endurance: Comprehensive Training

1. Kraemer, Ratamess, and French DN, "Resistance Training for Health and Performance,"165-171.
2. Fuzhong et al., "Tai Chi and Fall Reductions," 187-194.
3. Lai et al., "Two-year Trends in Cardiorespiratory Function," 1222-1227.
4. Song et al., "Effects of Tai Chi Exercise," 2039-2044.
5. Smith et al., "Crossfit-based High-intensity Power Training," 3159-3172.

6. Koziris, "Sprint Interval Exercise for Fat Loss," 41-42; Shing et al., "Circulating Adiponectin Concentrations," 2213-2218.
7. Gibala et al., "Short-term Sprint Interval v Traditional Endurance Training," 901-911; Burgomaster et al., "Similar Metabolic Adaptations," 151-160.
8. Hickson, "Interference of Strength Development," 255-264; Wilson et al., "Concurrent Training: Meta-analysis," 2293-2307.
9. Hawley, "Molecular Responses to Strength and Endurance Training," 355-361; Vissing et al., "Differentiated mTOR but not AMPK Signaling," 355-366; Atherton et al., "Selective Activation of AMPK-PGC-1a," 786-788.
10. Knowles, "Enzyme-catalyzed Phosphoryl Transfer," 877–919; Wells, Selvadurai, and Tein, "Bioenergetic Provision of Energy," 83-90.
11. Huxley and Niedergerke, "Structural Changes in Muscle Contraction," 971–973; Huxley and Hanson, "Changes in the Cross-striations of Muscle," 973–976.
12. Tyska and Warshaw, "The myosin Power Stroke," 1–15.
13. In the ETS, electrons are transferred from one protein to another, and flow from a high-energy to a low-energy state, culminating in the "final electron acceptor," which is oxygen. The corresponding change in free energy is used to drive protons against their electrochemical gradient into the intermembrane space of the mitochondrion. Therefore, the electrical potential created by the ETS is a *hydrogen ion gradient*, literally a *proton voltage*. The proton current driven by this voltage is used to power the process of ATP synthesis.
14. The oxidative phosphorylation step cannot operate without oxygen, because without oxygen to serve as a sort of chemical "electrode" (technically, the final electron acceptor), there is no electron current, no voltage, and no ATP production. The Krebs cycle does not use oxygen directly, but it's linked to oxidative phosphorylation through the electron carriers, and so has an indirect but absolute oxygen requirement.
15. Kraemer, Ratamess, and French, "Resistance Training for Health and Performance," 165-171; Wikipedia, "Efficiency of ATP Production"; The actual yield of metabolism is less than this theoretical threshold, with as few as 32 or less ATPs/glucose; Brooks, Fahey, and Baldwin, *Exercise Physiology*.
16. Kraemer WJ, Ratamess NA, French DN. "Resistance Training for Health and Performance," 165-171.
17. Brooks, Fahey, and Baldwin, *Exercise Physiology*; Schulz, "Beta oxidation of Fatty Acids," 109-120.
18. The fragments from both beta oxidation and glycolysis enter the Krebs Cycle in exactly the same form: that of Acetyl CoA.
19. Brooks, Fahey, and Baldwin, *Exercise Physiology*; Hochachka, Neely, and Driedzic, "Integration of Lipid Utilization," 2009-2014.
20. Brooks, Fahey, and Baldwin, *Exercise Physiology*; Ellington, "Evolution and Physiological Roles," 289-325; This system is also called the ATP-CrP system or the immediate energy system. We will refer to it as the phosphagen system in this text.
21. Kraemer, Ratamess, and French, "Resistance Training for Health and Performance," 165-171.
22. Brooks, Fahey, and Baldwin, *Exercise Physiology*; Gollnick et al., "Enzyme Activity and Fiber Composition," 312-319.
23. Kraemer, Ratamess, and French, "Resistance Training for Tealth and Performance," 165-171; Wilson et al., "Endurance, Strength and Power Training," 1724-1729; Paddon-Jones et al., "Adaptation to Chronic Eccentric Exercise," 466-71; Staron et al., "Misclassification of Hybrid Fast Fibers," 2616-2622.
24. Kraemer, Ratamess, and French, "Resistance Training for Tealth and Performance," 165-171; Brooks, Fahey, and Baldwin, *Exercise Physiology*; Gollnick et al., "Enzyme Activity and Fiber Composition," 312-319.
25. Nilwik et al. "Decline in Skeletal Muscle Mass," 492-8; Deschenes, "Effects of Aging on Muscle Fiber Type," 809-824; Brunner et al., "Effects of Aging on Type II Muscle Fibers," 336-348; Doherty, "Aging and Sarcopenia," 1717-1727.
26. Reid and Fielding, "Skeletal Muscle Power," 4-12.

27. Nilwik et al. "Decline in Skeletal Muscle Mass," 492-8.
28. Verdijk et al., "Satellite Cells in Skeletal Muscle."
29. Frontera et al., "Strength Conditioning in Older Men," 1038-1044.
30. Thrash and Kelly, "Flexibility and Strength Training," 74-75; Beedlel, Jesee, and Stone, "Flexibility Characteristics Among Athletes," 150-154; Todd, "Myth of the Muscle-bound Lifter," 37-41.
31. Orr et al., "Power Training Improves Balance," 78-85; Holviala et al., "Effects of Strength Training on Muscle," 336-344; Judge et al., "Balance Improvements in Older Women," 254-262; A number of contrary studies are to be found on this point. Without exception, these studies used non-structural exercises and low-dose resistance training.
32. More correctly, the integration of proprioceptive and vestibular inputs.
33. Sequin and Nelson, "Benefits of Strength Training," 141-149; Treuth et al., "Effects of Strength Training on Body Composition," 614-620; Schwartz and Evans, "Effects of Exercise on Body Composition," 147-150.
34. Kraemer, Ratamess, and French, "Resistance Training for Health and Performance," 165-171
35. Alvehus et al., "Metabolic Adaptations in Skeletal Muscle," 1463-1471; Vincent et al., "Improved Cardiorespiratory Endurance," 673-678; Frontera et al., "Strength Training and $VO_2$max," 329-333; Hagerman et al., "Effects of High-intensity Resistance Training," B336-B346.
36. Ades et al., "Weight Training Improves Walking Endurance," 568-572; Anderson and Kearny, "Effects of Three Resistance Training Programs," 1-7; Hoff, Gran, and Helgerud, "Maximal Strength Training," 288-295; Paavoleinen et al., "Explosive-strength training improves 5-km," 1527-1533.
37. Kraemer, Ratamess, and French, "Resistance Training for Health and Performance," 165-171; Paavoleinen et al., "Explosive-strength Training Improves 5-km," 1527-1533.; Storen et al., "Strength Training Improves Running," 1089-1094; Sunde et al., "Strength Training Improves Cycling," 2157-2165.
38. Granata et al., "Training Intensity Modulates PGC-1a and p53"; Psilander, "Effect of Different Exercise Regimens."
39. Tabata et al., "Effects of Moderate-intensity Endurance," 1327-1330.
40. Wikipedia, "High-intensity Interval Training."
41. Gibala et al., "Short-term Sprint Interval," 901-911; Wikipedia, "High-intensity Interval Training."; Burgomaster et al., "Metabolic Adaptations During Exercise," 151-160; Medbo and Burgers, "Effect of Training on anaerobic Capacity," 501-507; Rodas et al., "Short Training Programme," 480-486; Laursen and Jenkins, "Scientific Basis for High-intensity," 53-73.
42. Aagaard and Andersen, "Effects of Strength Training on Endurance," 39-47.
43. Marcell, Hawkins, and Wiswell, "Leg Strength Declines with Age," 504-513.

## Chapter 5 – Specificity and Effectiveness: Your Physiological 401k

1. Everett, *Olympic Weightlifting for Sports*; Newton and Kraemer, "Developing Explosive Muscular Power," 20-31; Haff, Whitley, and Potteiger, "Explosive Exercise and Sports Performance," 13.
2. Radecki, "Pharmaceutical Sponsorship Bias," 435-8; Mendelson et al., "Conflicts of Interest in Cardiovascular," 577; Stamatakis et al., "Undue Industry Influences," 469.
3. Prasad et al., "A Decade of Reversal," 790-798; Altman, "Poor-quality Medical Research," 2765-2767; Cohn, "Medical Research: Good, Bad and the Underpowered," 15-16.
4. Kilgore, "Paradigm lost"; Sullivan, "Year in Strength Science 2011"; Sullivan, "Year in Strength Science 2012"; Sullivan, "Year in Strength Science 2013."
5. Tibana RA, Navalta J, Bottaro M, et al., "Eight Weeks of Resistance Training," 11-19.
6. Williams et al., "Resistance Exercise in Individuals," 572-584.

7. Rana et al., "Cardiovascular Metabolic Syndrome," 218-232.
8. Schaffler et al., "Adipose Tissue as an Inflammatory Organ," 449-467; Berg and Scherer, "Adipose Tissue, Inflammation, and Cardiovascular Disease," 939-949; Fontana et al., "Visceral Fat Adipokine Secretion," 1010-1013; Iacobellis and Barbaro, "Double Role of Epicardial Adipose," 442-445; Beavers et al., "Role of Metabolic Syndrome," 617-623.
9. Greiwe et al., "Resistance Exercise Decreases TNF-alpha," 475-482; Olson et al., "Changes in Inflammatory Viomarkers," 996-1003; Schmitz et al., "Strength Training for Obesity Prevention," 326-333; Hunter et al., "Resistance Training and Intra-abdominal Adipose," 1023-8; Ross et al., "Influence of Diet and Exercise," 2445–55.
10. Bruunsgaard et al., "Muscle Strength After Resistance Training," 237-241; Campbell et al., "Increased Energy Requirements," 167-175; Strasser, Arvandi, and Siebert, "Resistance Training, Visceral Obesity," 578-591.
11. Hurley and Roth, "Strength Training in the Elderly," 249-268; Stensvold et al., "Strength Training vs Aerobic Interval Training," 804-810.
12. Sundell, "Resistance Training is an Effective Tool."
13. Lehnen et al., "Changes in the GLUT 4 Expression," 10.
14. Kennedy et al., "Exercise Induces GLUT4 Translocation," 1192-1197; Rose and Richter, "Skeletal Muscle Glucose Uptake."
15. Ren et al., "Exercise Induces Rapid Increases in GLUT4," 14396-14401.
16. Hansen et al., "Increased GLUT-4 Translocation," 1218-1222; Christ-Roberts et al., "Exercise Training Increases Glycogen," 1233-1242.
17. Hutchinson, Summers, and Bengtsson, "Regulation of AMP-activated Protein Kinase," 291-310.
18. Youngren "Exercise and the Regulation of Blood Glucose."
19. Perseghin et al., "Increased Glucose Transport-phosphorylation," 1357-1362.
20. Erikkson, Taimela, and Koivisto, "Exercise and the Metabolic Syndrome," 125-135; Reed et al., "Effects of High- and Low-volume Resistance Exercise," 251-260; Croymans et al., "Resistance Training Improves Indices," 1245-1253; Malin et al., "Effect of Adiposity on Insulin Action," 2933-2941; Durak et al., "Randomized Crossover Study of Resistance Training," 1039-1043; Hansen et al., "Insulin Sensitivity after Maximal and Endurance Resistance Training," 327-334; Leenders et al., "Elderly Men and Women Benefit," 769-779; Conceicao et al., "Sixteen Weeks of Resistance Training," 1221-1228; Castaneda et al., "Randomized Controlled Trial of Resistance Exercise," 2335-41.
21. Marcus et al., "Comparison of Combined Aerobic," 1345–54.
22. Irvine and Taylor, "Progressive Resistance Exercise Improves," 237-246.
23. Soukup and Kovaleski, "Effects of Resistance Training," 307-312; Tzankoff and Norris, "Effect of Muscle Mass Decrease," 1001-1006; Erikkson, Taimela, and Koivisto, "Exercise and the Metabolic Syndrome," 125-153; American College of Sports Medicine, "Recommended Quantity and Quality of Exercise," 265-274.
24. Jurca et al., "Association of Muscular Strength with Metabolic Syndrome," 1849-1855; Wijndaele et al., "Muscular Strength, Aerobic Fitness," 233-240.
25. Strasser, Siebert, and Schobersberger, "Resistance Training in the Treatment of Metabolic Syndrome," 397-415.
26. Grontved et al., "Prospective Study of Weight Training," 1306-1312.
27. Castaneda et al., "Randomized Controlled Trial of Resistance Exercise," 2335-2341; Dunstan et al., "High-intensity Resistance Training," 1729-1736; Eves and Plotnikoff, "Resistance Training and Type 2 Diabetes," 1933-1941; Sparks, Johannsen, and Church, "Nine Months of Combined Training," 1694-1702.
28. Utomi et al., "Systematic Review and Meta-analysis of Training Mode."
29. Saltin and Astrand, "Maximal Oxygen Uptake in Athletes," 353-358.

30. Saltin and Astrand, "Maximal Oxygen Uptake in Athletes," 353-358; Laursen and Jenkins , "Scientific Basis for High-intensity Interval Training," 53-73; Saltin and Astrand, "Maximal Oxygen Uptake and Heart Rate," 353-358.
31. Hurley, Hagberg, and Goldberg, "Resistive Training Reduce Coronary Risk," 150-154; Vincent and Vincent, "Resistance Training for Individuals," 207-216.
32. Hurley, Hagberg, and Goldberg, "Resistive Training Reduce Coronary Risk," 150-154; Blumenthal, Siegel, and Appelbaum, "Failure of Exercise to Reduce Blood Pressure," 2098-2104; Habberg et al., "Effect of Weight Training on Blood Pressure," 147-151; Harris and Holly, "Physiological Response to Circuit Weight Training," 246-252.
33. Pescatello et al., "Exercise and Hypertension," 533-53; Sousa et al., "Long-term Effects of Aerobic Training"; Hefferman et al., "Resistance Exercise Reduces Arterial Pressure"; Moraes et al., "Chronic Conventional Resistance Exercise," 1122-1129; Cornellisen and Fagard RH, "Effect of Resistance Training on resting Blood Pressure," 251-259.
34. Artero et al., "Prospective Study of Muscular Strength," 1831-7.
35. Braith and Stewart, "Resistance Exercise Training," 2642-2650.
36. Vincent and Vincent, "Resistance Training for Individuals," 207-216; Vincent et al., "Homocysteine Levels Following Resistance Training," 197-203; Maeda et al., "Resistance Training Reduces Plasma Endothelin-1," S443-446; Nash et al., "Circuit Resistance Training Improves Lipid Profile," 2-9; Ho et al., "Effect of 12 weeks of Aerobic, Resistance or Combination," 704
37. Braith and Stewart, "Resistance Exercise Training," 2642-2650;
38. Chen, Zhu, and Zhang, "Combined Endurance-resistance Training."; Servantes et al., "Home-based Exercise Training," 45-57; Savage et al., "Effect of Resistance Training on Physical Disability," 1379-1386; Toth et al. Resistance training alters skeletal muscle structure," 1243-1259.
39. Smart, Dieberg, and Giallauria, "Intermittent v Continuous Exercise," 352-358.
40. Ghilarducci, Holly, and Amsterdam, "High Resistance Training in Coronary Artery Disease," 866-870.
41. White et al., "Brain Ischemia and Reperfusion," 1-33, 2000.
42. White and Sullivan, "Apoptosis," 1019-29; Renehan, Booth, and Potten CS, "What is Apoptosis," 1536-1538.
43. White and Sullivan, "Apoptosis," 1019-29.
44. Collins et al., Growth Factors as Survival Factors," 133-138.
45. Sanderson et al., "Insulin Activates PI3K-Akt," 947-58.
46. Letai, "Growth Factor Withdrawal and Apoptosis," 728-30. 2006; Russell et al., "Insulin-like Growth factor-I Prevents Apoptosis," 455-67.
47. Blackman et al., "Growth Hormone and Sex Steroid," 2282-2292.
48. Dupont-Versteegden, "Apoptosis in Muscle Atrophy," 473-81.
49. Janssen et al., "Healthcare Costs of Sarcopenia," 80-85; Fielding et al., "Sarcopenia" 249-256.
50. Marzetti and Leeuwenburgh, "Skeletal Muscle Apoptosis," 1234-8; Ferreira et al., "Evidences of Apoptosis," 601-11.
51. Sharafi and Rahimi, "Effect of Resistance Exercise," 1142-1148; Peterson, Johannsen and Ravussin. "Skeletal Muscle Mitochondria and Aging.".
52. Whitman et al., "Contributions of the Ubiquitin-proteasome Pathway," 437-46.
53. Nelson et al., "High-intensity Strength Training,"1909-1914.
54. Larsson, "Histochemical Characteristics of Human Skeletal Muscle," 469-471; Nilwik et al. "Decline in Skeletal Muscle Mass," 492-8
55. Phillipou et al., "Type 1 Insulin-like Growth Factor," 208-18; Kostek et al., "Muscle Strength Response to

Training," 2147-2154; Boonen et al., "Musculoskeletal Effects of IGF-1/IGF Binding Protein-3," 1593-1599.

56. Janssen et al., "Healthcare costs of Sarcopenia," 80-85; Munzer et al., "Growth Hormone and Sex Steroid," 3833-41; Liu et al., "Safety and Efficacy of Growth Hormone," 104-15.
57. Munzer et al., "Growth Hormone and Sex Steroid," 3833-41; Liu et al., "Safety and Efficacy of Growth Hormone," 104-15.
58. American College of Sports Medicine Position Stand, "Recommended Quantity and Quality of Exercise," 975-991; Banz et al., "Effects of Resistance v Aerobic Training," 434-440; Hurley and Roth, "Strength Training in the Elderly," 249-268.
59. Nilwik et al. "Decline in Skeletal Muscle Mass," 492-8.
60. Liu and Latham, "Progressive Resistance Strength Training"; Pederson et al., "Resistance Exercise for Muscular Strength," 226-237.
61. Marques et al., "Multicomponent Training with Weight-bearing Exercises," 117-29.
62. Serra-Rexach et al., "Short-term, Light- to Moderate-intensity Exercise," 594-602; Liu and Latham, "Progressive Resistance Strength Training."
63. Singh et al., "Study of Mental and Resistance Training," 873-880.
64. Brooks, Fahey, and Baldwin, *Exercise Physiology.*
65. Pollock et al., "AHA Science Advisory," 828-833.
66. Pescatello et al., "ACSM Position, Exercise and Hypertension," 533-553.
67. Sigal et al., "Physical Activity/exercise and Type 2 Diabetes," 2518-2539.

## Chapter 6 – Simplicity and Efficiency: From Black Iron to Grey Steel

1. Smith et al., "Crossfit-based High-intensity Power Training," 3159-3172.

## Chapter 7 – Elementary Iron

1. Rippetoe, "Knee Wraps."
2. Reynolds and McNeely, "Barbell Safety."
3. Hamilton, Woodbury, and Harper, "Arterial, Cerebrospinal and Venous Pressure," 42-50; Prabhakar et al., "Intracranial Pressure During Valsalva," 98-101; Niewiadomski et al., "Effects of a Brief Valsalva,"145-157.
4. Vlak et al., "Rupture of Intracranial Aneurysms," 878-1882.
5. de Rooij et al., "Incidence of Subarachnoid Hemorrhage," 1365-1372; Haykowsky, Findlay, Ignaszeski, "Aneurysmal Subarachnoid Hemorrhage," 52-55; Matsuda et al., "Precipitating Aneurysmal Subarachnoid Hemorrhage,"55-29.
6. Sullivan, "The Valsalva and Stroke."
7. Ibid.

## Chapter 8 – A Brief Overview of the Squat

1. Hartmann, Wirth, and Kluseman, "Analysis of the Load on Knee Joint," 993-1008.
2. Hartmann et al., "Squatting depth on Jumping Performance," 3243-61; Rippetoe, *Starting Strength: Basic Barbell Training.*
3. Rippetoe, *Starting Strength: Basic Barbell Training.*
4. Rippetoe and Bradford, "Active Hip 2.0: Director's Cut."
5. Clemente, *Anatomy: Regional Atlas of the Human Body.*

6. Ibid.
7. Ibid.
8. Ibid.
9. Hartmann, Wirth, and Kluseman, "Analysis of the Load on Knee Joint," 993-1008; Hartmann et al., "Squatting depth on Jumping Performance," 3243-61.

## Chapter 10 – A Brief Overview of the Press

1. Feigenbaum, Goodmurphy, and Scheider, "Gripping Matters"
2. Zuckerman et al., "Interobserver Reliability of Acromial Morphology," 286-7; Chang et al., "Shoulder Impingement," 497-505; Ozaki et al., "Tears of the Rotator Cuff" 1224–30.

## Chapter 11 – A Brief Overview of the Bench Press

1. Lombardi and Troxel, "US Deaths and Injuries," S203; Hamill, "Relative Safety of Weightlifting," 53-57.

## Chapter 12 – A Brief Overview of the Power Clean and Power Snatch

1. Hamill, "Relative Safety of Weightlifting," 53-57; Calhoon and Fry, "Injury Rates and Profiles," 232-238.
2. Most of the American weightlifting coaches who read this just had an aneurysm.

## Chapter 15 – Adaptation

1. Selye, "Syndrome Produced by Diverse Nocuous Agents," 32.
2. Selye, "Physiology and Pathology of Exposure to Stress"; Szabo, Taeche, and Somogyi, "Legacy of Hans Selye," 472-478.
3. Kraemer and Ratamess, "Fundamentals of Resistance Training"; Rippetoe and Baker, *Practical Programming for Strength Training*; Verkoshansky, "General Adaptation Syndrome and its Applications."
4. Matveev, "The Problem of Periodization."
5. That would seem to be rather missing the point.

## Chapter 16 – Recovery: The Forgotten Training Variables

1. Churchward-Venne, Breen, and Phillips, "Alterations in Muscle Protein Metabolism,"199-205.
2. Davis and Aykroyd, *Coneheads: The Life and Times of Beldar Conehead.*
3. Eknoyan, "Average Man and Indices of Obesity," 47-51; Schneider et al., Predictive Value of Measures of Obesity," 1777-85.
4. Dickinson, Volpi, and Rasmussen, "Exercise and Nutrition to Target Protein Synthesis," 216-223.
5. Bilsborough and Mann, "Dietary Protein Intake," 129-152; Kreider and Campbell, "Protein for Exercise and Recovery," 13-21.
6. Schoenfeld, Aragon, and Krieger, "Effect of Protein Timing."
7. Taubes, "What if it's All Been a Big Fat Lie?"; Harcombe et al., "Evidence from Randomised Controlled Trials"; Schwab et al., "Effect of the amount and type of dietary fat"; Hooper et al., "Reduced or Modified Dietary Fat"; Siri-Tarino et al., "Association of Saturated Fat with Cardiovascular Disease," 535–546.
8. Kris-Etherton, Harris, and Appel, "Fish Consumption, Fish Oil, Omega-3 Fatty Acids," 2747-2757.
9. Tartibian, Maleki, and Abbasi, "Effects of Ingestion of Omega-3 Fatty Acids," 115-119.

10. Lenn et al., "Effects of Fish Oil and Isoflavones,"1605-1613.
11. Pittas et al., "Vitamin D and Calcium in Diabetes."
12. Grant and Holick, "Benefits and Requirements of Vitamin D," 94-111; Erikson and Glerup, "Vitamin D Deficiency and Aging," 73-77; Holic, "High Prevalence of Vitamin D Inadequacy," 353-373.
13. Tang et al., "Calcium in Combination with Vitamin D," 657-666; Bunout et al., "Vitamin D Supplementation," 746-752; Dawson-Hughes et al., "Calcium and Vtamin D supplementation," 670-676; Stockton et al., "Effect of Vitamin Supplementation on Muscle Strength," 859-871.
14. Palmer, "Coffee is Neither Good nor Bad."
15. Higdon and Frei, "Coffee and Health," 101-123; Ranheim and Halverson, "Coffee Consumption and Human Health," 274-284.
16. Del Coso et al., "Effects of a Caffeine-containing Energy Drink," 21; Duncan et al., "Acute Effect of a Caffeine-Containing Energy Erink," 2858-2865.
17. Mora-Rodriguez et al., "Caffeine Ingestion Reverses the Circadian Rhythm," e33807.
18. Duncan and Oxford, "Effect of Caffeine Ingestion," 178-85.
19. Smits, Pieters, and Thien. "Role of Epinephrine in Effects of Coffee," 431-437; Nehlig and Debry, "Caffeine and Sports Activity," 215-223.
20. Maughan and Griffin, "Caffeine Ingestion and Fluid Balance," 411-420; Wemple, Lamb, and McKeever, "Caffeine vs. Caffeine-free Sports Drinks," 40-46; Grandjean et al., "Effect of Beverages on Hydration," 591-600.
21. Zuniga et al., "Creatine Monohydrate Loading," 1651-1656; Jagim et al., "Buffered Form of Creatine"; Spradly et al., "Ingesting a Pre-workout Supplement," 28; Favero et al., "Creatine but not Betaine Supplementation."
22. Tarnopolsky and Safdar, "Potential Benefits of Creatine and Conjugated Linoleic Acid," 213-27.
23. Zuniga et al., "Creatine Monohydrate Loading," 1651-1656.
24. Jagim et al., "Buffered Creatine Does not Promote Greater Changes."
25. Panel members, "Opinion on Food Additives," 1-12; Gualano et al., "Effects of Creatine Supplementation on Renal Function," 33-40; Kreider et al., "Long-term Creatine Supplementation," 95-104.
26. Sawka et al., "Exercise and Fluid Replacement," 377-90.
27. Mendias, Tatsumi, and Allen, "Role of Cyclooxygenase-1 and -2," 497-500.
28. Novak *et al.*, "COX-2 Inhibitor Reduces Skeletal Muscle Hypertrophy," R1132-1139.
29. Mikkelson *et al.*, "NSAID Infusion Inhibits Satellite Cell," 1600-11; Trappe et al., "Effect of Ibuprofen and Acetaminophen," E551-56.
30. Trappe *et al.*, "Acetaminophen and Ibuprofen on Skeletal Muscle Adaptations," R655-62.
31. Sullivan , "Stopping Spread of Misinflammation."
32. Takahashi, Kipnis, and Daughaday, "Growth Hormone Secretion During Sleep," 2079–90.

## Chapter 17 – Elements of Program Design and Execution

1. ***Intensity*** has become a contentious term in exercise science circles, in our opinion unnecessarily so. Some have argued that the term is confusing or vague. It is true that *intensity* as applied to strength training and *intensity* as applied to running or swimming or sprinting will denote different quantities. But in each circumstance, *intensity* will always be more-or-less proportional to the athlete's power output, as opposed to the total amount of work (volume) in an exercise bout. We find the term useful, in part precisely because it *can* be applied to a diverse range of training situations. So we're not confused at all.
2. Campos et al., "Muscular Adaptations in Resistance-training Regimens," 50-60.
3. Carpinelli and Otto RN, "Strength Training," 73-84; Baggenhammar and Hansson, "Repeated Sets or a Single

Set," 154-160.

## Chapter 19 – The Novice Master

1. Rippetoe, *Starting Strength: Basic Barbell Training.*
2. Rippetoe and Baker, *Practical Programming for Strength Training.*
3. Evagrio, *Gli Otto Spiriti Malvagi,* 11-12.
4. Some Masters over 50 may be able to train in the power variants of the Olympic lifts. This is an individual matter to be decided (judiciously!) by coach and trainee. Intermediate athletes may also train power with dynamic effort sets, described in the Intermediate Chapters .

## Chapter 26 – Conditioning

1. Ho et al., "12 weeks of Aerobic, Resistance or Combination," 704; Marcus et al., "Comparison of Combined Aerobic and High-force Eccentric Resistance," 1345–54; Sparks, Johannsen, and Church, "Nine Months of Combined Training," 1694-1702.
2. The question of whether golf is a "sport" or a "game" is a point of perennial contention. We're not going to go there.
3. Gibala, "Molecular Responses to High-intensity Interval Exercise," 428-32; Helgerud et al., "Aerobic High-intensity Intervals," 665-71.
4. Wisløff, Ellingsen, and Kemi, "High-intensity Interval Training," 139-46.
5. Gibala et al., "Sprint Interval v Traditional Endurance," 901-911.
6. LaForgia, Withers, and Gore, "Effects of Exercise Intensity and Duration," 1247-1264; Skelly et al., "High-intensity Interval Exercise Induces 24-h Energy Expenditure," 845-848.
7. Reynolds and Bradford, "Death by Prowler."
8. Hickson, "Interference of Strength Development," 255-264; Wilson et al., "Concurrent Training: Meta-analysis," 2293-2307; Hawley , "Molecular Responses to Strength and Endurance Training," 355-361; Vissing et al., "Differentiated mTOR but not AMPK Signaling," 355-366; Atherton et al., "Selective Activation of AMPK-PGC-1a or PKB-TSC2-mTOR," 786-788.
9. Koziris, "Sprint Interval Exercise for Fat Loss," 41-42; Shing et al., "Adiponectin Concentrations and Body Composition," 2213-2218; Gibala et al., "Sprint interval v Traditional Endurance," 901-911; Burgomaster et al., "Metabolic Adaptations During Exercise," 151-160.

## Chapter 27 – The Female Master

1. At least, we sincerely hope so.
2. Murray et al., "Shoulder Motion and Muscle Strength," 268-273; Lindle et al., "Age and Gender Comparisons of Muscle Strength," 1581-1587; Frontera et al., "Cross-sectional Study of Muscle Strength," 644-650.
3. Kraemer et al., "Endogenous Anabolic Hormonal and Growth Factor Responses," 228-235.
4. Claflin, Larkin, and Cederna, "Effects of High- and Low-velocity Resistance Training," 1021-1030.

# Glossary

**Accumulation:** The phase of advanced programming in which heavy work at high volume is used over multiple workouts to impose an overload event.

**Actin:** A protein in muscle tissue. Actin (thin filaments) and myosin (thick filaments) are the protein myofilaments that slide across each other to produce muscular contraction.

**Active Hip:** A critical feature of the properly-performed low-bar back squat (the squat). External femoral rotation and abduction prevent impingement of abdominal tissue on the anterior thigh and promote recruitment of a vast amount of lower extremity, hip, and paraspinal muscle tissue.

**Active Rest:** Unstructured, low-intensity physical activity on non-training days. See Chapter 16 for details and examples.

**Adaptation:** Metabolic, structural, and behavioral changes expressed by an organism in response to the application of environmental and other stressors. Adaptation in the Stress-Recovery-Adaptation Cycle is stimulated by a correctly applied overload event and occurs as the athlete recovers from the training stress during this period.

**Adipokine:** A signaling molecule (hormone or cytokine) of fat tissue origin.

**ADP:** Adenosine diphosphate. When ATP is used to provide energy for living processes, it loses its terminal phosphate and becomes ADP. ADP must be "recharged" by the creatine phosphate system or by catabolism of food energy to maintain tissue ATP levels.

**Advanced:** An athlete who has progressed beyond the intermediate level of training to a phase where progress occurs on a slower timeline (monthly or longer). Also the program utilized by such an athlete.

**Advanced Novice:** An athlete who has progressed far enough in the novice program to require the introduction of light squat days and other modifications to maintain novice progression prior to the transition to intermediate status.

**Aerobic:** The part of metabolism which utilizes oxygen for the final extraction of energy from food substrates. Also loosely used to describe low-power, repetitive exercise in which this part of metabolism dominates energy delivery.

**Amino Acids:** A family of nitrogenous organic molecules that form the building blocks of proteins.

**AMPK-Akt Switch:** A putative molecular mechanism for the biological interference effect. In this model, resistance training primarily activates the Akt-mTOR pathway that leads to muscle hypertrophy and increased strength, while endurance training primarily activates the AMPK pathway, leading to increased mitochondrial biogenesis and improved oxidative efficiency, but more muscle protein breakdown. Each pathway inhibits the other, and concurrent training favors a more "aerobic" phenotype over strength.

**Anabolism:** The part of metabolism that results in the accumulation of larger molecules and tissue mass. Contrast with catabolism.

**Anabolic Resistance:** A multi-factorial state, endemic in Masters, in which the growth and addition of new tissue, particularly muscle and bone, is *relatively* resistant to stimulation by training, rest, and nutrition.

**Anaerobic:** May refer to that part of metabolism which does not directly utilize oxygen for the extraction of energy from food substrates. May also refer (imprecisely) to high-intensity physical activity (exercise) in which non-oxidative processes dominate energy delivery to muscle.

**Anthropometry:** The measurement and description of variations in human physical dimensions; also refers to the variations themselves. Individual anthropometric variations have a significant impact on the proper performance of barbell exercises. Conversely, barbell exercises allow for the proper expression of human movement independent of anthropometric variation, in stark contrast to machine-based exercises.

**Apoptosis:** A complex, regulated process by which cells destroy themselves in response to various external and internal stresses and triggers. Also known as programmed cell death or "cell suicide."

**Ascending Sets:** Sets performed at successively higher weights, culminating in a single target set performed at high intensity. May be performed as warm-ups or as a work set variant, depending on the program. To be distinguished from sets across.

**Athlete:** In this text, we use an explicitly and deliberately expansive definition of "athlete" as any individual who engages in long-term, programmed *training* designed to *progressively* develop and improve General Fitness Attributes.

**ATP:** Adenosine Triphosphate. A high-energy molecule that mediates energy exchange in all living systems. ATP consists of a ribose sugar bound to adenosine, attached to a chain of phosphates. The last or terminal phosphate is in a high-energy state. Food energy must be converted to ATP to be useful to the cell.

**Back Squat:** A squat exercise in which the barbell is carried on the back, in either the high-bar (high-bar squat) or low-bar (squat) position.

**Back-Off Sets:** Sets performed at lower intensity after a heavy work set. Back-off sets are useful for accumulation of volume and for the refinement of technique at lower weight.

**Balance:** A General Fitness Attribute. The ability to statically or dynamically maintain a stable position over the center of gravity.

**Bench Press:** A barbell exercise in which the athlete lies supine on a bench with the bar over his shoulder joints, lowers the bar to his chest, and presses it back up. Bench press variants are named according to modification (eg dumbbell bench press).

**Beta Oxidation:** A series of biochemical reactions that oxidizes free fatty acids, producing acetyl Co-A and electron carriers. These products can be used for the aerobic generation of ATP by the Krebs Cycle and the electron transport chain.

**Bioenergetics:** The study of energy transformations in living systems.

**Biomarker:** A measurable indicator or surrogate marker of some biological state or condition.

**Body Composition:** A General Fitness Attribute, most crudely expressed as some ratio of lean (fat-free) to fat mass.

**Bodybuilding:** The rather strange pursuit of an idealized (usually grotesque) physique through resistance training, self-mortification, and semi-starvation. Not recommended for Masters.

**Bracketing:** A nutritional strategy in which higher caloric-density ("starchy") carbohydrates are consumed primarily around training times, with more restricted carbohydrate intake at other times.

**Bulking-Up:** The ghastly prospect of an innocent but misguided female acquiring a grotesque, hypertrophic, absurdly masculine physique by engaging in a rational barbell training program for health and fitness. This phenomenon never actualizes in practice, but it does provide a convenient excuse for not training.

**Capacity:** In our discussion of bioenergetics, we use the term capacity to refer to the ability of a particular energy system to deliver power in a sustained fashion. Mitochondrial (low-power, "aerobic") energy systems have high capacity, while cytosolic (high-power, "anaerobic") energy systems have low capacity.

**Carbohydrate:** An organic molecule consisting of carbon, hydrogen, and oxygen; one of the principle macronutrients. Sugars, starches, and alcohols are examples of carbohydrates.

**Catabolism:** A metabolic state in which macromolecules and tissues are broken down to supply food energy to the organism.

**Cerebrovascular Disease:** A degenerative condition characterized by the accumulation of atherosclerotic plaques in the arteries that supply blood to brain tissue. This condition predisposes to cerebral infarction, or stroke.

**Chronic Program Hopping:** A common behavioral disorder in which the athlete constantly changes training goals, programs, exercise selection, and other training variables in an heroic but ultimately tragic quest to go nowhere. Easily diagnosed by inspection of the training log.

**Circuit Training:** A popular but misguided training approach in which one moves from one (usually machine-based) exercise to another in a "circuit" with minimal rest, in order to simultaneously train the attributes of strength and endurance. Not recommended for the vast majority of Master Athletes.

**Circus:** A commercial franchise gym, where one may observe all manner of entertaining, counterproductive, and downright dangerous tomfoolery with barbells, machines, dumbbells, and incompetent personal trainers in their little clown cars.

**Clean:** A barbell exercise in which the weight is lifted from the floor to the shoulders in a single movement. In one of the two contested movements in Olympic Weightlifting, the clean is followed by the jerk, in which the bar is propelled overhead and racked on fully extended arms (the *clean and jerk*).

**Collars:** Clamps attached to the sleeve of a barbell to secure the plates. Recommended for all exercises except the bench press.

**Concurrent Training:** An approach in which both resistance training for strength and conditioning training for endurance are simultaneously emphasized, in an attempt to progressively develop both attributes. When employing aerobic long-slow-distance (LSD) work, concurrent training appears to demonstrate biological and practical interference effects to the detriment of strength. Concurrent training with HIIT confers the benefits of conditioning work without interference.

**Conditioning:** A word that means "to bring something into the desired state for use." In the context of fitness, the term generally refers to training for stamina or endurance. This training can take on many forms, but may be viewed as falling into two general categories: high-intensity, low-volume conditioning (as in HIIT) and low-intensity, high-volume conditioning (as in LSD).

**Coronary Artery Disease:** A medical condition characterized by the accumulation of atherosclerotic plaques in the arteries that supply blood to the heart muscle. This condition predisposes to myocardial infarction, or heart attack.

**Creatine, Creatine Phosphate:** A small nitrogenous molecule found in muscle, brain, and kidney, which can store high-energy phosphate and permit the rapid replenishment of ATP during high-intensity work. Creatine is synthesized by the liver and kidney, as well as obtained from the diet and/or supplementation with commercial creatine products. Not to be confused with creatinine, a nitrogenous waste product of protein catabolism.

**Crossfit:** An extremely popular form of high-intensity power training and conditioning, characterized by workouts we find difficult to reconcile with the Stress-Recovery-Adaptation structure. The authors do not recommend this form of training for Masters.

**Cue:** A verbal, tactile, or gestural signal from coach to athlete to promote proper performance of a movement.

**Deadlift:** A barbell exercise in which the weight is lifted from the floor in the hands straight up the legs to a standing position.

**Detraining:** A situation in which the interruption of training leads to the progressive degradation of a previously developed fitness attribute.

**Diabetes:** From the Greek for "sweet urine." A group of pathological conditions in which either insulin secretion or insulin signaling is disrupted, resulting in elevated serum glucose and a range of systemic complications. Type I or juvenile onset diabetes is due to the loss of pancreatic islet cells and an inability to produce insulin. Type II diabetes usually appears in adulthood, is associated with obesity and metabolic syndrome, and is due to derangements in insulin signaling.

**Diagnostic Angles:** The set of anthropometric angles that manifest at a particular phase of a particular barbell movement. For example, an athlete in the proper setup for a deadlift will demonstrate a set of hip, back, knee, and ankle angles peculiar to his individual anthropometry.

**DOMS:** Delayed onset muscle soreness, a common phenomenon experienced 1-2 days after heavy strength training.

**Dynamic Effort Sets:** Low-volume, high-power sets in which barbell movements (usually squats and bench presses) are performed at low intensity but very high speed. See Chapter 23 for details on indication and use.

**Dyslipidemia:** A range of conditions and abnormalities characterized by altered (usually elevated) levels of serum fats and cholesterol (in the form of lipoproteins). Dyslipidemia is a feature of the metabolic syndrome and is believed by most medical authorities to promote the development of coronary artery disease.

**Electron Transport System:** A series of enzymatic and carrier proteins located on the inner mitochondrial membrane, capable of sequentially transferring high energy electrons from NADH and $FADH_2$ to oxygen. The energy released in this process is used to create a proton gradient ("voltage") that drives the production of ATP.

**Endocrine:** Refers to the production of hormones (signaling molecules) by non-ducted organs and tissues.

**Endurance:** The General Fitness Attribute that permits an individual to engage in sustained physical activity. Aerobic endurance or "stamina" is strongly correlated with maximal oxygen uptake ($VO_2max$) and cardiorespiratory fitness.

**Enzyme:** A biological molecule that catalyzes (facilitates) a biochemical reaction by reducing the activation energy of the process.

**EPOC:** Excess Post-Exercise Oxygen Consumption. Oxygen consumption remains elevated even after exercise ceases, indicating a prolonged increase in energy utilization.

**Exercise:** Any sort of physical activity.

**Exercise Order:** A training variable specifying the order in which exercises are to be performed.

**Fitness:** The capacity and readiness of an organism to meet the demands of its environment.

**Force:** In mechanics, force is an interaction that will affect the motion of (accelerate) an object with mass. Strength is the ability to generate a force against a resistance.

**Frailty:** A long-recognized feature of dysfunctional aging. Various conceptual models and frailty scores exist, but a frail individual is, quite simply, one who is increasingly easy to break. Frailty is a key component of the Sick Aging Phenotype.

**Frequency:** A training variable that specifies the rate of recurrence of a particular exercise or workout in a training program, e.g., 3 times per week, once per month, etc.

**Front Squat:** A squat variant in which the bar is held on the anterior deltoids. Characterized by a vertical back, open hip angle and closed (acute) knee angles.

**General Adaptation Syndrome:** Hans Selye's classic model of the organism's variable responses to stress.

**General Exercise Prescription:** An exercise prescription that is generally applicable to the Masters population by virtue of meeting the criteria of safety, wide therapeutic window, comprehensive impacts on fitness attributes, specificity to and effectiveness against the Sick Aging Phenotype, simplicity and efficiency.

**General Fitness Attributes:** The physical characteristics that positively impact the capacity and readiness of the organism to meet the physical demands of its life and environment. Different authors have presented more-or-less extensive lists of such attributes. In this text, we capture these attributes with the terms *strength, power, endurance, mobility, balance,* and *body composition.* See individual terms in the glossary for more detail.

**Genetic Potential:** The physical performance limitations imposed by the individual's genetic endowment.

**Glucose:** A simple six-carbon sugar. Carbohydrate is catabolized almost entirely in the form of glucose.

**Glucose Transporter:** A protein that permits translocation of glucose across the cell membrane, from the serum to the interior of a cell. Glucose transporters may function in response to insulin stimulation or in an insulin-independent manner, as in the case of skeletal muscle during exercise.

**Glycogen:** A storage form of carbohydrate found in muscle and liver tissue, sometimes called "animal starch." Glycogen is a branched chain (polymer) of glucose molecules.

**Glycolysis:** A phase of carbohydrate metabolism in which glucose is split into smaller fragments, releasing chemical energy. One molecule of glucose subjected to glycolysis will yield two molecules of ATP, two molecules of pyruvate, and two molecules of NADH (an electron carrier).

**Growth Factor:** Any of a number of steroid or peptide hormones capable of stimulating cellular growth, proliferation, healing, differentiation, and survival. Examples include insulin, IGF-1, HGH, and testosterone.

**Gym:** A facility equipped for physical training.

**Heart Failure:** A condition in which a structural, hydrodynamic, or metabolic derangement impedes the heart's ability to maintain cardiac output and maintain tissue perfusion. The most common causes of heart failure are coronary artery disease, high blood pressure, and valve disease.

**High-Bar Squat:** A back squat variant in which the barbell is carried high on the traps, characterized by a more vertical back angle, more open hip angle and more closed (acute) angles relative to the low-bar squat (the squat).

**HIIT:** High-Intensity Interval Training, a form of conditioning in which brief bouts of very high-intensity exercise are alternated with brief periods of rest.

**Homeostasis:** The maintenance of stable physical, biochemical, and functional conditions by living systems. For example, organisms maintain pH, temperature, and ATP concentrations within very narrow limits unless a stress perturbs one or more of these variables.

**Hooks:** Movable implements that hold a barbell on the rack.

**Hyperglycemia:** Elevated serum blood glucose ("high blood sugar").

**Hypertension:** Elevated blood pressure.

**Hypertrophy:** The growth and accumulation of tissue.

**IGF-1:** Insulin-like Growth Factor I, an important peptide growth factor. IGF-1 and similar molecules promote tissue growth, including muscle growth, and inhibit apoptosis or "cell suicide."

**Inflammation:** The complex and sometimes maladaptive biological response of organisms or tissues to harmful or stressful stimuli.

**Insulin:** A peptide growth factor and regulatory hormone, best known for its role in the regulation of glucose transport into cells. Insulin also has important effects on cell growth and survival.

**Insulin Resistance:** A state in which tissues are relatively insensitive to insulin stimulation. Insulin resistance constitutes a spectrum ranging from relatively mild, subclinical disease to full-blown diabetes.

**Intensification:** The phase of advanced programming in which increasingly heavy work at low volume is used over multiple workouts to display a strength adaptation.

**Intensity:** A measure of the power output or difficulty of an exercise. In the context of strength training, intensity refers to the load relative to the athlete's maximum for that lift.

**Intensity-Dependence:** An important characteristic of the Masters Athlete. Masters require more frequent exposure than younger athletes to high-intensity loading to maintain strength.

**Interference:** The phenomenon in which concurrent strength and aerobic endurance training eventually results in an inability to maintain strength gains over time, and may even lead to loss of strength. The *biological* interference effect has been observed in many studies and meta-analyses, although its underlying mechanisms and even its existence still remain somewhat controversial. *Practical* interference effects are frequently observed by fitness professionals. See Chapter 4 for more details.

**Intermediate:** An athlete who is strong enough to produce a training stress from which he cannot recover within 48-72 hours (before the next workout). Intermediate athletes require more complex and protracted training periods, generally of a week or more. Also refers to the programs used by such athletes.

**Interset Rest:** A training variable specifying the amount of time taken to recover between sets. Essential for the realization of immediate training objectives.

**Krebs Cycle:** A series of biochemical reactions in the mitochondrion, in which acetyl Co-A (formed from pyruvate or fatty acid) is broken down, yielding ATP, carbon dioxide, and high-energy electrons.

**Lactate:** One of the end products of glycolysis. Lactate, an organic acid, has multiple metabolic fates, depending on the energy demands of the organism. Many incorrectly consider it a waste product and a source of muscle soreness, neither of which are correct. Lactate is an energy source for many tissue types, and its contribution to muscle soreness has been discounted by research.

**Ligament:** Connective tissue that binds one bone to another.

**Limit set:** A set at the edge of the athlete's performance ability.

**Linear Progression:** Linear progression occurs when the overload increment at each training session is the same for each successive increase.

**Low-Bar Squat:** A barbell back squat performed with the bar just beneath the spines of scapulas. In this text, we assert that this type of squat, when performed below parallel, should be taken as the standard for training, and refer to it as ***the*** squat.

**LSD:** Long Slow Distance exercise – running, cross-country skiing or biking, and other endurance exercises.

**Macronutrient:** A class of chemically similar substances that form a substantial component of dietary intake. Proteins, carbohydrates, and fats are macronutrients.

**Masters Athlete:** In this text, we define a Masters Athlete as any individual aged forty and above who engages in long-term, explicitly programmed physical training for the optimization of health and General Fitness Attributes.

**Membrane:** In biology, a membrane is a double-layered sheet of phospholipid (fatty) molecules that encases a cell or cellular components. Membranes are fundamental to the organization of living matter.

**Metabolic Syndrome:** A cluster of physiological derangements including obesity, increased visceral fat, hyperglycemia, hypertension, and dyslipidemia. Systemic inflammation is frequently associated with the syndrome, but not part of the accepted definition. The metabolic syndrome is strongly associated with the development of diabetes, cardiovascular disease, stroke, and frailty.

**Metabolism:** The totality of biochemical processes that constitute the steady state of a living system. See also anabolism and catabolism.

**Micronutrient:** Dietary components which, while required only in very small amounts, are nevertheless essential for health. Usually divided into "vitamins" (B12, vitamin D, etc.) and "minerals" (calcium, magnesium, zinc, etc.).

**Mitochondrion:** A membrane-bound cellular organelle in which many critical metabolic processes occur, including the Krebs cycle and oxidative phosphorylation, which produce ATP.

**Mobility:** A General Fitness Attribute. In this text, we use the term to include flexibility, agility, and coordination.

**Moment:** In physics, the combination of a distance and a physical quantity. The moment of a physical force, or torque, is the product of a force and its distance from an axis of rotation – the moment or lever arm – which causes rotation around that axis.

**Motor Neuron:** A neuron (nerve cell) that sends control signals to various tissues and organs. Alpha motor neurons activate muscle cells and signal them to contract.

**Motor Unit:** An alpha motor neuron and all of the muscle fibers it activates (innervates). All of the muscle fibers of a motor unit are of the same fiber type. When a motor unit is activated, all of the muscle fibers are activated, and all contract. In vertebrates, the force of muscle contraction is a function of the number of motor units recruited into the movement, a property that is modified by training.

**Muscle:** A soft tissue in which contractile proteins (myosin and actin) are arranged in a hierarchical structure such that an action potential in the cell membrane results in contraction (shortening) of the cell. Also refers to individual structures made up of such tissue, e.g., biceps, triceps, gastrocnemius, etc.

**Muscle fascicle:** A collection of muscle fibers (muscle cells) in a connective tissue sheath. Skeletal muscles are usually a collection of muscle fascicles.

**Muscle Fiber:** A muscle cell. Muscle cells, or myocytes, are elongated, multinucleate cells with an elaborate hierarchical structure built up from protein filaments which allows them to contract when properly stimulated.

**Myocyte:** A muscle cell. See also Muscle Fiber.

**Myofibril:** A component of the muscle fiber or muscle cell. Myofibrils are bundles of myofilaments – actin and myosin – which produce movement.

**Myofilament:** Filaments composed of actin or myosin, which are essential for the function of muscle tissue.

**Myokine:** A signaling molecule (hormone or cytokine) of muscle tissue origin.

**Myosin:** A protein in muscle tissue. Actin (thin filaments) and myosin (thick filaments) are the protein myofilaments that slide across each other to produce muscular contraction.

**NADH:** A carrier of high-energy electrons yielded by catabolic processes. NADH can deliver these electrons to the electron transport chain in the mitochondrion for the production of ATP.

**Novice:** An athlete who is capable of recovering from and adapting to a training stress from one workout to the next, typically within 48-72 hr. Also the programs used by such athletes.

**Novice Effect:** In an untrained individual, virtually any physical stress will produce adaptations across a range of fitness attributes, including strength. So a rank novice may observe that going for a walk improves his squat strength. The benefits of the novice effect last only long enough to promote the sale of useless programs and exercise gizmos.

**NSAID:** Nonsteroidal Anti-Inflammatory Drug. NSAIDs decrease inflammation by inhibiting enzymes that produce inflammatory signals. Examples include ibuprofen, naproxen, and aspirin.

**Nucleus:** An organelle found in the cells of most organisms more advanced than bacteria. The nucleus contains the genetic material (DNA) that directs the structure and function of the cell.

**Obesity:** A medical condition in which body fat has accumulated sufficiently to have a negative impact on health and function.

**Osteopenia:** A medical condition characterized by low bone mineral density. A precursor to osteoporosis, in which the loss of bone mineral density is so advanced as to invite bone failure and pathologic fracture.

**Overload Event:** The specific training stress or accumulated stresses that disrupt homeostasis, applied over the training period of a Stress-Recovery-Adaptation Cycle, and programmed to drive progressive performance improvement.

**Overtraining:** A situation in which the accumulation of excessive training stress drives the athlete out of the Stress-Recovery-Adaptation cycle and into Selye's Stage III – exhaustion and collapse.

**Oxidative Phosphorylation:** Metabolic process occurring in the mitochondrion, in which high-energy electrons from glycolysis, the Krebs cycle, fatty-acid breakdown and other processes are combined with oxygen to generate a proton "voltage." This voltage is then used to power the production of ATP.

**Phosphagen:** The energy system in which high-energy phosphate is delivered directly to cellular processes and/or recharged without intervening metabolism. Use of the ATP already present in the cell, immediate regeneration of ATP by the creatine phosphate system, and the adenylate kinase system (not described) constitute the phosphagen system. Also known as *substrate-level phosphorylation* or the *immediate energy system.*

**Phosphate:** A chemical group composed of one phosphorous and four oxygen atoms. Phosphate groups can be used to transfer chemical energy for biological processes, e.g., ATP and creatine phosphate.

**Plates:** Disks of iron, plastic or (rarely) other materials used to load the barbell.

**Platform:** A sturdy construction of plywood or other durable material, possibly covered in full or in part by heavy rubber or vinyl matting, upon which the bar may rest and/or an athlete may stand during the performance of barbell exercises.

**Polypharmacy:** A disease in which the patient takes a large number of different medications, many if not most of which are unnecessary or even harmful. Rampant in industrialized societies.

**Power:** The first derivative of strength. Technically, power is the amount of physical work done per unit time (P=W/t) or the product of force and velocity (P=Fv).

**Power Clean:** A variant of the clean portion of the clean and jerk, one of the contested movements in Olympic weightlifting. In the power variant, the clean in received in a high quarter-squat position rather than a front squat or split position.

**Power Rack:** Also known as a power cage. A rigid structure in which barbell exercises may be performed safely. Required when bench presses or maximally heavy squats are performed without spotters.

**Power Snatch:** A variant of the snatch, one of the contested movements in Olympic weightlifting. In the power variant, the snatch is received in a high quarter-squat position rather than a full squat or split position.

**Powerlifting:** A sport in which athletes attempt to lift as much weight as possible for single repetitions in the squat, bench press, and deadlift. Placing is determined by the combined total of best successful attempt for each lift.

**Practice:** Exercise devoted to the progressive development and improvement of sport- or profession-specific skills. We follow Rippetoe in differentiating practice from training. General fitness attributes such as strength and endurance are trained. Triple axels, parries, javelin throws, and baseball bat swings are practiced. To be distinguished from training, which is directed at the development of General Fitness Attributes.

**Press:** A barbell exercise in which the weight is held at the shoulders while standing and pushed overhead. Press variants are qualified by their modifications (eg seated press, alternate dumbbell press).

**Programming:** The explicit and rational manipulation of training variables over time for the progressive development of targeted fitness or performance attributes.

**Program Templates:** In this text, basic program structures are presented as program templates. These structures are not to be taken as invariant, but rather as foundations upon which a large variety of individualized program variants can be constructed, to meet the needs of athletes and their particular training situations.

**Progressive Overload:** The addition of increasing levels of physical stress in training to produce adaptive improvements in fitness attributes. See also Stress-Recovery-Adaptation cycle and Overload Event.

**Protein:** A biological molecule formed by stringing amino acids in a chain in a specific, genetically-determined sequence. Proteins serve as signaling molecules, structural components, enzymes, metabolic regulators, and defense components, among other functions.

**Pull:** Refers to any exercise in which the barbell is lifted ("pulled") from the floor: deadlifts, cleans, and snatches.

**Pyruvate:** One of the end products of glycolysis. Pyruvate, an organic acid, has multiple metabolic fates, depending on the energy demands of the organism.

**Rank Novice**: An untrained individual at the very beginning of training.

**Recovery:** The part of the Stress-Recovery-Adaptation Cycle, in which a disruption of homeostasis is resolved and the organism returns to or exceeds its previous capacity to withstand stress. In the context of training, active rest, sleep, and nutrition support recovery from the stress created by the overload event over the training period.

**Recovery Interval:** A training variable specifying the duration (usually in days) between prescribed workouts.

**Reduced Frequency Model:** A programming approach that reduces training frequency (and usually volume) to accommodate the physical or logistical requirements of a particular athlete.

**Repetition Progression (Rep Progression):** A programming approach that allows the athlete to slowly achieve new performance increases over time by advancing the number of reps that can be performed at a particular weight before more weight is added. See Chapters 22, 23, and 24 for details and variations.

**Repetition Totals:** A programming approach that allows the athlete to slowly achieve new performance increases over time by advancing the total number of reps that can be performed in a workout over multiple sets. A particularly useful progression metric for pull-ups, chin-ups, and other assistance exercises. See Chapter 13 for details.

**Rest Interval:** A training variable specifying the duration of rest between sets or conditioning bouts.

**Safety Pins:** Heavy metal rods inserted into a power rack at a selected height to prevent a failed rep from crushing the lifter.

**Sarcomere:** The contractile unit – a bundle of myofilaments arranged in an elaborate pattern within a muscle cell. Muscle cells contract because their sarcomeres contract.

**Sarcopenia:** The degenerative loss of muscle tissue and strength associated with aging.

**Sets Across:** The performance of all sets for a particular exercise before moving to another exercise. The programs in this book prescribe sets across – for example, the athlete will complete all squat sets before moving on to the press, etc.

**Sick Aging Phenotype:** A meta-syndrome of pathological aging characterized by metabolic syndrome, sarcopenia and osteopenia, frailty, and polypharmacy. Detailed in Chapter 1.

**Sick Fat:** See Visceral Fat.

**Sleep Hygiene:** The set of practices, habits, and environmental preparations that promote regular, sustained, healthy, restorative sleep for optimal recovery.

**Snatch:** An exercise in which a barbell is rapidly lifted from the floor to an overhead position on locked elbows in a single movement. One of the two contested movements in Olympic Weightlifting.

**Specificity:** Refers to the relative tendency of a particular stress to produce a specific adaptation.

**Speed of Movement:** A training variable prescribing the relative speed at which a movement is to be performed, as in Dynamic Effort Sets.

**Split Routine:** A programming approach that splits upper- and lower-body work into different training sessions.

**Spotter:** One who watches and assists the athlete in the event of a missed repetition. In usual practice, a spotter is indicated only for the bench press performed outside a rack. The deadlift and press cannot and need not be spotted. Safely spotting the squat is challenging (see Rippetoe, *Starting Strength: Basic Barbell Training, 3rd edition*).

**Squat:** An exercise in which a weight is carried in the hands or on the body and the hips are lowered and raised.

**Stage I:** The first stage of Selye's General Adaptation Syndrome, *alarm,* in which an environmental stress disrupts the organism's homeostasis. Corresponds to the Stress – the Overload Event – of the Stress-Recovery-Adaptation cycle.

**Stage II:** The second stage of Selye's General Adaptation Syndrome, *resistance,* in which the organism responds to the stress of Stage I by elaborating manifold biological responses to the challenge. If the stress of Stage I lies within the organism's adaptive range, Stage II will result in a return to homeostasis and, for a brief interval, a condition in which the organism is actually stronger than before. Stage II encompasses the Recovery and Adaptation aspects of the Stress-Recovery-Adaptation cycle.

**Stage III:** The third stage of Selye's General Adaptation Syndrome, *exhaustion* or *collapse*. If the stress of Stage I lies outside the organism's adaptive range, the disruption of homeostasis will result in a state chronic derangement, disease, distress, or death. From the perspective of the athlete, this corresponds to the condition of overtraining.

**Standard Teaching Progression:** A fixed approach or "script" for teaching a barbell exercise that produces good performance of the movement with a minimum of time and attention to extraneous or irrelevant details, and begins the introduction of useful cues for real-time correction and optimization. Standard teaching progressions for all the major barbell exercises in this book have been developed and refined by Rippetoe and are detailed in *Starting Strength: Basic Barbell Training, 3rd Edition.*

**Steroid:** A broad and diverse group of molecules characterized by a "steroid ring" structure. Cholesterol, glucocorticoid hormones, and sex and anabolic hormones are all steroid molecules, affecting a diversity of biological functions.

**Strength:** The ability to produce force against an external resistance.

**Stress:** The component of the Stress-Recovery-Adaptation Cycle which disrupts homeostasis. In the context of training, the Overload Event delivers the necessary stress to produce an adaptive response.

**Stress-Recovery-Adaptation Cycle:** The fundamental structure of all rational physical training. Impose a training stress (overload event), recover and adapt. Repeat.

**Structural Exercise:** For our purposes, a barbell exercise that imposes a training stress on the spine and hips. From a practical perspective, this means exercises that are performed while standing.

**Sumo Deadlift:** A deadlift variant in which the athlete lifts the bar with a wide stance, a grip inside the legs, and a relatively vertical back. Almost never indicated.

**Syncope:** A brief and self-limited loss of consciousness and postural tone (a "faint").

**Tendon:** A connective tissue structure that joins a muscle to a bone.

**Texas Method:** An intermediate-level programming model where the overload event delivers the stress across the week in volume-, recovery- and intensity-focused sessions.

**Therapeutic Window:** The dose range that will safely produce a therapeutic response. Usually defined as the ratio of the minimum effective dose to the minimum toxic dose.

**Thrashabout:** An unstructured exercise bout that involves a lot of movement, sweat, strain, yelling, cheering, and self-congratulation, but not the rational manipulation of training variables for the realization of long-term progressive improvements in fitness attributes. Most often seen in the context of sessions with personal trainers, DVD exercise programs, and fitness "boot camps."

**Training:** An explicitly and rationally structured form of exercise that manipulates training variables in a long-term program aimed at the improvement of one or more General Fitness Attributes.

**Training Density:** The ratio of training work and the time taken to perform it. Three sets of 5 over 30 minutes represents a higher training density than 3 sets of 5 over 60 minutes.

**Transfer:** The realization of a meaningful performance improvement as a result of training one or more fitness attributes. For example, if training for strength improves a wrestler's ability to pin an opponent, we may say that the training demonstrates transfer.

**Triglyceride:** A complex molecule consisting of glycerol and fatty acids; the storage form of fat.

**Type I Fibers:** Muscle fibers with relatively low cross-sectional area, low power, low strength, and high oxidative capacity.

**Type IIa Fibers:** Muscle fibers with relatively high cross-sectional area, moderately high power and strength, and moderately high oxidative capacity.

**Type IIx Fibers:** Muscle fibers with high cross-sectional area, power, and strength, but low oxidative capacity.

**Uprights:** The vertical beams of a power rack or pressing bench.

**Visceral Fat:** Fat (adipose tissue) accumulated around the internal organs. Excess accumulation of visceral fat is strongly linked to the development of the metabolic syndrome and cardiovascular disease.

**Visceral Obesity:** The accumulation of excess visceral fat.

**$VO_2$:** The rate at which the organism takes up and uses oxygen. Measured in ml of oxygen per kilogram of bodyweight per minute.

**$VO_2$max:** The maximum sustainable rate at which oxygen can be delivered to tissues. $VO_2$max is strongly correlated with aerobic capacity, and is generally regarded as a marker of cardiovascular function and health.

**Volume:** A loose synonym for "quantity." In strength programming, the volume of a workout is a function of the total repetitions of that workout.

**Volume-Sensitivity:** An important characteristic of the Masters Athlete. Masters do not benefit from high-volume work to the same degree as younger athletes, and are more sensitive to volume-induced overtraining.

**Warm-up Sets:** Sets performed at low but gradually-increasing weight to prepare the athlete for work sets.

**Weightlifting (Olympic):** A strength sport in which the athlete attempts to lift as much weight as possible for single repetitions in the snatch and the clean and jerk. The best attempts for each lift are combined to determine competition placing.

**Work:** In mechanics, work is a force acting through a distance: $W = Fd$.

**Work Interval:** A training variable specifying the duration of a training task. Most frequently used in association with HIIT.

**Work sets:** Sets performed to provide the training stress of a workout. Work sets produce the prescribed volume and intensity that the athlete must accomplish *today* to move training forward.

# Bibliography

Aagaard P, Andersen JL. Effects of strength training on endurance capacity in top-level endurance athletes. *Scand J Med Sci Sports* 2010;20:39-47.

Aarsland D, Sardahaee FS, Anderssen S, et al. Is physical activity a potential preventive factor for vascular dementia? A systematic review. *Aging Mental Health* 2010;14(4):386-395.

Abramson J, Wright JM. Are lipid-lowering agents evidence-based? *Lancet* 2007;369(9557):168-169.

Ades PA, Ballor DL, Ashikaga T, et al. Weight training improves walking endurance in healthy elderly persons. *Ann Intern Med* 1996;124(6):568-572.

Ahlskog JE, Geda YE, Graff-Radford NR, Peterson RC. Physical exercise as a preventative or disease-modifying treatment of dementia and aging. *Mayo Clinic Proced* 2011;86(9):876-884.

Ahlskog JE. Does vigorous exercise have a neuroprotective effect in Parkinson disease? *Neurology* 2011;77(3):288-94.

Ahmed H, Blaha MJ, Nasir K, et al. Effects of physical activity on cardiovascular disease. *Am J Cardiol* 2012;109(2):288-295.

Albright A, Franz M, Hornsby G, et al. American College of Sports Medicine Position Stand. Exercise and type 2 diabetes. *Med Sci Sports Exerc* 2000;32(7):1345-1360.

Altman D. Poor-quality medical research: what can the journal do? *JAMA* 2002;287:2765-2767.

Alvehus M, Boman N, Soderlund K, et al. Metabolic adaptations in skeletal muscle, adipose tissue, and whole-body oxidative capacity in response to resistance training. *Eur J Appl Physiol* 2014;114(7):1463-1471.

American College of Sports Medicine Position Stand. The recommended quantity and quality of exercise for developing and maintaining cardiorespiratory and muscular fitness and flexibility in healthy adults. *Med Sci Sports Exerc* 1998;30:975-991.

American College of Sports Medicine. The recommended quantity and quality of exercise for developing and maintaining cardiorespiratory and muscular fitness in healthy adults. *Med Sci Sports Exerc* 1990;22:265-274.

Amidu N, Owiredu WKBA, Alidu H, et al. Association between the metabolic syndrome and sexual dysfunction among men with clinically diagnosed diabetes. *Diabetology Metab Synd* 2013;5:42-50.

Anderson T, Kearny JT. Effects of three resistance training programs on muscular strength and absolute and relative endurance. *Res Quart Exerc Sport* 1982;53(1):1-7.

Armstrong GL, Conn LA, Pinner RW. Trends in infectious diseases mortality in the United States during the 20th century. *JAMA* 1999;281(1):61-66.

Artero EG, Duck-chul L, Ruiz Jr, et al. A prospective study of muscular strength and all-cause mortality in men with hypertension. *JACC* 2011;57(18):1831-7.

Atherton PJ, Babraj J, Smith K, et al. Selective activation of AMPK-PGC-1a or PKB-TSC2-mTOR signaling can explain specific adaptive responses to endurance or resistance training-like electrical muscle stimulation. *FASEB J* 2005;19(7):786-788.

Baggenhammar S, Hansson EE. Repeated sets or a single set of resistance training—a systematic review. *Adv Physioth* 2007;9(4):154-160.

Banz WJ, Maher MA, Thompson WG, et al. Effects of resistance versus aerobic training on coronary artery disease risk factors. *Exp Biol Med* (Maywood) 2003;228:434-440.

Barzilay JI, Blaum C, Moore T, et al. Insulin resistance and inflammation as precursors of frailty. The Cardiovascular Health Study. *Arch Intern Med* 2007;167(7):635-641.

Batsis JA, Sahakyan KR, Rodriguez-Escudero JP, et al. Normal weight obesity and mortality in the United States Subjects > 60 years of age (from the Third National Health and Nutrition Examination Survey). *Am J Cardiol* 2013;112(10):1592-1598.

Beavers KM, Hsu FC, Houston DK, et al. The role of metabolic syndrome, adiposity and inflammation in physical performance in the Health ABC Study. *J Gerontol Med Sci* 2013;68(5):617-623.

Bibliography


Beedlel B, Jesee C, Stone MH. Flexibility characteristics among athletes who strength train. *JSCR* 1991;5(3):150-154.

Beltran VMR, Dimauro I, Brunelli A, et al. Explosive-type of moderate resistance training induces functional cardiovascular and molecular adaptations in the elderly. *Age* 2014;36(2):759-772.

Berg AH, Scherer PE. Adipose tissue, inflammation, and cardiovascular disease. *Circ Res* 2005;96:939-949.

Berg, Jeremy M., John L. Tymoczko, and Lubert Stryer. *Biochemistry* (5th Ed), 2002. W. H. Freeman, New York.

Berryman JW. Exercise is medicine: a historical perspective. *Curr Sports Med Rpts* 2010;9(4):195-201.

Bilsborough S, Mann N. A review of issues of dietary protein intake in humans. *Int J Sport Nut ExercMetab* 2006; 16:129-152.

Blackman MR, Sorkin JD, Munzer T, et al. Growth hormone and sex steroid administration in healthy aged women and men. A randomized controlled trial. *JAMA* 2002;228:2282-2292.

Blaum CS, Xue QL, Michelon E, et al. The association between obesity and the frailty syndrome in older women: the women's health and aging studies. *J Am Ger Soc* 2005;53(6):927-934.

Blumenthal JA, Siegel WC, Appelbaum M. Failure of exercise to reduce blood pressure in patients with mild hypertension. *JAMA* 1991;266:2098-2104.

Bonanno JA, Lies JE. Effects of physical training on coronary risk factors. *Am J Cardiol* 1974;33(6):760-764.

Boonen S, Rosen C, Bouillon R et al. Musculoskeletal effects of the recombinant human IGF-1/IGF binding protein-3 complex in osteoporotic patients with proximal femoral fracture: a double-blind, placebo-controlled study. *J Clin Endocrinol Metab* 2002;87:1593-1599.

Borghouts LB, Keizer HA. Exercise and insulin sensitivity: a review. *Int J Sports Med* 2000;21(1):1-12.

Bozaoglu K, Bolton K, McMillan J, et al. Chemerin is a novel adipokine associated with obesity and the metabolic syndrome. *Endocrinology* 2007;148(10):4687-4694.

Brach JS, Simonsicki EM, Kritchevsy S, et al. The association between physical function and lifestyle activity and exercise in the health, aging and body composition study. *J Am Geriat Soc* 2004;52(4):502-509.

Braith RW, Stewart KJ. Resistance exercise training: its role in the prevention of cardiovascular disease. *Circulation* 2006;113:2642-2650.

Bridle C, Spanjers K, Patel S, et al. Effect of exercise on depression severity in older people: systematic review and meta-analysis of randomized controlled trials. *Br J Psych* 2012;201:180-185.

Brooks GA, Fahey TD, Baldwin KM. *Exercise Physiology: Human Bioenergetics and Its Applications* (4th Ed). 2005; McGraw Hill, New York, NY.

Brunner F, Schmid A, Sheikhzadeh A, et al. Effects of aging on Type II muscle fibers: a systematic review of the literature. *J Aging Physical Act* 2007;15:336-348.

Bruunsgaard H, Bjerregaard E, Schroll M, Pedersen BK. Muscle strength after resistance training is inversely correlated with baseline levels of soluble tumor necrosis factor receptors in the oldest old. *J Am Geriatr Soc* 2004;52(2):237-241.

Bucchanna CI, Marsh RL. Effects of exercise on the biomechanical, biochemical and structural properties of tendons. *Comp Bioch Physiol A* 2002;133(4):1101-1107.

Bunout D, Barrerra G, Leiva L, et al. Effects of vitamin D supplementation and exercise training on physical performance in Chilean vitamin D-deficient elderly subjects. *Exp Geront* 2006;41(8):746-752.

Burgomaster KA, Howarth KR, Phillips SM, et al. Similar metabolic adaptations during exercise after low volume sprint interval and traditional endurance training in humans. *J Physiol* 2008;586.1:151-160.

Calhoon G, Fry AC. Injury rates and profiles of elite competitive weightlifters. *J Athl Train* 1999;34(3):232-238.

Campbell WW, Crim MC, Young VR, Evans WJ. Increased energy requirements and changes in body composition with resistance training in older adults. *Am J Clin Nutr* 1994;60:167-175.

Campos ER, Luecke TJ, Wendeln HK, et al. Muscular adaptations in response to three different resistance-training regimens: specificity of repetition maximum training zones. *Eur J Appl Physiol* 2002;88:50-60.

Campos P, Suguy A, Ernsberger P, et al. The epidemiology of overweight and obesity: public health crisis or moral panic? *Int J Epidem* 2006;35(1):55-60.

Campos P. *The Obesity Myth: Why America's Obsession with Fat is Hazardous to Your Health.* 2004, Gotham-Penguin.

Carek PJ, Laibstain SE, Carek SM, et al. Exercise for the treatment of depression and anxiety. *Int J Psych Med* 2011; 41(1):15-28.

Carpinelli RN, Otto RN. Strength training. *Sports Med* 1998;26(2):73-84.

Carter JG, Potter AW, Brooks KA. Overtraining syndrome: causes, consequences and methods for prevention. *J Sport Human Perf* 2014;2(1).

Castaneda C, Layne JE, Munoz-Orians L, et al. A randomized-controlled trial of resistance exercise training to improve glycemic control in older adults with type 2 diabetes. *Diabetes Care* 2002;25:2335-2341.

Castaneda C, Layne JE, Munoz-Orians L, et al. A randomized controlled trial of resistance exercise training to improve glycemic control in older adults with type 2 diabetes. *Diabetes Care* 2002;25(12):2335-41.

Chang EY, Moses DA, Babb JS, Schweitzer ME. Shoulder impingement: objective 3D shape analysis of acromial morphologic features. *Radiology* 2006; 239:497-505.

Cheema B, Gaul CA, Lane K, Singh MAF. Progressive resistance training in breast cancer: a systematic review of clinical trials. *Br Ca Res Treat* 2008;109(1):9-26.

Chen Y, Zhu M, Zhang Y. Combined endurance-resistance training improves submaximal exercise capacity in elderly heart-failure patients: a systematic review of controlled trials. *Int J Cardiol* 2012;http://dx.doi.org/10.1016/j.ijcard.2012.09.114.

Cho KY, Park H, Seo JW. The relationship between lifestyle and metabolic syndrome in obese children and adolescents. *Korean J Pediatr Gastroenterol Nutr* 2008;11(2):150-159.

Chowdury R, Warnakula S, Kunutsor S, et al. Association of dietary, circulating and supplemental fatty acids with coronary risk: a systematic review and meta-analysis. *Ann Intern Med* 2014;160(6):398-406.

Christ-Roberts CY, Pratipanawatr T, Pratinpanawatr W, et al. Exercise training increases glycogen synthase activity and GLUT4 expression but not insulin signaling in overweight nondiabetic and type 2 diabetic subjects. *Metabolism* 2004;53(9):1233-1242.

Chrysohoou C, Pitsavos C, Tsitsinakis G, et al. High intensity, interval exercise improves quality of life, ventricular diastolic function, ergometric capacity and psychological status of patients with chronic heart failure: a phase III randomized clinical trial. *J Am Coll Cardiol* 2014;63:12-S:1303-1306.

Churchward-Venne TA, Breen L, Phillips SM. Alterations in human muscle protein metabolism with aging: Protein and exercise as countermeasures to offset sarcopenia. *Biofactors* 201;40(2):199-205.

Ciloglu F, Peker I, Pehlivan A, et al. Exercise intensity and its effects on thyroid hormones. *Neuroend Lett* 2005; 26(6):830-834.

Claflin DR, Larkin LM, Cederna PS. Effects of high- and low-velocity resistance training on the contractile properties of skeletal muscle fibers from young and older humans. *J Appl Physiol* 2011;111:1021-1030.

Clemente CD. *Anatomy: Regional Atlas of the Human Body* (6th Ed). 2010 Lippincott, Williams and Wilkins, Baltimore, MD.

Cohn B. Medical research: the good, the bad and the underpowered. *Emerg Phys Monthly* 2014;21(1):15-16.

Colcombe SJ, Erickson KI, Scaif PE, et al. Aerobic exercise training increases brain volume in aging humans. *J Gerontol A Biol Sci Med Sci* 2006;61(11):1166-1170.

Collins MK, Perkins GR et al. Growth factors as survival factors: regulation of apoptosis. *Bioessays* 1994;15(2):133-8.

Conceicao MS, Bonganha V, Vecchin FC, et al. Sixteen weeks of resistance training can decrease the risk of metabolic syndrome in healthy postmenopausal women. *Clin Intervent Aging* 2013;8:1221-1228.

Convit A. Links between cognitive impairment in insulin resistance: an explanatory model. *Neurobiol Aging* 2005; 26(1):31-35.

Cooney GM, Dwan K, Greig CA, et al. Exercise for depression. *Cochrane Database Syst Rev* 2013; doi: 10.1002/14651858.CD004366.pub6

Cornelissen VA, Fagard RH, Coeckelberghs E, Vanhees L. Impact of resistance training on blood pressure and other cardiovascular risk factors: a meta-analysis of randomized controlled trials. *Hypertension* 2011;58:950-958.

Cornellisen VA, Fagard RH. Effect of resistance training on resting blood pressure: a meta-analysis of randomized controlled trials. *J Hypertension* 2005;23(2):251-259.

Cotman CW, Berchtold NC, Christie LA. Exercise builds brain health: key roles of growth factor cascades and inflammation. *Trends Neurosci* 2007;30(9):464-472.

Cotman CW, Berchtold NC. Exercise: a behavioral intervention to enhance brain health and plasticity. *Trends Neurosci* 2002;25(6):295-301.

Bibliography

Croymans DM, Paparisto E, Lee MM, et al. Resistance training improves indices of muscle insulin sensitivity and β-cell function in overweight/obese, sedentary young men. *J Appl Physiol* 2013;115:1245-1253.

Culver AL, Ockene IS, Balasubramanian R, et al. Statin use and risk of diabetes mellitus in postmenopausal women in the women's health initiative. *Arch Int Med* 2012;172(2):144-152.

Dai DF, Chiao YA, Marcinek DJ, et al. Mitochondrial oxidative stress in aging and healthspan. *Long Healthspan* 2014;3:6.

Danielson L, Noras AM, Waern M, Carlsson J. Exercise in the treatment of major depression: a systematic review grading the quality of the evidence. *Physioth Theory Pract* 2013;29(8):573-585.

Dawson-Hughes B, Harris SS, Krall EA, et al. Effect of calcium and vitamin D supplementation on bone density in men and women 65 years of age or older. *New Engl J Med* 1997;337:670-676.

de Rooij NK, Linn FHH, van der Plas JA et al. Incidence of subarachnoid hemorrhage : a systematic review with emphasis on region, gender, age and time trends. *J Neurol Neurosurg Psychiatry* 2007;78:1365-1372.

Del Coso JD, Salinero JJ, Gonzalaz-Milan CG, et al. Dose response effects of a caffeine-containing energy drink on muscle performance: a repeated-measures design. *J InternatSoc Sports Nutr* 2012;9:21.

den Heijer T, Vermeer SE, van Dijk EJ, et al. Type 2 diabetes and atrophy of temporal lobe structures on brain MRI. *Diabetologica* 2003;46:1604-1610.

Deschenes MR. Effects of aging on muscle fiber type and size. *Sports Med* 2004;34(12):809-824.

Despres JP, Lemieux I. Abdominal obesity and metabolic syndrome. *Nature* 2006;444:881-887.

Dickinson JM, Volpi E, Rasmussen BB. Exercise and nutrition to target protein synthesis impairments in aging skeletal muscle. *Exerc Sport Sci Rev* 2013;41(4):216-223.

Doherty TJ. Aging and sarcopenia. *J Appl Physiol* 2003;95(4):1717-1727.

Dominguez LJ, Barbagello M. The cardiometabolic syndrome and sarcopenic obesity in older persons. *J Cardiomet Synd* 2007;2(3):183-189.

Dornerman TM, McMurray RG, Renner JB, Anderson JJ. Effects of high-intensity resistance exercise on bone mineral density and muscle strength 40-50 year-old women. *J Sports Med Phys Fit* 1997;37(4):246-251.

Duncan MJ, Smith M, Cook K, James RS. The acute effect of a caffeine-containing energy drink on mood state, readiness to invest effort, and resistance exercise to failure. *JSCR* 2012;26(10):2858-2865.

Duncan MJ,Oxford SW. The effect of caffeine ingestion on mood state and bench press performance to failure. *JSCR* 2011;25(1): 178-85.

Duncan P, Richards L, Wallace D, et al. A randomized, controlled pilot study of a home-based exercise program for individuals with mild and moderate stroke. *Stroke* 1998;29:2055-2060.

Dunstan DW, Daly RM, Owen N, et al. High-intensity resistance training improves glycemic control in older patients with Type 2 diabetes. *Diabetes Care* 2002;25(10):1729-1736.

Dupont-Versteegden EE. Apoptosis in muscle atrophy: relevance to sarcopenia. *Exp Gerontol* 2005;40(6):473-81.

Durak EP, Jovanovic-Peterson L, Peterson CM. Randomized crossover study of effect of resistance training on glycemic control, muscular strength, and cholesterol in type I diabetic men. *Diabetes Care* 1990;13:1039-1043.

Eggerston L. Lancet retracts 12-year-old article linking autism to MMR vaccines. *CMAJ* 2010;182(4):doi:10.1503/cmaj.109-3179.

Eghbalzadeh K, Brixius K, Bloch W, Brinkmann C. Skeletal muscle nitric oxide (NO) synthases and NO-signaling in "diabesity"— What about the relevance of exercise training interventions? *Nitric Oxide* 2013;doi:10.1016/j.niox.2013.2009

Eknoyan G. AdopheQuetelet (1796-1874)—the average man and indices of obesity. *Nephrol Dial Transplant* 2008; 23(1):47-51.

Ellington WR. Evolution and physiological roles of phosphagen systems. *Ann Rev Physiol* 2001;63:289-325.

Engelke K, Kemmler W, Lauber D, et al. Exercise maintains bone density at spine and hip EFOPS: a 3-year longitudinal study in early postmenopausal women. *Osteoporosis Int* 2006;17:133-142.

Erikkson J, Taimela S, Koivisto VA. Exercise and the metabolic syndrome. *Diabetalogica* 1997;40:125-135.

Erikson EF, Glerup H. Vitamin D deficiency and aging: implications for general health and osteoporosis. *Biogerontology* 2002;3:73-77.

Esposito K, Giugliano F, Martedi E, et al. High proportions of erectile dysfunction in men with the metabolic syndrome. *Diabetes Care* 2005;28(5):1201-1203.

Evagrio Pontico, *Gli Otto Spiriti Malvagi*, trans., Felice Comello, Pratiche Editrice, Parma, 1990, p.11-12.

Everett G. *Olympic Weightlifting for Sports.* 2012; Catalyst Athletics Inc.

Eves ND, Plotnikoff RC. Resistance training and type 2 diabetes. *Diabetes Care* 2006;29(8):1933-1941.

Farinatti P, Neto AGC, da Silva NL. Influence of resistance training variables on excess postexercise oxygen consumption: a systematic review. *ISRN Physiol* 2013; http://dx.doi.org/10.1155/2013/825026.

Fauci AS, Morens DM. The perpetual challenge of infectious diseases. *N Engl J Med* 2012;366:454-461.

Favero S, Roschel H, Artioli R et al. Creatine but not betaine supplementation increases muscle phosphoryl-creatine content and strength performance. *Amino Acids* 2011;epub ahead of print.

Feigenbaum J, Goodmurphy C, Scheider C. Gripping matters: Anatomy 501 for the press. 2013 The Aasgaard Company. http://startingstrength.com/article/gripping_matters

Ferreira I, Twisk JS, van Mechelen W et al. Development of fitness, fatness and lifestyle from adolescence to the age of 36 years. Determinants of the metabolic syndrome in young adults: the Amsterdam Growth and Health Longitudinal Study. *Arch Intern Med* 2005;165(1):42-48.

Ferreira R, Neuparth MJ, Vitorino R, et al. Evidences of apoptosis during the early phases of soleus muscle atrophy in hindlimb suspended mice. *Physiol Res* 2008;57:601-11.

Ferris LT, Williams JS, Shen CL. The effect of acute exercise on serum brain-derived neurotrophic factor levels and cognitive function. *Med Sci Sports Exerc* 2007;39(4):728-734.

Fielding RA, Vellas B, Evans WJ, et al. Sarcopenia: an Undiagnosed condition in Older Adults. Current consensus definition: Prevalence, Etiology and Consequences. International Working Group on Sarcopenia. *J Am Med Dir Assoc* 2011;12(4):249-256.

Fischer-Wellman KH, Bloomer RJ. Oxidative stress and exercise in cardiopulmonary and metabolic disorders. *Systems Biology of Free Radicals and Antioxidants* 2014;Springer Berlin Heidelberg 3805-3830.

Fontana L, Eagon JC, Trujillo ME, et al. Visceral fat adipokine secretion is associated with systemic inflammation in obese humans. *Diabetes* 2007;56(4):1010-1013.

Ford ES, Giles WH, Dietz WH. Prevalence of metabolic syndrome among US adults: findings from the third National Health and Nutrition Examination Survey. *JAMA* 2002;287(3):356–359.

Fried LP, Tangen CM, Walston J, et al. Frailty in older adults: Evidence for a phenotype. *J Gerontol A Biol Sci Med Sci* 2001;55(3):M146-M157.

Fries JF, Bruce B, Chakravarty E. Compression of morbidity 1980-2011: a focused review of paradigms and progress. *J Aging Res* 2011; http://dx.doi.org/10.4061/2011/261702

Frontera WR, Hughes VA, Lutz KJ, Evans WJ. A cross-sectional study of muscle strength and mass in 48-72-yr-old men and women. *J Appl Physiol* 1991;71(2):644-650.

Frontera WR, Meredith CN, O'Reilly KP, et al. Strength conditioning in older men: skeletal muscle hypertrophy and improved function. *J Appl Physiol* 1988;65(3):1038-1044.

Frontera WR, Meredith CN, O'Reilly KP, Evans WJ. Strength training and determinants of $VO_2$max in older men. *J Appl Physiol* 1990;68:329-333.

Fulginiti V. The millennium in infectious diseases: Focus on the last century 1900-2000. *Medscape Gen Med* 2000;2(1): http://www.medscape.com/viewarticle/408050_3

Fuzhong L, Harmer P, Fisher KJ, et al. Tai Chi and fall reductions in older adults: a randomized controlled trial. J *Gerontol Biol Sci* 2005;60(2):187-194.

Ghilarducci LEC, Holly RG, Amsterdam EA. Effects of high resistance training in coronary artery disease. *Am J Cardiol* 1989;65(14):866-870.

Gibala MJ, Little JP, van Essen M, et al. Short-term sprint interval versus traditional endurance training: similar adaptations in human skeletal muscle and exercise performance. *J Physiol* 2006;575.3;901-911.

Gibala, M. 2009. Molecular responses to high-intensity interval exercise. *App Phys Nut Metab* 2009;34(3):428-32.

Gollnick PD, Armstrong RB, Saubert IV, et al. Enzyme activity and fiber composition in skeletal muscle of untrained and trained men. *J Appl Physiol* 1972;33(3):312-319.

Graff-Radford NR. Can aerobic exercise protect against dementia? *Alzh Res Therapy* 2011;3(6):2-6.

Granata C, Oliveira RSF, Little JP, et al. Training intensity modulates changes in PGC-1a and p53 protein content and mitochondrial respiration, but not markers of mitochondrial content in human skeletal muscle. *FASEB J* 2015; fj-15.

Grandjean AC, Reimers KJ, Bennick KE, Haven MC. The effect of caffeinated, non-caffeinated, caloric and non-caloric beverages on hydration. *J Am CollNutr* 2000;19(5):591-600.

Grant WB, Holick MF. Benefits and requirements of vitamin D for optimal health: a review. *Alt Med Rev* 2005; 10(2):94-111.

Greiwe JS, Cheng B, Rubin DC, et al. Resistance exercise decreases skeletal muscle tumor necrosis factor alpha in frail elderly humans. *FASEB J* 2001;15(2):475-482.

Grontved A, Rimm EB, Willet WC, et al. A prospective study of weight training and risk of type 2 diabetes in men. *Arch Int Med* 2012;172(17):1306-1312.

Gross L. A Broken Trust: Lessons from the Vaccine–Autism Wars. *PLoS Biol* 2009;7(5): e1000114.

Grundy SM. Obesity, metabolic syndrome, and cardiovascular disease. *J Clinic Endocrin Metab* 2004;89(6):2595-2600.

Gualano B, Ugrinowitsch C, Novaes RB, et al. Effects of creatine supplementation on renal function: a randomized, double-blind, placebo-controlled clinical trial. *Eur J App Physiol* 2008;103(1):33-40.

Guasch E, Mont L. Exercise and the heart: unmasking Mr. Hyde. *Heart J* 2014;doi:10.1136/heartjnl-2014-305780

Habberg JM, Ehsani AA, Foldring O, et al. Effect of weight training on blood pressure and hemodynamics in hypertensive adolescents. *J Pediatrics* 1984;19:147-151.

Haff G, Whitley A, Potteiger J. A brief review: explosive exercise and sports performance. *Strength and Cond J* 2001; 23(3):13.

Hagerman FC, Walsh SJ, Staron RS, et al. Effects of high-intensity resistance training on untrained older men. I. Strength, cardiovascular and metabolic responses. *J Gerontol A Biol Sci Med Sci* 2000;55A(7)B336-B346.

Hajjar ER, Cafiero AC, Hanlon JT. Polypharmacy in elderly patients. *Am J Ger Pharm* 2007;5(4):345-351.

Hamill BP. Relative safety of weightlifting and weight training. *JSCR* 1994;8(1):53-57.

Hamilton WF, Woodbury RA, Harper HT. Arterial, cerebrospinal and venous pressure changes in man during cough and strain. *Am J Physiol* 1944;141(1):42-50.

Hansen E, Landstad BJ, Gundersen KT, et al. Insulin sensitivity after maximal and endurance resistance training. *JSCR* 2012;26(2):327-334.

Hansen PA, Noite LA, Chen MH, Holloszy MO. Increased GLUT-4 translocation mediates enhanced insulin sensitivity of muscle glucose transport after exercise. *J Appl Physiol* (1985)1998;85(4):1218-1222.

Harcombe Z, Baker JS, Cooper SM, et al. Evidence from randomised controlled trials did not support the introduction of dietary fat guidelines in 1977 and 1983: a systematic review and meta-analysis. *Open Heart* 2014;doi:10.1136/openhrt-2014-000196

Harris KA, Holly RG. Physiological response to circuit weight training in borderline hypertensive subjects. *Med Sci Sports Exerc* 1987;19:246-252.

Hartmann H, Kluseman WK, Dalic J, et al. Influence of squatting depth on jumping performance. *J Strength Cond Res* 2012;26(12):3243-61.

Hartmann H, Wirth K, Kluseman M. Analysis of the load on knee joint and vertebral column with changes in squatting depth and weight load. *Sports Med* 2013;43(10):993-1008.

Hawley JA. Molecular responses to strength and endurance training: are they compatible? *Appl Physiol Nut Metab* 2009;34:355-361.

Haykowsky MJ, Findlay JM, Ignaszeski MD. Aneurysmal subarachnoid hemorrhage associated with weight training: three case reports. *Clin J Sport Med* 1996;6(1):52-55.

Headley S, Germain M, Mailloux P, et al. Resistance training improves strength and functional measures in patients with end-stage renal disease. *Am J Kidney Dis* 2002;40(2):355-364.

Hefferman KS, Yoon ES, Sharman JE, et al. Resistance exercise training reduces arterial reservoir pressure in older adults with prehypertension and hypertension. *Hyperten Res* 2012;Epub ahead of print.

Helgerud, J., et al. Aerobic high-intensity intervals improve $VO_2$max more than moderate training. *Med Sci Sports Ex* 2007;39(4):665-71.

Heyn P, Abreu BC, Ottenbacher KJ. The effects of exercise training on elderly persons with cognitive impairment and dementia: a meta-analysis. *Arch Phys Med Rehab* 2004;85(10):1694-1704.

Hickson RC. Interference of strength development by simultaneously training for strength and endurance. *Eur J Appl Physiol* 1980;45:255-264.

Higdon JV, Frei B. Coffee and health: A review of recent human research. *Crit Rev Food SciNutr* 2006;46(2):101-123.

Hill DJ, Milner RDG. Insulin as a growth factor. *Pediatr Res* 1985;19:879-886.

Hillman CH, Erickson KI, Kramer AF. Be smart, exercise your heart: exercise effects on brain and cognition. *Nature Rev Neurosci* 2008;9:58-65.

Hirano A, Suzuki Y, Kuzuya M, et al. Influence of regular exercise on subjective sense of burden and physical symptoms in community-dwelling caregivers of dementia patients: a randomized controlled trial. *Arch Geront Geriat* 2011;53(2):e158-e163.

Ho SS, Dhaliwal SS, Hills AP, Pal S. The effect of 12 weeks of aerobic, resistance or combination exercise training on cardiovascular risk factors in the overweight and obese in a randomized trial. *BMC Public Health* 2012;12:704.

Hochachka PW, Neely JR, Driedzic WR. Integration of lipid utilization with Krebs cycle activity in muscle. *Federation proceedings* 1977;36(7):2009-2014.

Hoff J, Gran A, Helgerud J. Maximal strength training improves aerobic endurance performance. *Scand J Med Sci Sports* 2002;12(5):288-295.

Hoffman DF. Arthritis and exercise. *Prim Care* 1993;20(4):895-810.

Holic MF. High prevalence of vitamin D inadequacy and implications for health. *Mayo ClinProc* 2006;81(3):353-73.

Holviala JHS, Sallinen JM, Kraemer WJ, et al. Effects of strength training on muscle strength characteristics, functional capabilities, and balance in middle-aged and older women. *JSCR* 2006;20(2):336-344.

Hooper L, Summerbell CD, Thompson R, et al. Reduced or modified dietary fat for preventing cardiovascular disease. Cochrane heart group 2012; doi:10.1002/14651858.CD002137.pub3

Horwich TB, Fonarow GC. Glucose, obesity, metabolic syndrome and diabetes: relevance to incidence of heart failure. *J Am Coll Cardiol* 2010; 55:283-293.

Hunter GR, Bryan DR, Wetzstein CJ, et al. Resistance training and intra-abdominal adipose tissue in older men and women. *Med Sci Sports Exerc* 2002 Jun;34(6):1023-8.

Hurley BF, Hagberg JM, Goldberg AP. Resistive training can reduce coronary risk factors without altering $VO_2$max or percent body fat. *Med Sci Sports Exerc* 20;150-154.

Hurley BF, Roth SM. Strength training in the elderly. *Sports Med* 2000;30:249-268.

Hurley BF, Roth SM. Strength training in the elderly: effects on risk factors for age-related diseases. *Sports Med* 2000; 30:249-268.

Hutchinson DS, Summers RJ, Bengtsson T. Regulation of AMP-activated protein kinase activity by G-coupled protein receptors: potential utility in treatment of diabetes and heart disease. *Pharmacol Therap* 2008;119(3):291-310.

Huxley AF, Niedergerke R. Structural changes in muscle during contraction: interference microscopy of living muscle fibres. *Nature* 1954;173(4412):971–973.

Huxley H, Hanson J. Changes in the cross-striations of muscle during contraction and stretch and their structural interpretation. *Nature* 1954;173(4412):973–976.

Iacobellis G, Barbaro G. The double role of epicardial adipose tissue as pro- and anti-inflammatory organ. *Horm Metab Res* 2008;40(7):442-445.

Inelman EM, Sergi G, Coin A, et al. Can obesity be a risk factor for elderly people? *Obesity Rev* 2003;4(3):147-55.

International Diabetes Federation. The IDF consensus worldwide definition of the metabolic syndrome. *IDF Communications* 2006;http://www.idf.org/webdata/docs/IDF_Meta_def_final.pdf

Irvine C, Taylor NF. Progressive resistance exercise improves glycaemic control in people with Type 2 diabetes mellitus: a systematic review. *Aust J Physiotherapy* 2009;55:237-246.

Jagim AR, Oliver JM, Sanchez A, et al. A buffered form of creatine does not promote greater changes in muscle creatine content, body composition, or training adaptations than creatine monohydrate. *J Int Soc Sports Nut* 2012;9(43).

Jahnke R, Larkey L, Rogers C, et al. A comprehensive review of health benefits of Qigong and Tai Chi. *Am J Health Prom* 2010;24(6):e1-e25.

Janssen I, Shepard DS, Katzmarzyk PT, Roubenoff R. The healthcare costs of sarcopenia in the United States. *J Am Geriatrics Soc* 2004;52(1):80-85.

Johannson SE, Sundquist J. Change in lifestyle factors and their influence on health status and all-cause mortality. *Internat J Epidem* 1999;28:1073-1080.

Jones DS, Podolsky SH, Greene JA. The burden of disease and the changing task of medicine. *N Engl J Med* 2012; 366:2333-2338.

Judge JO, Lindsey C, Underwood M, Winsemius D. Balance improvements in older women: effects of exercise training. *Physical Therapy* 1993;73(4):254-262.

Jurca R, Lamonte MJ, Barlow CE, et al. Association of muscular strength with metabolic syndrome in men. *Med Sci Sports Exerc* 2005;37(11):1849-1855.

Kalitesi EvY. Exercise and quality of life. *Trakya Univ Tip Fak Derg* 2010;27(S1):54-56.

Kata A. Anti-vaccine activists, Web 2.0, and the postmodern paradigm—An overview of the tactics and tropes used online by the anti-vaccination movement. *Vaccine* 2012;30(25):3778-3789.

Kavanagh T. Exercise in cardiac rehabilitation. *Br J Sports Med* 2000;34:3-6.

Kelley GA, Kelley KS, Tran ZV. Resistance training and bone mineral density in women: a meta-analysis of controlled trials. *Phys Med Rehab* 2001;80(1):65-77.

Kemmler W, Lauber D, Weineck J, et al. Benefits of 2 years of intense exercise on bone density, physical fitness, and blood lipids in early postmenopausal osteopenic women. *Arch Intern Med* 2004;164(10):1084-1091.

Kennedy JW, Hirschman MF, Gervino EV, et al. Acute exercise induces GLUT4 translocation in skeletal muscle of normal human subjects and subjects with type 2 diabetes. *Diabetes* 1999;48:1192-1197.

Kilgore, L., & Rippetoe, M. (2007). Redefining Fitness For Health and Fitness Professionals. *J Ex Phys Online*, 2007;10(2),34-39.

Kim S, Popkin BM. Commentary: Understanding the epidemiology of overweight and obesity – a real global public health concern. *Int J Epidem* 2006;35(1):60-67.

Knowles JR. Enzyme-catalyzed phosphoryl transfer reactions. *Ann Rev Biochem* 1980;49: 877–919.

Kostek MC, Delmonico MJ, Reichel JB, et al. Muscle strength response to strength training is influenced by insulin-like growth factor 1 genotype in older adults. *J Appl Physiol* 2005;98:2147-2154.

Koziris LP. Sprint interval exercise for fat loss: good return on investment. *Strength and Cond J* 2013;35(5):41-42.

Kraemer WJ, Gordon SE, Fleck SJ, et al. Endogenous anabolic hormonal and growth factor responses to heavy resistance exercise in male and females. *Int J Sports Med* 1991;12:228-235.

Kraemer WJ, Ratamess NA, French DN. Resistance training for health and performance. *Curr Sports Med Rep* 2002; 1(3):165-171.

Kraemer WJ, Ratamess NA. Fundamentals of resistance training: Progression and exercise prescription. *Med Sci Sports Exerc* 2004;36(4):674-688.

Kraemer WJ, Ratamess NA. Hormonal responses and adaptations to resistance exercise and training. *Sports Med* 2006; 35(4):339-361.

Kreider RB, Campbell B. Protein for exercise and recovery. *Physician Sports Med* 2009;37(2):13-21.

Kreider RB, Melton C, Rasmussen CJ, et al. Long-term creatine supplementation does not significantly affect clinical markers of health in athletes. *Mol Cell Biochem* 2003;244(1-2):95-104.

Kris-Etherton PM, Harris WS, Appel LJ. AHA Scientific Statement: fish consumption, fish oil, omega-3 fatty acids, and cardiovascular disease. *Circulation* 2002;106:2747-2757.

Kubo K, Kanehisa H, Miyatani M et al. Effect of low-load resistance training on the tendon properties in middle-aged and elderly women. *Acta Physiol Scand* 2003;178(1):25-32.

Kurella M, Lo JC, Chertow GM. Metabolic syndrome and the risk for chronic kidney disease among nondiabetic adults. *J Am Soc Nephrol* 2005;16:2134-2140.

LaForgia J, Withers RT, Gore CJ. Effects of exercise intensity and duration on the excess post-exercise oxygen consumption. *Journal of Sports Science* 2006;24(12):1247-1264.

Lai JS, Lan C, Wong MK, Teng SH. Two-year trends in cardiorespiratory function among older Tai Chi Chuan practitioners and sedentary subjects. *J Am Geriatr Soc* 1995;43(11):1222-1227.

Lakka TA, Laaksonen DE, Lakka HM, et al. Sedentary lifestyle, poor cardiorespiratory fitness, and the metabolic syndrome. *Med Sci Sports Exerc* 2003;35(8):1279-1286.

Lange-Aschenfeldt, Kojda G. Alzheimer's disease, cerebrovascular dysfunction and the benefits of exercise: From vessels to neurons. *Exp Gerontol* 2008;43(6):499-504.

Larsson L. Histochemical characteristics of human skeletal muscle during aging. *Acta Physiol Scand* 1983;117:469-71.

Laursen PB, Jenkins DG. The scientific basis for high-intensity interval training. *Sports Med* 2002;32(1):53-73.

Leenders M, Verdijk LB, van der Hoeven L, et al. Elderly men and women benefit equally from prolonged resistance-type exercise training. *J Gerontol* 2012;68(7):769-779.

Lehnen AM, De Angelis K, Markoski MM, D'Agord Schaan B. Changes in the GLUT 4 expression by acute exercise, exercise training and detraining in experimental models. *J Diabet Metab* 2012;S:10.

Lemmey AB, Marcora SM, Chester K, et al. Effects of high-intensity resistance training in patients with rheumatoid arthritis: a randomized controlled trial. *Arthritis Care Res* 2009;61(12):1726-1734.

Lenn J, Uhl T, Mattacola C, et al. The effects of fish oil and isoflavones on delayed onset muscle soreness. *Med Sci Sports Exerc* 2002;34(10):1605-1613.

Letai A. Growth factor withdrawal and apoptosis: the middle game. *Mol Cell* 2006;17;21(6):728-30.

Li J, Siegrist J. Physical activity and risk of cardiovascular disease—a meta-analysis of prospective cohort studies. *Int J Environ Res Public Health* 2012;92(2):391-407.

Lindle RS, Metter EJ, Lynch NA, et al. Age and gender comparisons of muscle strength in 655 women and men aged 20-93 yr. *J Appl Physiol* 1997;83(5):1581-1587.

Liu CJ, Latham NK. Progressive resistance strength training for improving physical function in older adults. *Cochrane Database of Systematic Reviews* 2009, Issue 3. Art No: CD002759.

Liu H, Bravata DM, Olkin I, et al. Systematic review: the safety and efficacy of growth hormone in the healthy elderly. *Ann Intern Med* 2007;146(2):104-15.

Loeser RF, Gandhi U, Long DL, et al. Aging and oxidative stress reduce the response of human articular chondrocytes to insulin-like growth factor 1 and osteogenic protein 1. *Arth Rheum* 2014;66(8):2201-2209.

Lombardi VP, Troxel RK. US deaths and injuries associated with weight training. *Med Sci Sports Exerc* 2003; 35(5):pS203.

Mackenbach JP. The epidemiologic transition theory. *J Epidemiol Community Health* 1994;48:329-331.

Maeda S, Miyauchi T, Iemitsu M, et al. Resistance exercise training reduces plasma endothelin-1 concentration in healthy young humans. *J Cardiovasc Pharmacol* 2004;44:S443-446.

Mahdavi H, Kim JB, Safarpour S, et al. Dyslipidemia and cardiovascular disease. *Curr Op Lipid* 2009;20:157-158.

Malik S, Wong ND, Franklin SS, et al. Impact of the metabolic syndrome on mortality from coronary artery disease, cardiovascular disease, and all causes in United States adults. *Circulation* 2004;110:1245-1250.

Malin SK, Hinnerichs KR, Echtenkamp BG, et al. Effect of adiposity on insulin action after acute and chronic resistance exercise in non-diabetic women. *Eur J Appl Phsyiol* 2013;113:2933-2941.

Marcell TJ, Hawkins SA, Wiswell RA. Leg strength declines with advancing age despite habitual endurance exercise in active older adults. *JSCR* 2014;28(2):504-513.

Marcus RL, Smith S, Morrell G, et al. Comparison of combined aerobic and high-force eccentric resistance exercise with aerobic exercise only for people with type 2 diabetes mellitus. *Phys Ther* 2008;88(11):1345–54.

Marques EA, Mota J, Machado L, et al. Multicomponent training program with weight-bearing exercises elicits favorable bone density, muscle strength, and balance adaptations in older women. *Calcif Tissue Int* 2011;88(2):117-29.

Marzetti E, Leeuwenburgh C. Skeletal muscle apoptosis, sarcopenia and frailty at old age. *Exp Gerontol* 2006;41(12):1234-8.

Matsuda M, Watanabe K, Saito A, et al. Circumstances, activities and events precipitating aneurysmal subarachnoid hemorrhage. *J Stroke Cerebrovasc Dis* 2007;16(1):55-29.

Maughan RJ, Griffin J. Caffeine ingestion and fluid balance: a review. *J Human Nutr Diet* 2003;16(6):411-420.

Bibliography


Maury E, Brichard SM. Adipokine dysregulation, adipose tissue inflammation and metabolic syndrome. *Mol Cell Endocrin* 2010;314(1):1-16.

McCartney N. Acute responses to resistance training and safety. *Med Sci Sports Exerc* 1999;32(1):31-37.

Medbo JI, Burgers S. Effect of training on anaerobic capacity. *Med Sci Sports Med* 1990;22(4):501-507.

Mendelson TB, et al. Conflicts of interest in cardiovascular clinical practice guidelines. *Arch Intern Med* 2011; 171(6):577.

Mendias CL, Tatsumi R, Allen RE. Role of cyclooxygenase-1 and -2 in satellite cell proliferation, differentiation and fusion. *Muscle and Nerve* 2004;30(4):497-500.

Menon, Ram K., and Mark A. Sperling. Insulin as a growth factor. *Endocrinol Metab Clin N Amer* 1996;25(3): 633-47.

Mikkelson UR, Langberg H, Helmark IC, et al. Local NSAID infusion inhibits satellite cell proliferation in human skeletal muscle after eccentric exercise. *J ApplPhysiol* 2009;107:1600-11.

Mokdad AH, Ford ES, Bowman BA et al. Type 2 diabetes trends in the US: 1990-1998. *Diabetes Care* 2000;23:1278-1283.

Monteiro R, Azevedo I. Chronic inflammation in obesity and the metabolic syndrome. *Nutr Metab Cardiovasc Dis* 2004;14(5):228-32.

Moraes MR, Bacurau RFP, Casarini DE, et al. Chronic conventional resistance exercise reduces blood pressure in stage 1 hypertensive men. *JSCR* 2012;26(4):1122-1129.

Mora-Rodriguez R, Pallares JG, Lopez-Samanas A, et al. Caffeine ingestion reverses the circadian rhythm effects on neuromuscular performance in highly resistance-trained men. *PLOS One* 2012;7(4):e33807.

Morrisey MC, Harman EA, Johnson MJ. Resistance training modes: specificity and effectiveness. *Med Sci Sports Exerc* 1995;27(5):648-660.

Morriss JN, Chave SPW, Adam C et al. Vigorous exercise in leisure-time and the incidence of coronary artery disease. *Lancet* 1973;301(7799):333-339.

Munzer T, Harman SM, Sorkin JD, Blackman MR. Growth hormone and sex steroid effects on serum glucose, insulin, and lipid concentrations in healthy older women and men. *J Clin Endocrinol Metab* 2009;94(10);3833-41.

Murray MP, Gore DR, Gardner GM, Mollinger LA. Shoulder motion and muscle strength of normal men and women in two age groups. *Clin Ortho Rel Res* 1985;192:268-273.

Myers J. Exercise and cardiovascular health. *Circulation* 2003;107:e2-e5.

Nash MS, Jacobs PL, Mendez AJ, Goldberg RB. Circuit resistance training improves the atherogenic lipid profile of persons with chronic paraplegia. *J Spinal Cord Med* 2001;24:2-9.

Nash MS, Mendez AJ, Goldberg RB. Circuit resistance training improves the atherogenic lipid profiles of persons with chronic paraplegia. *J Spinal Cord Med* 2001;24(1):2-9.

National Vital Statistics Report 2002;50:15, September 16, 2002.

Navarro-Yepes J, Burns M, Anandhan A, et al. Oxidative stress, redox signaling and autophagy: cell death versus survival. *Antiox Redox Signal* 2014;21(1):66-85.

Nehlig A, Debry G. Caffeine and sports activity: a review. *Int J Sports Med* 1994;15(5):215-223.

Nelson ME, Fiatorone MA, Morganti CM, et al. Effects of high-intensity strength training on multiple risk factors for osteoporotic fractures: a randomized controlled trial. *JAMA* 1994;272:1909-1914.

Newton R, Kraemer W. Developing explosive muscular power: implications for a mixed methods training strategy. *Strength and Cond* 1994;16(5):20-31.

Nied RJ, Franklin B. Promoting and prescribing exercise for the elderly. *Am Fam Phys* 2002;65(3):419-426.

Niewiadomski W, Pills W, Laskowsak D, et al. Effects of a brief Valsalva maneoeuvre on hemodynamic response to strength exercise. *Clin Physiol Funct Imaging* 2012;32:145-157.

Nilwik R, Snijders T, Leenders M, et al. The decline in skeletal muscle mass with aging is mainly attributed to a reduction in type II muscle fiber size. *Exp Gerontol* 2013;492-8.

NNT, Statin Drugs Given for 5 Years for Heart Disease Prevention (Without Known Heart Disease) http://www.thennt.com/nnt/statins-for-heart-disease-prevention-without-prior-heart-disease

Novak ML, Billich W, Smith SM, et al. COX-2 inhibitor reduces skeletal muscle hypertrophy in mice. *Am J PhysiolRegulIntegr Comp Physiol* 2009;296:R1132-1139.

O'Gara PT, Kushner FG, Ascheim DD, et al. 2013 ACCF/AHA Guideline for the management of ST-elevation myocardial infarction : A report of the American College of Cardiology Foundation/American Heart Association Task Force on Practice Guidelines. *Circulation* 2013;127(4):e362-345.

Ogden CL, Carroll MD, Kit BK, Flegal KM. Prevalence of obesity in the United States, 2009-2010. NCHS Data brief 2012, No. 82.

Oka RK, De Marco T, Haskell W, et al. Impact of a home-based walking and resistance training program on quality of life in patients with heart failure. *Am J Cardiol* 2000;85(3):365-369.

Omran AR. The epidemiological transition: a theory of the epidemiology of population change. *Milbank Q* 1971; 49:509-538.

Orr R, deVos NJ, Singh NA, et al. Power training improves balance in healthy older adults. *J Gerontol Med Sci* 2006; 61(1):78-85.

Ottenbacher KJ, Ostire GV, Peck MK, et al. Diabetes mellitus as a risk factor for hip fracture in Mexican American older adults. *J Gerontol Med Sci* 2002;57A:M658-M653.

Ozaki J, Fujimoto S, Nakagawa Y, et al. Tears of the rotator cuff of the shoulder associated with pathological changes in the acromion. A study *in cadavera*. *J Bone Joint Surg Am* 1988;70:1224–30.

Paavoleinen L, Hakkinen K, Hamalainen I et al. Explosive-strength training improves 5-km running time by improving running economy and muscle power. *J Appl Physiol* 1999;86:1527-1533.

Paddon-Jones D, Leveritt M, Lonergan A, Abernethy P. Adaptation to chronic eccentric exercise in humans: the influence of contraction velocity. Eur *J Appl Physiol* 2001;85:466-71.

Palmer B. Shut Up and Sip. Coffee is neither good nor bad for you. Now you may go. http://www.slate.com/articles/health_and_science/medical_examiner/2015/06/is_coffee_good_or_bad_for_you_the_answer_is_neither.html

Panagiotakos DB, Pitsavos C, Chrysohoou C, et al. Impact of lifestyle habits on the prevalence of the metabolic syndrome among Greek adults from the ATTICA study. *Am Heart J* 2004;147(1):106-112.

Panel members. Opinion of the Scientific Panel on food additives, flavourings, processing aids and materials in contact with food (AFC) on a request from the Commission related to creatine monohydrate for use in foods for particular nutritional uses. *EFSA Journal* 2004;36:1-12.

Paracelsus (Phillippus Aureolus Threophastus Bombastus von Hohenheim). *Die Dosis macht das Gift*. "The dose makes the poison." 1538; *Dritte Defensio*.

Park YW, Shankuan Z, Palaniappan L, et al. The metabolic syndrome: Prevalence and associated risk factor findings in the US population from the Third National Health and Nutrition Examination Survey, 1988-1994. *Arch Intern Med* 2003;163(4): 427-436.

Pedersen BK. Exercise-induced myokines and their role in chronic diseases. *Brain Behav Immun* 2011;25(5):811-816.

Pedersen BK. Muscles and their myokines. *J Exp Biol* 2011;214:337-346.

Pederson MD, Rhea MR, Sen A, Gordon PM. Resistance exercise for muscular strength in older adults: a meta-analysis. *Ageing Res Rev* 2010;9(3):226-237.

Penninx BWJH, Nicklas BJ, Newman AB, et al. Metabolic syndrome and physical decline in older persons: results from the health, aging and body composition study. *J Gerontol: Med Sci* 2009;64A(1):96-102.

Perseghin,G, Price,TB, Petersen,KF, et al. Increased glucose transport-phosphorylation and muscle glycogen synthesis after exercise training in insulin-resistant subjects. *N Engl J Med* 1996;335:1357-1362.

Pescatello LS, Franklin BA, Fagard R, et al. American College of Sports Medicine position stand: Exercise and hypertension. *Med Sci Sports Exerc* 2004;36(3):533-53.

Peterson CM, Johannsen DL, Ravussin E. Skeletal muscle mitochondria and aging: a review. *J Aging Research* 2012; http://dx.doi.org/10.1155/2012/194821

Petrides JS, Mueller GP, Kalogeras KT, et al. Exercise-induced activation of the hypothalamic-pituitary-adrenal axis: marked differences in the sensitivity to glucocorticoid suppression. *J Clin Endocrin Met* 1994;79(2):377-383.

Pittas AG, Lau J, Hu FB, Dawson-Hughes B. The role of vitamin D and calcium in type 2 diabetes: a systematic review and meta-analysis. *J ClinEndocrinMetab* 2013;http://dx.doi.org/10.1210/jc.2007-0298

Phillipou A, Halapas A, Maridaki M, Koutsilieras M. Type 1 insulin-like growth factor receptor signaling in skeletal muscle regeneration and hypertrophy. *J Musculoskelet Neuronal Interact* 7(3);208-18, 2007.

Pleket, H. W. "On the Sociology of Ancient Sport." *Sport in the Greek and Roman Worlds: Greek Athletic Identities and Roman Sports and Spectacle* 2 (2014): 29.

Pollack ML, Franklin BA, Balady GJ, et al. Resistance exercise in individuals with and without cardiovascular disease: benefits, rationale, safety and description. AHA Science Advisory. *Circulation* 2000;101:828-833.

Pollak M. Insulin and insulin-like growth factor signaling in neoplasia. *Nat Rev Cancer* 2008;8(12):915-928.

Pollock ML, Franklin BA, Balady GJ, et al. Resistance exercise in individuals with and without cardiovascular disease: Benefits, rationale, safety and prescription. An advisory from the Committee on Exercise, Rehabilitation, and Prevention, Council on Clinical Cardiology, American Heart Association. *Circulation* 2000;101:828-833.

Potter R, Ellard D, Reese K, Thorogood M. A systematic review of the effects of physical activity on physical functioning, quality of life and depression in older people with dementia. *Int J Geriatr Psych* 26(10):1000-1011.

Prabhakar H, Bithal PK, Surl A, et al. Intracranial pressure changes during Valsalva manoeuvre in patients undergoing a neuroendoscopic procedure. *Minim Invas Neurosurg* 2007;50:98-101.

Prasad V, Vandross A, Toomey C, et al. A decade of reversal: An analysis of 146 contradicted medical practices. *Mayo Clin Proc* 2013;88(8):790-798.

Psilander N. The effect of different exercise regimens on mitochondrial biogenesis and performance. (Dissertation). Karolinska Institutet, Stockholm, Sweden.

Qiang MA. Beneficial effects of moderate voluntary physical exercise and its biological mechanisms on brain health. *Neurosci Bull* 2008;24(4):265-270.

Radak Z, Hart N, Marton O, Koltai E. Regular exercise results in systemic adaptation against oxidative stress. *Systems Biology of Free Radicals and Antioxidants* 2014; Springer Berlin Heidelberg 3855-3869.

Radak Z, Taylor AW, Ohno H, Goto S. Adaptation to exercise-induced oxidative stress: from muscle to brain. *Exerc Immun Rev* 2001;7:90-107.

Radecki R. Pharmaceutical sponsorship bias influences thrombolytic literature in acute ischemic stroke. *West J Med* 2011;12(4):435-8.

Rana JS, Nieuwdorp M, Jukema JW, Kastelein JJ. Cardiovascular metabolic syndrome – an interplay of obesity, inflammation, diabetes and coronary heart disease. *Diab Obes Metab* 2007;9:218-232.

Ranheim T, Halverson B. Coffee consumption and human health—beneficial or detrimental? Mechanisms for effects of coffee consumption on different risk factors for cardiovascular disease and type 2 diabetes mellitus. *Mol Nutr Food Res* 2005;49(3):274-284.

Rasgon N, Jarvik L. Insulin resistance, affective disorders, and Alzheimer's disease: review and hypothesis. *J Gerontol Med Sci* 2004;59A:178-183.

Ray KK, Seshasai SR, Ergou S, et al. Statins and all-cause mortality in high-risk primary prevention: a meta-analysis of 11 randomized controlled trials involving 65,229 participants. *Arch Intern Med* 2010;170(12):1024-1031.

Reed ME, Ben-Ezra V, Biggerstaff KD, Nichols DL. The effects of two bouts of high- and low-volume resistance exercise on glucose tolerance in normoglycemic women. *JSCR* 2012;26(1):251-260.

Reid K, Fielding R. Skeletal muscle power: a critical determinant of physical functioning in older adults. *Exerc Sport Sci Rev* 2012; 40(1):4-12.

Ren JM, Semenkovich CF, Gulve EA, et al. Exercise induces rapid increases in GLUT4 expression, glucose transport capacity, and insulin-stimulated glycogen storage in muscle. *J Biol Chem* 1994;269:20:14396-14401.

Renehan AG, Booth C, Potten CS. What is apoptosis, and why is it important? *BMJ* 2001;322(7301):1536-1538.

Reynolds M, Bradford S. Death by prowler. 2011 The Aasgaard Company. http://startingstrength.com/article/death_by_prowler

Reynolds M, McNeely W. Barbell Safety. 2014 The Aasgaard Company. http://startingstrength.com/article/barbell_safety

Riedner CE, Rhoden EL, Ribeiro EP, Fuchs SC. Central obesity is an independent predictor of erectile dysfunction in older men. *J Urol* 2006;176(4 Pt1):1519-1523.

Rigby N. Commentary: Counterpoint to Campos et al. *In J Epidemiol* 2006;35(1):79-80.

Rippetoe M. *Starting Strength: Basic Barbell Training* (3rd Ed). 2011 The Aasgaard Company, Wichita Falls, TX.

Rippetoe M. Knee Wraps. 2011 The Aasgaard Company. http://startingstrength.com/video/platform_knee_wraps

Rippetoe M, Baker A. *Practical Programming for Strength Training* (3rd Ed). 2013 The Aasgaard Company, Wichita Falls, TX.

Rippetoe M, Bradford S. Active hip 2.0: The director's cut. 2010 The Aasgaard Company. http://startingstrength.com/article/active_hip_2

Rodas G, Ventura JL, Cadefau JA, et al. A short training programme for the rapid improvement of both aerobic and anaerobic metabolism. *Eur J Appl Physiol* 2000;82:480-486.

Roger V, et al. Heart disease and stroke statistics-2011 Update. *Circulation* 2011;123:e18-e209.

Rose AJ, Richter EK. Skeletal muscle glucose uptake during exercise: How is it regulated? *Physiology* 2005; 20:doi:10.1152/physiol.00012.2005.

Ross RJ, Rissanan H, Pedwek J, Clifford P, Shagge L. Influence of diet and exercise on skeletal muscle and visceral adipose tissue in men. *J Appl Physiol* 1996;81:2445–55.

Russell JW, Windebank AJ, Schenone A, Feldman EL. Insulin-like growth factor-I prevents apoptosis in neurons after nerve growth factor withdrawal. *J Neurobiol* 15;36(4):455-67, 1998.

Saeterbakken AH, Fimland MS. Electromyographic activity and 6RM strength in bench press on stable and unstable surfaces. *JSCR* 2013;27(4):1101-1107.

Saeterbakken AH, Fimland MS. Muscle force output and electromyographic activity in squats with various unstable surfaces. *JSCR* 2013;27(1):130-136.

Sallis RE. Exercise is medicine and physicians need to prescribe it. *Br J Sports Med* 2009;43:3-4.

Saltin B, Astrand PO. Maximal oxygen uptake and heart rate in various types of muscular activity. *J Appl Physiol* 1967; 23:353-358.

Saltin B, Astrand PO. Maximal oxygen uptake in athletes. *J Appl Physiol* 1967;23:353-358.

Sanderson TH, Kumar R, Sullivan JM et al. Insulin activates the PI3K-Akt survival pathway in vulnerable neurons following global brain ischemia. *Neurol Res* 2009;31(9):947-58.

Sattar N, Preiss D, Murray HM, et al. Statins and risk of incident diabetes: a collaborative meta-analysis of randomized statin trials. *Lancet* 2010; 375(9716):735-742.

Sattelmair J, Pertman J, Ding EL, et al. Dose-response between physical activity and risk of coronary heart disease: a meta-analysis. *Circulation* 2011;124:789-795.

Savage P, Shaw AO, Miller MS, et al. Effect of resistance training on physical disability in chronic heart failure. *Med Sci Sports Exerc* 2011;43(8):1379-1386.

Sawka MN, Burke LM, Eichner ER, et al. American College of Sports Medicine position stand. Exercise and fluid replacement. *Med Sci Sports Exerc* 2007;39(2):377-90.

Schaffler A, Muller-Ladner U, Scholmerich J, Buchler C. Role of adipose tissue as an inflammatory organ in human diseases. *Endocrine Rev* 2013;27(5):449-467.

Schmitz KH, Jensen MD, Kugler KC et al. Strength training for obesity prevention in midlife women. *Internat J Obesity* 2003;27:326-333.

Schneider HJ, Friedrich N, Klotsche J, et al. The predictive value of different measures of obesity for incident cardiovascular events and mortality. *J Clin Endocrin Metab* 2009;95(4):1777-85.

Schoenfeld BJ, Aragon AA, Krieger JW. The effect of protein timing on muscle strength and hypertrophy: a meta-analysis. *J Internat Soc Sports Nut* 2013;10:53: doi: 10.1186/1550-2783-10-53.

Schulz, H. Beta oxidation of fatty acids. *Biochimica et Biophysica Acta* (BBA)-Lipids and Lipid Metabolism 1991; 1081(2):109-120.

Schwab, U; Lauritzen, L; Tholstrup, et al. Effect of the amount and type of dietary fat on cardiometabolic risk factors and risk of developing type 2 diabetes, cardiovascular diseases, and cancer: a systematic review. *Food Nutr Res* 2014; 58. doi:10.3402/fnr.v58.25145

Schwartz RS, Evans WJ. Effects of exercise on body composition and functional capacity in the elderly. *J Gerontol Med Sci* 1995;50A:147-150.

Selye H. A syndrome produced by diverse nocuous agents. *Nature* 1936;138:32.

Selye H. The physiology and pathology of exposure to stress, a treatise based on the concepts of the general-adaptation-syndrome and the diseases of adaptation. 1950; ACTA Medical Publishers, Montreal.

Sequin R, Nelson ME. The benefits of strength training for older adults. *Am J Prev Med* 2003;24(3):141-149.

Serra-Rexach JA, Bustamante-Ara N, Hierro Villarán M, et al. Short-term, light- to moderate-intensity exercise training improves leg muscle strength in the oldest old: a randomized controlled trial. *J Am Geriatr Soc* 2011;59(4):594-602.

Servantes DM, Pelcerman A, Salvetti XM, et al. Effects of home-based exercise training for patients with chronic heart failure and sleep apnoea: a randomized comparison of two different programmes. *Clin Rehab* 2012;26:45-57.

Sharafi H, Rahimi R. The effect of resistance exercise on p53, caspase-9, and caspase-3 in trained and untrained men. *JSCR* 2012;26(4):1142-1148.

Shephard RJ, Balady GJ. Exercise as cardiovascular therapy. *Circulation* 1999;99:963-972.

Shing CM, Webb JJ, Driller MW et al. Circulating adiponectin concentrations and body composition are altered in response to high-intensity interval training. *JSCR* 2013;27(8):2213-2218.

Sigal RJ, Kenny GP, Wasserman DH, Castaneda-Sceppa C. Physical activity/exercise and type 2 diabetes. *Diabetes Care* 2004;27:2518-2539.

Singh MAF, Gates N, Saigal N, et al. The study of mental and resistance training (SMART) study—resistance training and/or cognitive training in mild cognitive impairment: a randomized, double-blind, double-sham controlled trial. *JAMDA* 2014;15:873-880.

Singh NA, Clements KM, Fiatarone MA. A randomized controlled trial of progressive resistance trianing in depressed elders. *J Gerontol A Biol Sci Med Sci* 1997;52A(1):M27-M25.

Siri-Tarino PW, Sun Q, Hu FB, et al. Meta-analysis of prospective cohort studies evaluating the association of saturated fat with cardiovascular disease. *Am J Clin Nut* 2010;91(3):535–546.

Siri-Tarino PW, Sun Q, Hu FB, Kraus RM. Saturated fat, carbohydrate, and cardiovascular disease. *Am J Clin Nutr* 2010;91(3):502-509.

Skelly LE, Andrews PC, Gillen JB, et al. High-intensity interval exercise induces 24-h energy expenditure similar to traditional endurance exercise despite reduced time commitment. *App Physiol Nut Metab* 2014;39(7):845-848.

Smart NA, Dieberg G, Giallauria F. Intermittent versus continuous exercise training in chronic heart failure: A meta-analysis. *Int J Cardiol* 2011;166(2):352-358.

Smith MM, Sommer AJ, Starkoff BE, Devor ST. Crossfit-based high-intensity power training improves maximal aerobic fitness and body composition. *JSCR* 2013; 27(11):3159-3172.

Smith SM, Schroeder K, Fahey T. Over-the-counter (OTC) medications for acute cough in children and adults in ambulatory settings. *The Cochrane database of systematic reviews* 8:CD001831.doi:10.1002/14651858.CD001831

Smits P, Pieters G, Thien T. The role of epinephrine in the circulatory effects of coffee. *Clin Pharm Therap* 1986; 40(4):431-437.

Soleyn N. Training and performance for the novice athlete. 2014 The Aasgaard Company. http://startingstrength.com/article/training_performance_for_the_novice_athlete

Song R, Lee EO, Lam P, Bae SC. Effects of tai chi exercise on pain, balance, muscle strength, and perceived difficulties in physical functioning in older women with osteoarthritis: a randomized clinical trial. *J Rheum* 2003;30(9):2039-2044.

Soukup JT, Kovaleski JE. A review of the effects of resistance training for individuals with diabetes mellitus. *Diabetes Educ* 1993;19(4):307-312.

Sousa N, Mendes R, Abrantes C, et al. Long-term effects of aerobic training versus combined aerobic and resistance training in modifying cardiovascular disease risk factors in elderly men. *Geriatr Gerontol Int* 2013;13(4):928-935.

Sparks LM, Johannsen NM, Church TS. Nine months of combined training improves ex vivo skeletal muscle metabolism in individuals with type 2 diabetes. *J Clin Endocrinol Metab* 2013;98:1694-1702.

Spradly BD, Crowley KR, Tai CY, et al. Ingesting a pre-workout supplement containing caffeine, B-vitamins, amino acids, creatine and beta-alanine before exercise delays fatigue while improving reaction time and muscular endurance. *Nutr Metab* 2012;9:28.

Stamatakis E, et al. Undue industry influences that distort healthcare research, strategy, expenditure and practice: a review. *Eur J Clin Invest* 2013;43(5):469.

Staron RS, Herman JR, Schuencke MD, et al. Misclassification of hybrid fast fibers in resistance-trained human skeletal muscle using histochemical and immunohistochemical methods. *JSCR* 2012:26(1);2616-2622.

Stener JL, Murphy A, McClellan JL, et al. Exercise training increases mitochondrial biogenesis in the brain. *J Appl Physiol* 2011;111:1066-1071.

Stensvold D, Tjonna AE, Skaug EA, et al. Strength training vs aerobic interval training to modify risk factors of metabolic syndrome. *J Appl Physiol* 2010;108:804-810.

Stevens J, McClain JE, Truesdale KP. Commentary: Obesity claims and controversies. *In J Epidemiol* 2006;35(1): 77-78.

Stockton KA, Mengerson K, Paratz JD, et al. Effect of vitamin supplementation on muscle strength: a systematic review and meta-analysis. *Osteoporosis* 2011;22:859-871.

Storen O, Helgerud J, Stoa EM, Hoff J. Maximal strength training improves running economy in distance runners. *Med Sci Sports Exerc* 2008;40(6):1089-1094.

Strasser B, Arvandi M, Siebert U. Resistance training, visceral obesity and inflammatory response: a review of the evidence. *Obesity Rev* 2012;13:578-591.

Strasser B, Siebert U, Schobersberger W. Resistance training in the treatment of metabolic syndrome. A systematic review and meta-analysis of the effect of resistance training on metabolic clustering in patients with abnormal glucose metabolism. *Sports Med* 2010;40(4):397-415.

Sullivan JM. The year in strength science. 2011 The Aasgaard Company. http://startingstrength.com/article/the_year_in_strength_science_2011

——The year in strength science. 2012 The Aasgaard Company. http://startingstrength.com/article/the_year_in_strength_science_2012

——The year in strength science. 2013 The Aasgaard Company. http://startingstrength.com/article/the_year_in_strength_science_2013

——Stopping the spread of misinflammation. 2012 The Aasgaard Company. http://startingstrength.com/article/inflammation_sullivan

——The Valsalva and stroke: Time for everyone to take a deep breath. 2012 The Aasgaard Company. http://startingstrength.com/article/the_valsalva_and_stroke

Sunde A, Storen O, Bjerkaas M, et al. Maximal strength training improves cycling economy in competitive cyclists. *JSCR* 2010;24(8):2157-2165.

Sundell J. Resistance training is an effective tool against metabolic and frailty syndromes. Advances Prev Med 2001; doi:10.4061/2011/9846833.

Szabo S, Taeche Y, Somogyi A. The legacy of Hans Selye and the origins of stress research: A retrospective 75 years after his landmark brief "letter" to the Editor of Nature. *Stress* 2012;15(5):472-478.

Tabata I, Nishimura K, Kouzaki M, et al. Effects of moderate-intensity endurance and high-intensity intermittent training on anaerobic capacity and $VO_2$max. *Med Sci Sports Exerc* 1996;38(10):1327-1330.

Takahashi Y, Kipnis D, Daughaday W. Growth hormone secretion during sleep. *J Clin Invest* 1968;47(9):2079–90.

Tang BMP, Eslick GD, Nowson C, et al. Use of calcium in combination with vitamin D supplementation to prevent fractures and bone loss in people aged 50 years and older: a meta-analysis. *Lancet* 2007;370(9588):657-666.

Tarnopolsky MA, Safdar A. The potential benefits of creatine and conjugated linoleic acid as adjuncts to resistance training in older adults. *Appl Physiol Nutr Metab* 2008;33(1):213-27.

Tartibian B, Maleki B, Abbasi A. The effects of ingestion of omega-3 fatty acids on perceived pain and external symptoms of delayed onset muscle soreness in untrained men. *Clin J Sports Med* 2009;19(2):115-119.

Taubes G. *Good Calories, Bad Calories*. 2007 Random House LLC.

Taubes G. What if it's all been a big fat lie? New York Times 2002 July 7.

Taylor F, Ward K, Moore TH, et al. Statins for the primary prevention of cardiovascular disease. *Cochr Database Syste Rev* 2011;19(1):CD004816.

Teicholz T. The questionable link between saturated fat and heart disease. http://online.wsj.com/news/articles/SB10001424052702303678404579533760760481486

ten Have M, de Graaf R, Monshouwer K. Physical exercise and mental health status: findings from the Netherlands Mental Health Survey and Incidence Study (NEMESIS). *J Psychosom Res* 2011;71(5):342-348.

Thompson PD, Clarkson P, Karas RH. Statin-associated myopathy. JAMA 2003;289(13):1681-1690.

Thrash K, Kelly B. Flexibility and strength training. *JSCR* 1987;1(4):74-75.

Tibana RA, Navalta J, Bottaro M, et al. Effects of eight weeks of resistance training on the risk factors of metabolic syndrome in overweight/obese women – "A Pilot Study." *Diabet and Met Syndr* 2013;5:11-19.

Tilk, Maria. "Educational Narratives as a Pedagogical Paradigm: the Epics of Homer." *Acta Paedagogica Vilnensia* 32 (2014).

Todd T. Historical perspective: The myth of the muscle-bound lifter. *Natl Strength Cond J* 1985;7(3):37-41.

Toth MJ, Miller MS, VanBuren P, et al. Resistance training alters skeletal muscle structure and function in human heart failure: effects at the tissue, cellular and molecular levels. *J Physiol* 2012;590.5:1243-1259.

OlsonTP, Dengel DR, Leon AS, Schmitz KH. Changes in inflammatory biomarkers following one year of moderate resistance training in overweight women. *Internat J Obesity* 2007;31:996-1003.

Trappe TA, Carroll CC, Dickinson JM, et al. Influence of acetaminophen and ibuprofen on skeletal muscle adaptations to resistance exercises in older adults. *Am J PhysiolRegulIntegr Comp Physiol* 2011;300(3):R655-62.

Trappe TA, White F, Lambert CP, et al. Effect of ibuprofen and acetaminophen on post-exercise muscle protein synthesis. *Am J Physiol Endocrinol Metab* 2001;282: E551-56.

Treuth MS, Ryan AS, Pratley RE, et al. Effects of strength training on total and regional body composition in older men. *J App Physiol* 1994;77(2):614-620.

Tyska, Matthew J.; Warshaw, David M. The myosin power stroke. *Cell Motility and the Cytoskeleton* 2002;51(1):1–15.

Tzankoff SP, Norris AH. Effect of muscle mass decrease on age-related BMR changes. *J Appl Phyisol* 1977;43: 1001-1006.

Utomi V, Oxborough D, Whyte GP, et al. Systematic review and meta-analysis of training mode, imaging modality and body size influences on the morphology and function of the male athlete's heart. *Heart* 2013(3); epub ahead of print.

van Dam RM, Li T, Spiegelman D, et al. Combined impact of lifestyle factors on mortality: prospective cohort study in US women. *BMJ* 2008;337:a1400, doi:10.1136/bmj.a1440

Vega SR, Knicker A, Hollman W, et al. Effect of resistance exercise on serum levels of growth factors in humans. *Horm Metab Res* 2010;42(13):982-986.

Verdijk LB, Snijders T, Drost M, et al. Satellite cells in human skeletal muscle; from birth to old age. *Age* 2013; doi: 10.1007/s11357-013-9583-2

Verkoshansky, "General adaptation syndrome and its applications in sport training. 2012 http://www.cvasps.com/wp-content/uploads/2012/04/GAS-NV-2012.ppt.

Vincent KR, Braith RW, Bottiglieri T, et al. Homocysteine levels following resistance training in older adults. *Prev Cardiol* 2003;6:197-203

Vincent KR, Braith RW, Felman RA, et al. Improved cardiorespiratory endurance following 6 months of resistance exercise in elderly men and women. *Arch Int Med* 2002;162(3):673-678.

Vincent KR, Vincent HK. Resistance training for individuals with cardiovascular disease. *J Cardiopulm Rehab* 2006; 25:207-216.

Vissing K, McGee SL, Farup J, et al. Differentiated mTOR but not AMPK signaling after strength vs. endurance exercise in training-accustomed individuals. *Scand J Med Sci Sport* 2013;23(3):355-366.

Vissing K, McGee SL, Farup J, et al. Differentiated mTOR but not AMPK signaling after strength vs. endurance exercise in training-accustomed individuals. *Scand J Med Sci Sport* 2013;23(3):355-366.

Vlak MHM, Rinkel GJE, Greebe P, et al. Trigger factors and their attributable risk for rupture of intracranial aneurysms. *Stroke* 2011;42:878-1882.

Voss MW, Nagamatsu LS, Liu-Ambrose T, Kramer AF. Exercise, brain and cognition across the life span. *J Appl Physiol* 2011;111:1505-1513.

Wayne PM, Berkowitz DL, Litrownik DE, et al. What do we really know about the safety of Tai Chi? A systematic review of adverse event reports in randomized trials. *Arch Phys Med Rehab* 2014; doi: 10.1016/ j.apmr. 2014. 05.005.

Wells GD, Selvadurai H, Tein I. Bioenergetic provision of energy for muscular activity. *Ped Resp Rev* 2009;10(3): 83-90.

Wemple RD, Lamb DR, McKeever KH. Caffeine vs. caffeine-free sports drinks: effects on urine production at rest and during prolonged exercise. *Int J Sports Med* 1997;18(1):40-46.

White BC, Sullivan JM, DeGracia DJ, et al. Brain ischemia and reperfusion: molecular mechanisms of neuronal injury. *J NeuroSci* 2000;179(S 1-2):1-33.

White BC, Sullivan JM. Apoptosis. *Acad Emerg Med* 1988;5(10):1019-1029.

Whitehead JP, Richards AA, Hickman IJ, et al. Adiponectin: a key adipokine in the metabolic syndrome. *Diab Obes Metab* 2006;8(3):264-280.

Whitman SA, Wacker MJ, Richmond SR, Godard MP. Contributions of the ubiquitin-proteasome pathway and apoptosis to human skeletal muscle wasting with age. *Pflugers Arch* 2005;450:437-46.

Wijndaele K, Duvigneud N, Matton L, et al. Muscular strength, aerobic fitness and metabolic risk syndrome risk in Flemish adults. *Med Sci Sports Sci* 2007;29:233-240.

Wikipedia. Efficiency of ATP production. https://en.wikipedia.org/wiki/Cellular_respiration#Efficiency_of_ATP_production

Wikipedia. High-intensity interval training. http://en.wikipedia.org/wiki/High-intensity_interval_training

Willette AA, Guofan X, Johnson SC, et al. Insulin resistance, brain atrophy, and cognitive performance in late middle-aged adults. *Diabetes Care* 2012;36(2):443-449.

Williams MA, Haskell WL, Ades PA, et al. Resistance exercise in individuals with and without cardiovascular disease: 2007 update. A scientific statement from the Amercian Heart Association Advisory Council on Clinical Cardiology and Council on Nutrition, Physical Activity and Metabolism. *Circulation* 2007;116:572-584.

Wilson JM, Loenneke JP, Jo E, et al. The effects of endurance, strength and power training on muscle fiber type shifting. *JSCR* 2012:26(6);1724-1729.

Wilson JM, Marin PJ, Rhea MR, et al. Concurrent training: a meta-analysis examining interference of aerobic and resistance exercises. *JSCR* 2012;26(8):2293-2307.

Wisløff, U., Ellingsen, Ø.,& Kemi, O. J. High-intensity interval training to maximize cardiac benefits of exercise training? *Ex Sport Sci Rev* 2009;37(3):139-46.

Wohlgemuth SE, Calvani R, Marzetti E. The interplay between autophagy and mitochondrial dysfunction in oxidative stress-induced cardiac signaling and pathology. *J Mol Cell Biol* 2014;71(6):62-70.

Yongming L, Cao C, Chen X. Similar electromyographic activities of lower limbs between squatting on a Reebok Core Board and ground. *JSCR* 2013;27(5):1349-1353.

Youngren JF, Exercise and the regulation of blood glucose. http://diabetesmanager.pbworks.com/w/page/17680187/Exercise%20and%20the%20Regulation%20of%20Blood%20Glucose

Zuckerman JD, Kummer FJ, Cuomo F, Greller M. Interobserver reliability of acromial morphology classification: an anatomic study. *J Shoulder Elbow Surg* 1997;6:286-7

Zuniga JM, Housh TJ, Camic CL, et al. The effects of creatine monohydrate loading on anaerobic performance and one-repetition max strength. *JSCR* 2012;26(6):1651-1656.

# Authors

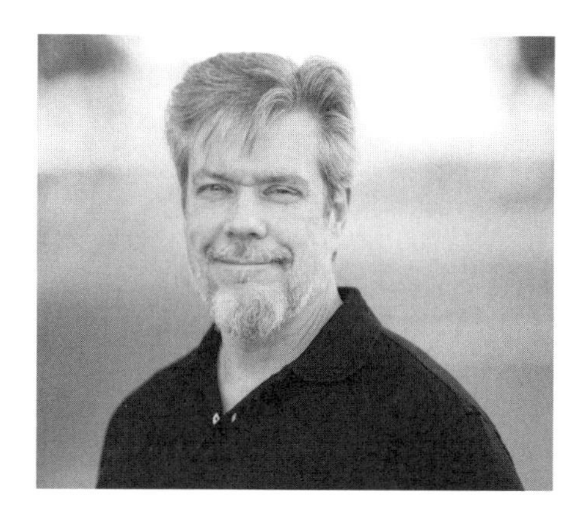

**Jonathon Sullivan MD, PhD, SSC** is the owner of Greysteel Strength and Conditioning, a coaching practice and Starting Strength Gym devoted to barbell-based training for Masters, in Farmington, MI. Dr. Sullivan conducts semi-private barbell coaching and programming for adults in their 50s, 60s, 70s and beyond. He is also Associate Professor of Emergency Medicine at Wayne State University/Detroit Receiving Hospital, a Level I Trauma Center where he has worked in patient care, teaching, and research for over twenty years. Until his retirement from basic research in 2012, he was Associate Director of the Cerebral Resuscitation Laboratory, where he conducted basic research in molecular mechanisms of neuronal salvage and repair in the setting of cardiac arrest, stroke, and trauma. He is the author of several dozen research articles, abstracts, and book chapters in the emergency medicine and neuroscience literature, as well as articles on strength training which can be found at www.startingstrength.com. He has served on several committees for the Starting Strength Coaches Association, and participated in the development of the Maintenance of Certification process for Starting Strength Coaches. He is a former US Marine, holds the rank of 3rd *Dan* in *Tang Soo Do*, and has been known to publish the occasional science fiction short story. He lives in Farmington Hills, MI, with his wife, three ungrateful cats, and a wooded lot full of raccoons, skunks, possums, foxes, herons, and ducks. His training website and contact information can be found at www.greysteel.org.

**Andy Baker, SSC** is the owner of Kingwood Strength & Conditioning (KSC), a private barbell training facility in Kingwood TX. Since opening KSC in 2007 Andy has provided coaching and personal training to clients ranging from Division I collegiate athletes and competitive powerlifters to average people of all ages and abilities who are interested in getting stronger.

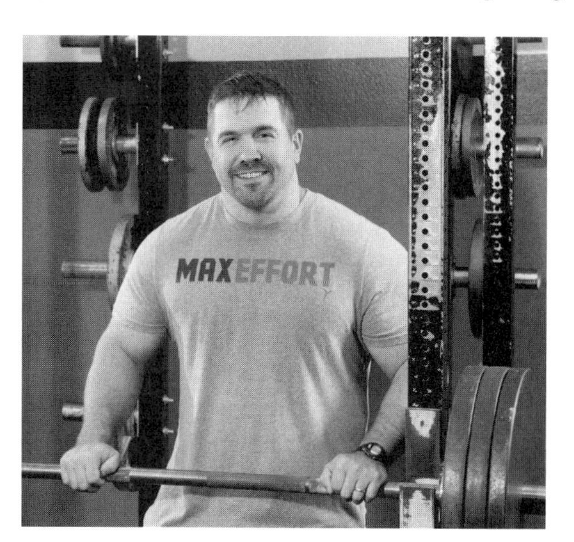


Andy is a former U.S. Marine and served multiple combat tours in support of Operation Iraqi Freedom between 2003-2007. While on active duty, Andy received his undergraduate degree in Health & Sport Science from the American Military University. He is a Starting Strength Coach, and is the co-author with Mark Rippetoe of the best-selling *Practical Programming for Strength Training 3rd edition.*

Andy is also a Raw and Drug Free Powerlifter in the Natural Athlete Strength Association. In 2010 Andy won N.A.S.A. Grand Nationals in the 198 lb raw division, with a 529 lb Squat, 380 lb Bench Press, and 562 lb Deadlift. He is a native of Kingwood Texas, and currently resides there with his wife and 3 children.

# Index